Intermediate Care
of Older People

Edited by

**SIÂN WADE RGN, DNCert, DPSN, BSc,
HAGerontology, PGDip Ed**

Lead Nurse for Older People, Oxford Radcliffe Hospitals Trust

W

WHURR PUBLISHERS
LONDON AND PHILADELPHIA

© 2004 Whurr Publishers

First published 2004 by
Whurr Publishers Ltd
19b Compton Terrace, London N1 2UN, England and
325 Chestnut Street, Philadelphia PA 19106, USA

British Library Cataloguing in Publication Data

A catalogue record for this book is available from the
British Library.

ISBN 1 86156 356 6

Printed and bound in the UK by Athenaeum Press Limited,
Gateshead, Tyne & Wear.

Contents

Preface

Intermediate care has become a buzzword within health and social care over the past few years as evidenced by the NHS Plan (DoH, 2000c), the HSC/LAC Intermediate Care Guidance circular (DoH, 2001e) and the National Service Framework for Older People (DoH, 2001h). Seen as the panacea for a number of woes, particularly for older people, intermediate care has been held up as a way forward within contemporary health and social care.

This book is written with the intention of exploring in more detail what is understood by the concept of intermediate care and, in particular, ways in which the needs of older people can best be met by this new range of services. We have tried to show how intermediate care can contribute effectively to providing a first-class service within a carefully managed continuum of care that is superior to the somewhat disparate services often experienced by older people within contemporary health and social care. This will occur, we suggest, only if careful attention is given to planning and resourcing such services and schemes within a whole system of service delivery and in partnership with all those involved. In addition, it is argued, it is imperative to pay attention to the preparation and development of staff. The potential of intermediate care to become either a Cinderella or a Rolls-Royce service will depend upon how these elements are addressed.

Part 1 centres on the concept of intermediate care and the motives for its development. This includes a summary of the range of intermediate care services that have been developed, with a discussion of some of the confusion that surrounds the concept. The debate then moves on to centre on older people, discussing first why older people have come to be perceived as one of the main client groups that may benefit from intermediate care, and then how intermediate care could be developed to serve their needs more fully. Part II provides an overview of ageing and the uniqueness of older people, followed by an exploration of some of the challenges faced by older people within society — and how this has extended into the delivery of health and social care.

Part III discusses the practicalities of planning and commissioning new intermediate care services and schemes, and some of the considerations that need to be made. When planning and commissioning new services it is important to seek the views of users and carers, and Penny Thewlis describes her involvement in facilitating older people to make their views and concerns heard so that they can influence these developments.

Some recent initiatives are seen to play a key role within intermediate care. The focus on care pathways and integrated care pathways is one such initiative. While the value of such initiatives in the care of older people is perhaps debatable, discussion is provided to examine how they might usefully be of benefit to older people transferring to intermediate care services; there is also an exploratory examination of the Single Assessment Process and its potential to act in the best interests of older people. Evaluation of previous intermediate care services has not always been easy, and so at this point there is a brief outline of the important role played by evaluation in the development of new services. This is followed by a report of a study undertaken to explore the experience of carers who have been involved in intermediate care services.

Throughout this book there is an emphasis on ensuring the careful planning and development of new intermediate care services, with due recognition of the unique and special needs of older people. We argue in Part IV that if these services are to be successful it is essential that staff are adequately prepared to provide this care, with structured education and development. For this reason a range of important practice-related issues are explored in some depth, emphasizing the skill and expertise required of staff if the ambition and potential of intermediate care is to be fulfilled. Those involved in developing these services are asked to consider carefully such preparation.

This book comes at a time when there are great changes in the health and social care system for older people. While it focuses on the introduction of intermediate care in relation to older people, it holds great relevance for those involved in the delivery of care for older people across the whole health and social care spectrum, including practitioners, managers, project workers and students. It is best read as a whole to appreciate fully the discussion and debate surrounding intermediate care and the care of older people. It does, however, also lend itself to the reader who wishes to 'dip in' to examine specific aspects or issues related to intermediate care, and has been written with this approach in mind. Each chapter is supported by summaries of key points or practice-related features, to ease reading and to highlight these points.

At the back of the book there is a glossary, which not only explains terms used in the text but also provides a quick reference guide for the reader.

Contributors

Sheila Begley is a Clinical Hospital Manager at Milton Keynes General Hospital and is involved in the development of intermediate care services in that area. Her interest in the area of intermediate care comes from a nursing background in both primary and secondary health care. She has been involved in research exploring public sector partnerships and friendship and befriending of older people. She undertakes some lecturing and has recently completed her PhD thesis.

Jon Glasby is a lecturer at the University of Birmingham Health Services Management Centre. Research and publication interests include services for older people, community care and the health/social care divide. Jon is a member of the national evaluation of intermediate care and is the author of introductory textbooks on partnership working and hospital discharge.

Liz Lees is a Consultant Nurse for Acute Medicine at Birmingham Heartlands and Solihull Hospital NHS Teaching Trust, a joint post with the Eastern Birmingham Primary Care Trust (previously Consultant Nurse for Intermediate Care at Birmingham Specialist Community Health NHS Trust). Liz has extensive experience in acute care, in the planning and delivery of intermediate care services and in working at the interface between organizations.

Penny Thewlis is a qualified teacher whose main focus was on teaching within health and social services. After working for a voluntary organization, she moved to work with the Community Health Council for ten years. Her work here highlighted the importance of involving older people in service development — hence her move to work with Age Concern and her current post facilitating the Older Persons Panel. She has a strong interest in collaborative working to produce more joined-up services.

Siân Wade is Lead Nurse for Older People at Oxford Radcliffe Hospitals Trust, and prior to this was a Consultant Nurse for Intermediate Care. Siân has worked with older people within a range of settings for over 20 years.

She is a qualified district nurse and has spent over ten years working within community settings. She is also a qualified teacher and taught at Oxford Brookes University for eight years, focusing her teaching on the older person, and leading a multi-level gerontology programme there.

PART I
The Concept and Context of Intermediate Care

1

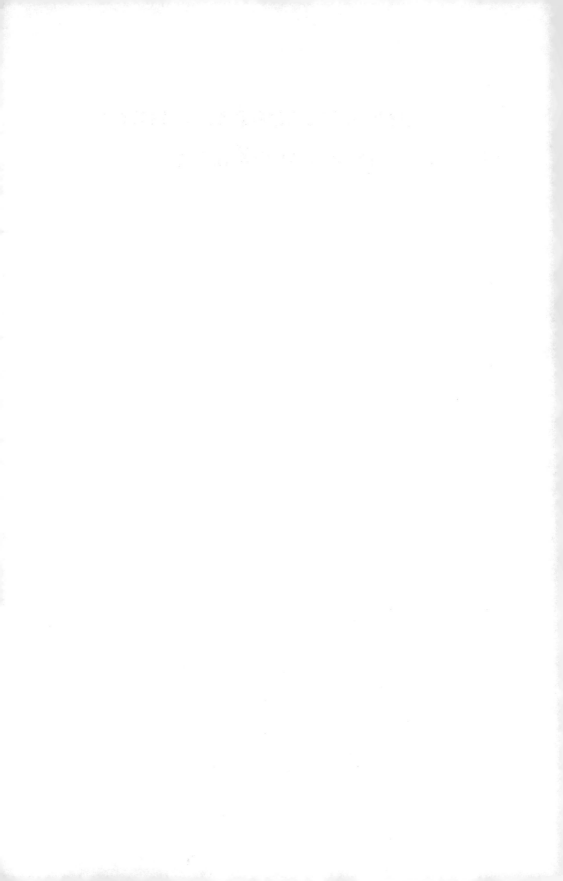

Intermediate care: what are we talking about?

SIÂN WADE AND LIZ LEES

Introduction

This chapter introduces the concept of intermediate care, setting the scene and providing the background for this book. Fundamental issues, concerns, challenges and opportunities are introduced that will be enlarged upon at various points throughout the book.

Background to intermediate care

Since 1997, government policy has focused on the modernization of health and social care services (DoH, 1997; DoH, 1998a; DoH, 1999b; DoH, 2000c; DoH, 2001e). A key goal within this modernization agenda has been the promotion of health and independence, and this was summed up in a statement made by Alan Milburn when speaking at the LSE on the 8 March 2000: 'investment now to prevent ill health and to promote fast effective treatment and rehabilitation may be as important economically as it is socially'.

A key strand within this policy directive was the introduction and development of intermediate care to support this drive. With this new interest in the concept, intermediate care seems to have taken on a new significance and meaning within contemporary health care delivery (DoH, 2000c; NHS Executive, 2000a; DoH, 2001e; DoH, 2001h). Intermediate care describes services that are just that – 'intermediate' and 'in the middle' – and represents a wide range and diversity of services.

This recent concentration and emphasis on intermediate care within contemporary health care suggests that it has been viewed as the panacea to solve all service ills, irrespective of the setting. Yet for many, the concept is not new. Emrys-Roberts (1991) eloquently described the chequered history of community hospitals (sometimes known as cottage hospitals), regarded by some in recent years as a model of intermediate care. Over the previous hundred years they experienced a rise and fall in popularity, struggling at times to survive against adversity. With pressure on beds and the recent annual winter crisis over the past few years, temporary injections of money have facilitated the development of a variety of community-based initiatives to be established throughout the UK to meet the needs of particular client groups. Examples of some innovations, in part replicated through these 'new services', were seen within the early work of nursing development units (Vaughan and Lathlean, 1999). The teams involved were clear about their services, funding, roles and responsibilities and over the years, for some, their relationships and services were redefined or redrawn to become accepted as 'the norm' (Vaughan et al., 1999). Yet it is exactly this kind of service that is now being 'rebranded' within the 'new concept' of intermediate care.

From a philosophical perspective it is perhaps inappropriate to suggest that community hospitals form an example of this new concept of intermediate care. For, rather like the care of older people – or 'geriatrics' – community hospitals have been steeped in a history of being marginalized, with the care they offered perceived as being of low skill and low status (Emrys-Roberts, 1991; Akid, 2001) and the services they provided as lacking proactivity. This would surely not be the image the government would wish to have associated with the modernization of the health service in this new millennium. Yet there is no doubt that much development work has been done in many of these settings over the years – take for example the Oxfordshire Community Hospitals Development Unit (McCormack, 1992). Working in such community settings and caring for older people requires highly skilled and expert care (RCN, 1999; Akid, 2001; Coombes, 2001) and this level of expertise will be paramount to the success of future intermediate care service developments (CSP, 2001). That this has long been unrecognized (Wade, 1999; Wade, 2000; Coombes, 2001) may not bode well, and it could be that the current notion of intermediate care is simply a temporary reprieve for these much maligned services.

Alternatively, with the stark reality of an ageing population (OPCS, 2001) and the need for more responsive care services, this field of work may perhaps at last see 'a coming of age' or 'the renaissance of geriatric medicine in the UK' as described by MacMahon (2001: 23). With this there is an opportunity to see the revival and emergence of services that will form the backbone of our future health service for some years to come. Hence, in part, 'reconfiguration' makes provision for 'redevelopment' of existing services and 'development' of the new. It may be in the guise of a new terminology, but it does provide the opportunity to develop current services together with new imaginative and needs-responsive services all under the umbrella of 'intermediate care', dismissing forever those much berated 'Cinderella services'.

What is intermediate care?

As suggested above, the concept of intermediate care has been around for some time, even if not under the guise of intermediate care. In recent years, with pressures on beds and escalating winter crises, the concept seems to have taken on a new meaning, with a range of different services evolving over the past decade or so. Along with these developments, a range of definitions has emerged that tries to describe the services involved and their purposes. These will be explored in more detail in Chapter 2.

It was not until January 2001 that central guidance was provided in the form of the HSC/LAC Circular released on 19 January (DoH, 2001e). The guiding principles outlined in this document have tended to form the foundation of developments planned and implemented since this date, although many previously developed services have retained their own characteristics. The HSC/LAC guidance provided an initial marker for intermediate care and was built upon with the publication of *The National Service Framework for Older People* in March 2001 (DoH, 2001h). This could be said to have sealed the place of intermediate care as a key arena of service development within contemporary health care, and to have established it as an early priority area for investment. It is notable that intermediate care was placed within the National Service Framework for older people, making a clear statement that intermediate care was seen to have a key place within the trajectory of care to be received by this client group.

In general, the service models outlined in the HSC/LAC Circular (DoH, 2001e) are quite wide-ranging – ranging from predominantly social models to more health-based models such as nurse-led early discharge and acute respiratory assessment services for managing exacerbations of COPD (chronic obstructive pulmonary disease) (see Table 1.1). These are examined in more detail in Chapter 2. More recently a range of models with similar features have been developed within the field of mental health and these have received recommendation (Nursing Older People, 2002).

Drivers for intermediate care

Over the past decade there has been a significant reduction in the number of hospital beds available. In 1948 the NHS national stock was 480 000 beds, while over 50 years later this had been reduced to 190 000 (DoH, 2000d). In particular, beds designated specifically for older people have seen an

Table 1.1 Range of services falling within the concept of intermediate care

Hospital-based intermediate care wards	• often with a focus on rehabilitation
Community-based intermediate care unit	• Nurse- or GP-led, often with a focus on slower stream rehabilitation
Day hospital	• community-based, e.g. within in-bed setting
Rapid response team	• focus of service may vary, from acute and technical intervention to more social care (services are time-limited – anything from 5 days to 6 weeks usually)
Supportive discharge	• supporting earlier discharge than would normally be possible with traditional services
'Hospital at home' care	• providing more intensive care than would normally be provided at home – usually related to planned surgery for specific conditions such as hip replacements
'Hospice at home'	• provides more intensive terminal care than would normally be available from community services
CART/CRT	• Community Assessment Rehabilitation Team – time limited
CCRT	• Continuous Community Rehabilitation Team – may reach into homes and nursing/residential homes.
Neuro-rehabilitation teams	• may reach into homes or other care settings, providing specialist expertise
'Step-down'/'step-up' schemes	• often utilizing beds in nursing homes – but service seems to vary
Outreach service	• often focused on therapy and rehabilitation to follow up and assess progress

unprecedented decline, with the model of integrated care seemingly to take precedence. At the same time, the number of admissions has constantly risen over these years, compensated by the dramatic reduction in the length of stay of patients (Martin, 2001). Concurrently, demographic changes have led to an ageing population, such that this client group tends to account for a large and growing proportion of patients occupying in-patient beds. The National Beds

Inquiry showed that two-thirds of hospital beds were occupied by people who were over 65 years of age, and half the recent growth in admissions comes from people over 75 years (DoH, 1999b).

Concern over bed-occupancy, delayed discharges and capacity management has focused the minds of many ministers and hospital managers over the past few years (Bagust et al., 1999; Mahoney, 2001; DoH, 1999b; NHS Executive, 2000a; DoH, 2001h). Challenged with annual concern about a winter bed crisis, a range of initiatives has emerged over the years to try to resolve and address this perennial problem. The situation has no doubt been exacerbated by the drive to reduce hospital waiting times for outpatients and elective surgery, along with the commitment to reduce trolley waits in A&E, and for patients to be seen in and admitted from A&E within specified timespans. All these pressures have led to the need to maximize the use of beds and demonstrate their effectiveness.

Sadly, much attention and criticism seems to have been directed towards older people, who for a range of reasons tend to account for the majority of those patients deemed to be inappropriately placed in these beds. Following publication of the NHS Plan (DoH, 2000c), the National Beds Inquiry (DoH, 1999b) and the National Service Framework for older people (DoH, 2001h), various new initiatives and targets have been introduced to try to resolve some of these problems. These have focused predominantly on measures devised to avoid the admission of older people to acute beds or institutionalized care, with targets to avert their admission and reduce the number of delayed discharges of people over 75 years. Indeed, many would argue that the Government's survival depends upon the success of these targets, as evidenced by the imperatives being placed on Chief Executives of Trusts that are not currently meeting them (DoH, 2000/2001).

The concept of intermediate care and the range of service initiatives being developed within it seem to have been embraced as the solution to many of the bed management problems experienced (DoH, 2000b; DoH, 2001e). According to the Department of Health review *Intermediate Care: Moving Forward* (DoH, 2002d), significant developments have been made over the two years since its 'official' initiation. As discussed above, the emphasis has been very much on promoting the independence of older people in a bid to prevent or reduce the use of beds in hospitals or institutions. Furthermore, the maximization of an individual's ability and hence independence is perceived to save a great deal economically – and, more importantly, can be argued to improve quality of life (DoH, 1999c). Although there is limited evidence to substantiate the benefits of many of these intermediate care initiatives to date (Shepperd and Illiffe, 1998a; Griffith et al., 2000; Steiner, 2001), there is a belief that the social well-being of an individual is best met at home or as near to home as possible.

A further justification for intermediate care developments is that hospitals are often regarded as 'dangerous places', associated with risks of infection and complications (Illich, 1975), where the risk of iatrogenic illness becomes greater than relapse (Steiner, 2001) – although as services develop, the risks of health-related infections in other settings will increase (Gould, 2002). This, however, should not be allowed to become an excuse for denying older people the facilities and focused expert skills often available only in an acute setting. The failure to ensure such services are appropriately available to, and accessed by, older people would result in intermediate care becoming a contemporary Cinderella service, to be treated with the same contempt associated with the long-stay/workhouse images of earlier years (Townsend, 1964; Means and Smith, 1985), where settings were situated away from the main diagnostic and treatment facilities, marginalizing the care older people received. This in turn could lead to patients and carers perceiving that the care they received was second-rate – the very situation that the National Service Framework for older people is supposedly trying to dispense with (DoH, 2001h).

Those involved in the care of any older person therefore face the challenge of making sure that older people receive those services that they rightly require and deserve. This in effect means ensuring that the patient is 'in the right place', 'at the right time', 'with the right skills'. Achieving this requires clarity about the outcomes expected of different services, management of the 'whole system' of services, together with a range of different expected activities within different sets of organizations. Most importantly, effective collaboration and partnership working is essential – which is no mean feat.

A key goal in maximizing independence is to meet the rehabilitation needs of patients as soon as they are able to benefit. With the current profile of hospital occupancy this requires that rehabilitation is readily available to patients within an acute hospital setting, including access to focused specialist rehabilitation. Intermediate care may well thus form part of the care pathway of some older people, but there will be those it does not suit and those who will not need it. Intermediate care is not, therefore, a substitute for providing specialist care and rehabilitation in acute care but it is one option that will meet the needs of a proportion of patients – especially older people.

Intermediate care and its challenges

Where is intermediate care?

The commitment to the principle of 'closer to home' drives the concept of intermediate care services being developed and provided in community settings. The Government refers to 5000 new intermediate care beds and 1700 intermediate care places in the NHS Plan. The interpretation of this may have been misleading (NHS Executive, 2000b) as it may have placed greater attention on the concept of beds, which may be self-limiting. As such, intermediate care risks becoming synonymous only with nurse-led units/community hospitals rather than with other more needs-responsive service developments. For those engaged in the work of intermediate care, the wide range and diversity of what this concept entails is probably very evident. However, for those less familiar with the concept, a more basic and one-dimensional interpretation may inform their understanding and practice and this could limit the potential and the opportunities available to develop a needs-responsive range of services. The notion of 'convalescence' is still referred to by some, while wards based in acute hospitals described as 'nurse-led' run the great risk of becoming interim beds used by bed management to transfer patients who are waiting for ongoing care or funding.

What is it for?

There were some key features within the HSC/LAC intermediate care guidance (DoH, 2001e) that need particular note. As outlined above, it focused on promoting independence based on active rehabilitation. This, it suggested, should be provided within a maximum of six weeks – often within only two weeks, and as such it would be funded from health. It advised that only in exceptional cases should the length of care be extended beyond this. This element of specifying that the service is time-limited has caused problems in both the design and use of some services, especially those newly created in line with the guidance document. In July 2002, the health secretary Alan Milburn announced the Government's intention to legislate that all intermediate care should be provided free of charge at the point of use, whether by the NHS or by councils. This suggested some giving way on this issue. While not specifically cited in the outlined criteria, there is a repeated reference to, and emphasis on, these services being primarily directed towards older people, although note is made that other age groups may benefit from it. It is recommended that care be provided on the basis of a comprehensive assessment which results in an individualized care plan involving therapy. Finally, it requires that service provision should involve cross-professional working, utilization of a single assessment, shared record-keeping and shared protocols.

In summary, intermediate care seems to have been increasingly associated with time-limited rehabilitation for older people, which will not be means-tested and which will be provided closer to home. It remains, however, according to Black and Pearson (2002), an ill-defined entity. It could, they suggest 'have an important role but requires resources, strong leadership and dedicated medical time to ensure that it is care of equivalent quality in an alternative environment, not simply a cheaper option' (2002: 611). There are many questions unanswered and a number of issues and concerns which will be revisited throughout this book.

The use or interpretation of criteria for referral to specific services may be constraining and may give rise to a number of challenges in the development of services. These criteria need to be guided in part by the outcomes expected of the service, and this does not always seem to be clear. While 'rapid response' and 'hospital at home' services seem to be flexible in the age range of their clients, in-patient bed facilities seem to be developing with the older person in mind and there is still a drive in many schemes for patients to complete their rehabilitation needs within six weeks or other time limits. Palliative care, those who need longer-term rehabilitation, and a range of other client needs seem to have been excluded from these criteria. There are many opportunities to be more pragmatic in what can be provided in these settings than simply the concept of rehabilitation, and it may be that, once established, new services will become more opportunistic and flexible as the range of possibilities present. Established services such as community hospitals, which have often had more flexible criteria for admission, may need to rethink their service provision, but this may impose unnecessary restrictions that limit what evolved as an effective local needs-responsive service.

The challenge of medical stability

A key challenge to the use of intermediate care services lies with the difficulty experienced in reaching agreement on what constitutes 'stability' or 'predictability'. This has been a point of debate in many forums, with any consensus being impossible to reach. This is hardly surprising, due to the complex, fragile and unstable status of many older people's health and the significance of professional judgment. As Steiner (2001) argues, at some point the balance of clinical risk needs to shift and as such it becomes more desirable for patients to be out of acute hospitals than in.

Partnership and inter-agency working

To facilitate the concept of 'closer to home' and the emphasis on a 'primary-care-led NHS', funding has been directed towards local authorities and PCTs. It has not always been clear either how the original money was made available or how it was spent, since one of the major controversies was the perceived 'loss' or 'invisibility' of the early money the Government claimed to have invested in intermediate care. A range of theories have been put forward, including the failure to ring-fence money, the need to allocate to other services, poor accountability with regard to its spending, and the belief that it has been double- or treble-counted with other service developments. One of the dilemmas being faced is that there is no legally binding arrangement that the Government can enforce to ensure money is spent by ring-fencing it. Only with a change in law could this be achieved. Doing this could have repercussions for the Government, especially when re-election is a concern. Also, although local government has been allocated additional resources (mostly through the Personal Social Services SSA), these are for a diverse range of services that are linked to intermediate care, such as home care. Judging by the current pressures faced by social services, the promised increases in SSA will have to be substantial if they are to be able to participate as actively as would be wished.

Thus, while the ethos of the NHS Plan is for health and social services to work in partnership, this contrast in funding creates a rather unequal footing for each party and could be seen to create an unfair balance of power and influence. This concern is further challenged by the statutory obligation for local councils to means-test and charge for their services. The solution provided by the Government in the HSC/LAC Circular Guidance (DoH, 2001e) was for local councils to agree with their health service partners that the NHS should take responsibility for these services, within the framework of a jointly planned and jointly funded intermediate care service. This, however, could be argued to give the health service an upper hand, and challenge effective partnership working. It could also challenge the potential to create more person-centred social models of care which take a socially inclusive and holistic perspective and thus clearly lend themselves to intermediate care services. The alternative is to create Care Trusts, but it would seem that the enthusiasm for these waned coming up to the 2001 General Election, and to date little progress seems to have been made. Steiner (2001) points out that little progress in financing can be made until the various stakeholders acknowledge the differences that exist in acute, primary, community and social service budgets. However, even where this is acknowledged, the logistics of overcoming these differences could be described as an uphill struggle.

Different cultures and working principles, as well as professional boundaries and roles, and geographical boundaries further challenge the concept of partnership working, creating considerable difficulties at an operational level. Inter-agency and professional working has traditionally not been a strength in the provision of health and social care. To achieve effective working and overcome some very fundamental barriers is a huge undertaking while planning and developing completely new services, as described by Jon Glasby in Chapter 6. This has been further challenged with the emergence of

PCTs, which have been preoccupied with addressing and overcoming early fundamental organizational arrangements, requirements and developments. This has taken considerable time and, since progress has been hampered by lack of resources, there have been delays in being able to develop strategic priorities for service provision and development (Banks-Smith et al., 2001).

Service and financial effectiveness

There is a misconception that intermediate care services and schemes, especially nurse/therapy-led units, are cheap and easy to set up. Nothing could be further from the truth, as demonstrated by a wide range of research (Shepperd and Illiffe, 1998a; Griffith et al., 2000; Steiner et al., 2001). Staffing levels and skill mix need to reflect the autonomous situation staff will work in, and the intensity of intervention required to promote effective proactive rehabilitation. Such services require very careful planning, preparation and induction of staff (Williams and Last, 1998; Steiner et al., 2001). Staff will often be working in isolation, across inter-agency and inter-disciplinary boundaries, with patients who have complex and demanding care needs. Here skilled care, case and risk management and decision-making skills are imperative. There is no doubt that this kind of setting provides many stimulating and demanding opportunities for staff seeking this challenge. There is almost certainly a labour force available nationally with much skill and experience (not withstanding current shortages) who would welcome these new roles that provide greater autonomy (Vaughan et al., 1999). Adequate preparation of staff, however, is essential, as personal experience has shown. It is not sufficient simply to transfer staff from an acute hospital setting with a medical model of care to work in an intermediate care service, for this involves a completely new cultural context. Issues need to be resolved regarding the composition of the professional team and their working philosophy and training needs.

Care pathways may well provide a structure for 'integration of care across professional and organizational boundaries' (Middleton and Roberts, 2000). They are, however, open to testing and validation, while not emulating a medical model and not detracting from the all-encompassing needs of those with complex needs and/or multiple pathology. In particular, there is a need to relinquish the more medical model of care, which tends to focus on one medical problem or on clinical intervention, in favour of adopting a more person-centred, holistic approach to care, more along the lines of a social model of care; such an approach could also encompass a more open-minded approach to risk assessment. As discussed above, this requires multi- and interdisciplinary teamwork that involves working across professional boundaries and adopting a range of activities and functions to meet patient needs in an effective, efficient and needs-responsive way (Steiner et al., 2000). Staff will need assistance in developing and adopting such an approach (see Chapter 16).

The crux of the financial argument may centre on the discussion in the Department of Health's intermediate care guidance (DoH, 2001e) related to length of stay and funding arrangements. As mentioned above, there is a repeated emphasis in this document on time-limited intermediate care, but it would appear that the rigidity of time limits has been relaxed and will be left more to professional discretion; however, this is in any case likely to need regular review and reassessment. This supports the notion of the 'whole continuum of care' mentioned within the document, so that as intermediate care services develop, patients will be transferred within particular routes of these services. These will legitimately direct patients' needs to their dependency at changing points in time, but nevertheless could extend over the overall period – possibly beyond six weeks. Reassessment should be an individual affair carried out at each indicative milestone integral to the kind of pathway the patient is following and their ultimate end-point destination. The difficulties in reassessing, six weeks being the original parameter, may give rise to 'exercising discretion' (paragraph 18) especially if there is an intention to try to levy charges after such a period. This should be free, however, if outcome measures are in place indicating intermediate care as the best choice of service for an individual's continued care needs – as would be the case if still in an Acute Trust bed.

Personal experience of working in these settings provides evidence of care extending beyond six weeks, especially when providing care for older frail people with complex and changing physical or mental health care needs, or those who have had a stroke and need extended time to allow recovery. An editorial published in the *BMJ* (Heath, 2000) took up this point, expressing concern that intermediate care would become a ruse for transferring health care to means testing and personal financing, in a similar way to that which occurred with the transfer of long-term care to residential and nursing homes after the NHS and Community Care Act (DoH, 1990a). It is therefore crucial that as we move towards developing further intermediate care services, we are fully apprised of the long-term financial implications for prospective patients.

Quality or expediency

While there is evidence to suggest that many of those services set up are no cheaper, or are in fact more expensive, than traditional services, there is limited evidence to demonstrate their effectiveness, since evaluation has been limited. Due to the funding arrangements and drivers behind many of the early intermediate care services, they were often developed in ad hoc and pressurized circumstances, using non-recurrent and sporadic monies. This often required time-limited bids with rapid service development responses, making it almost impossible to implement effective evaluation.

Where research has been undertaken, patients have been shown to appreciate the quality of care in a nurse/therapy-led service. However, in terms of outcomes such as length of stay and improved functional ability, there is limited evidence of significant improvements being demonstrated. In some cases it has been poorer than would have been expected if the patient had followed the usual plan of care. The cost has also been shown to be greater (Griffith et al., 2000; Steiner et al., 2001). Sheppard and Illiffe (1998a) have described studies of 'hospital at home' schemes where outcomes were no better although satisfaction was the same or better, but where cost was greater (see Chapter 11). It is important, however, not to use these studies to reject the development of intermediate care services. Each study needs its merits assessed, taking into consideration the range of multiple factors that will have influenced their outcomes, i.e. setting, focus and ultimate aim. What they do imply is that variable factors will impact on a new service and need to be carefully thought through when development is considered alongside evaluation. It is therefore of paramount importance to build in an effective evaluation strategy when developing a service: this is discussed in more detail in Chapter 11.

It is also vital to review all services (acute, intermediate, community and primary care) and ensure that they interface cohesively, providing an integrated whole that gives patients the experience of a 'seamless' transition as they progress from one service to another. This concept of a seamless service has great significance, but what may be necessary to achieve this cannot be overestimated: see Table 1.2.

Table 1.2 Factors for achieving seamless care delivery

- Set of problems
- Environmental factors
- Awareness of options
- Medical opinion
- Liaison with patients/relatives/carers
- Engage with all other services and agencies
- Social care provision
- Stages or steps

Accessing appropriate care

While the focus of care in intermediate care services may be on a more nurse-led and therapeutic approach, it is essential not to assume that intermediate care does not require medical input or that it is simply an extension of the general practitioner role. It is imperative that patients have access to specialist consultations and investigations as and when needed, either from a medical consultant or from other specialist health and social care professionals. The routes out of a service are often well defined, but the routes back in are often precarious and laden with the risk of fragmentation or inequity. The Royal College of Physicians warns of the risk of such intermediate care in the community becoming 'community neglect', where there are risks in simply transferring both costs and pressures to patients and carers through the inappropriate substitutions of hospital facilities (Black et al., 2000).

However, at a time when the context and culture of health care is changing (Vaughan at al., 1999), there is an ideal opportunity to take stock and review current health care delivery, with appropriate intermediate care services and schemes providing such an opportunity. These models of care open the door to more creative approaches to care; they allow for more inter-agency working and possibly create an opportunity to break down current barriers, such as those that are sometimes observed between secondary and primary care. The development of shared care and the concept of 'hub and spoke' care are examples of how more needs-responsive, person-centred care could develop, while there are many opportunities to develop in-reach and outreach working, or more importantly, joint working, to enhance the integration of care received (see Chapter 3). Any such development should occur only with due consideration of the impact not only on patients but also on carers, as discussed in Chapter 12. Due care also needs to be taken to ensure that in developing new services those that are already provided and effective are not destroyed without replacement.

Challenges to utilization

As already discussed, if intermediate care services and schemes are to be utilized effectively to provide integrated and seamless care, there is a need to develop a whole-systems approach. This is a new challenge to providers who have traditionally often worked in isolation.

With the development of ad hoc services due to non-recurrent funding as described above, this coherence and co-ordination of seamless care has often been lacking. The result has been the 'mushrooming' of a range of uncoordinated services that staff across organizations have found difficult to understand or to access. With the development of PCTs and the emerging picture of each one responding locally by providing its own perceived needs-responsive services, it becomes even more important to achieve an integrated service that interfaces with others. Effective partnership and whole-systems working are therefore essential in planning and developing services. In developing a range of needs-responsive services within individual localities, it can be difficult to ensure consistency in expectations while retaining local needs-responsive services. The alternative is to form confederations where decision-making power is delegated in agreed formats.

There are many members of staff involved in the care of patients, and it can be difficult to introduce new services and ensure that these staff are clear about the expectations of that service as well as familiar with the referral criteria, since the very breadth of what can be incorporated within a particular kind of service can cause misunderstanding (see Chapter 2). Confusion may occur as staff struggle to sort out which patient is suitable for which service: trying to ensure unsatisfactory situations do not arise and patients do not 'fall through cracks' is a challenge (MacMahon, 2001). There is thus a need for staff from all disciplines in Acute Trusts to have an understanding of discharge and transfer of care planning. They also need to be aware of the services available as they develop, in order to identify suitable patients. This will help them to have their 'finger on the pulse' in terms of assessing at which stage a patient is, in readiness for transfer or discharge. This requires alertness to predictors and the need to plan proactively from the point of admission.

There have been some creative approaches to assist with this process. In district general hospitals the appointment of a nurse for older and vulnerable people in A&E and medical assessment units provides expertise in assessing the older person and advising about the appropriate care pathway for this client group (Bridges et al., 2000). Similarly, the appointment of occupational therapists and/or social workers in these settings is proving invaluable (Bywaters et al., 2002). Discharge liaison or co-ordinating nurses can play an active part in assisting with the process without taking over the roles of ward staff. In particular, they can keep up to date with new service developments and assist staff in assessing and identifying appropriate patients for particular services by referring to the individual criteria, and matching needs with services. Developing a single point of access or transfer of care team for referrals from both wards and community settings could prove to be an effective means of managing these services.

Within hospitals, there is a need to be aware of patients who are 'in the system' so as to assist with their timely referral/transfer. The creation of a tracking system can be appropriate in supporting this, where patients are assessed and reassessed for their changing needs so that the most appropriate service is identified and accessed. This can be achieved by the creation of 'a Virtual Ward' whereby a team communicate and track via e-mail and a website, as described in Chapter 18, or by the creation of tracking teams with tracker nurses, as has occurred in the Liverpool area (Rosbotham-Williams, 2002). Comprehensive assessment and evaluation (including comprehensive geriatric assessment) are an effective means of identifying medical problems and other health and social care needs and seem to be a tool that ought to be used (MacMahon, 2001); the Single Assessment Process would be perceived as helping with this.

A key challenge in delivery is related to staffing issues, for there is presently a shortage of almost every professional group involved in providing care in intermediate care services. If staff are recruited to newly formed intermediate care service teams, they are likely simply to be poached from other services, so challenging the ability of these original services to provide the care required of them. Vaughan et al. (1999) identify the fact that intermediate care services provide both challenges and opportunities for nurses in what is a more autonomous service. This should not, however, be at the expense of other services, where the pace of activity has probably increased as a result of intermediate care service developments. There is a need to explore how the needs of staff in these services can best be addressed and a need to explore a range of new or more generic roles (see Chapters 3, 5 and 8), but there can be no doubt of the current challenge given the nationwide difficulties in recruitment and retention. There is also a challenge regarding the increased demands being made on traditional services such as district nursing, whose traditional roles are becoming overlaid with additional responsibilities as greater numbers of older people are enabled to remain at home and their care needs increase (Queens Nursing Institute, 2002).

Conclusion

Intermediate care has been conceived as the way forward in providing for a wide range of future health care needs. While it is not a totally new concept, and to some extent remains an ill-defined entity, future developments are open to many greater opportunities than have been realized in the past. Chapter 2 analyses further the concept of intermediate care and explores the service models that it encompasses. It is evident that there is considerable variety in the services that fall under the umbrella of each of these models. However, this very variety may well provide solutions to some of the current challenges faced in caring for sub-acutely ill and physiologically stable people. Any such new direction must be approached with care, taking account of previous research and recognizing potential pitfalls. Moreover, research, evaluation and audit cannot be adequately implemented without consistency and longevity of funding streams, so that short-termism can be turned into long-term strategic planning at the heart of the NHS Plan. The need to develop intermediate care is undoubtedly a tall order when there has been so much significant organizational change over the past few years –

with the shift towards PCT status, the creation of strategic health authorities and confederations along with policy drivers and their inherent performance indicators and milestones (DoH, 1997; DoH, 1998a; DoH, 2000/2001; DoH, 2002f). However, this should not prevent health care professionals grasping opportunities to be creative in developing much needed patient-centred and needs-responsive services.

KEY POINTS

• Intermediate care may be viewed as a 'new concept' or just another name designed to deal with an age-old problem.
• Intermediate care can involve a wide range of services and functions providing needs-responsive services for a wide range of patients.
• Older people have been identified as a key client group to benefit from intermediate care.
• Intermediate care demands that we break down inter-professional and interdisciplinary boundaries, adopt 'new ways of working', and take a new approach to care.
• The complexity of intermediate care can lead to misunderstanding and misuse of services.
• Intermediate care is not a quick solution: it is costly, requires great expertise, careful planning of the service and preparation of staff.
• Intermediate care could be another Cinderella service; if managed well, however, it could provide many opportunities to develop needs-responsive services, and put the care of older people in the forefront of public awareness.

CHAPTER 2

Spotlight on intermediate care: a deeper analysis

LIZ LEES

Introduction

This chapter examines relevant literature to explore in more depth the concept of intermediate care. Definitions are identified and analysed in order to develop practitioners' detailed understanding of what intermediate care actually is. This is important since it appears from experience that there is confusion about the whole concept (Black and Pearson, 2002). There is confusion about what intermediate care encompasses, and at an operational level there is often ongoing difficulty in finding appropriate referrals for many of the intermediate care beds and services that have been developed. This is despite the impetus to develop these new services (DoH, 2001a) at a time when secondary care is under considerable pressure with seemingly unremitting or increasingly extensive trolley waits and capacity problems, as discussed in Chapter 1.

Terminology

There is a plethora of interchangeable terminology related to the concept of intermediate care. Most notable are the following:

- admission prevention and admission avoidance;
- therapeutic care and therapy;
- early discharge and supported discharge;
- 'hospital from home' and 'hospital at home';
- 'step-up' and 'step-down' units;
- nurse-led, post-acute and intermediate care units.

On examining the literature, the most extensive research seems to have been attributed to examining service models designed to speed up discharges, such as nurse-led units and 'hospital at home' teams (Shepperd and Illiffe, 1998c; Griffiths et al., 2001; Steiner, 2001). This may be because these were the earlier models of care created, and the early focus of service development concentrated on this element of care. On the other hand it is apparent that there is a dearth of research exploring admission prevention, such as rapid response and community assessment/rehabilitation teams.

The literature appears to be divided into distinctive methods for researching different models. Randomized controlled trials (RCTs), are the predominant method used for nurse-led units and 'hospital at home' teams (Steiner, 1997; Shepperd and Illiffe, 1998c; Griffiths et al., 2001; Steiner, 2001). While rapid response teams and community assessment rehabilitation teams are scrutinized from a naturalistic (qualitative/phenomenological) perspective, RCTs tend to be regarded as the gold standard, allowing rigorous, replicable study (Polit and Hungler, 1999). Some researchers consider this latter approach inhibitory to the intuitive (artistic) concepts of intermediate care (Vaughan, 1998). For example, the naturalistic literature explored tends to characterize intermediate care through clinical decision-making skills, interdisciplinary and inter-agency working practices, with the emphasis diverted away from the need for medical support (Vaughan, 1998; Steiner, 1997). There is therefore the argument that measurement through reductionism (limiting variables) perhaps best befits the medical model found in secondary care rather than intermediate care settings (Polit and Hungler, 1999).

Examining the concept

In 1997 Steiner conducted a comprehensive literature review with an apparent emphasis on models in practice, while Newman's literature review (1998) analysed the literature from an organizational and somewhat pragmatic perspective 'in order to help decision-makers plan services'. A comprehensive book and service directory expanded this further with 'models in practice' (Vaughan and Lathlean, 1999). By 2001, Steiner published a stimulating research-based review exploring models and functions, offering a new definition for intermediate care. Given such multi-dimensional complexity, this review of definitions will be analysed under several headings':

- intermediate perspectives
- broad definitions
- political perspectives
- individual model definitions.

These perspectives and their objectives will be examined so as to build an incremental picture of current service provision. Ultimately, however, because intermediate care overlaps with services designed specifically for older people and has many professional and organizational interfaces (Steiner, 1997; Vaughan and Lathlean, 1999), there would appear to be no single, perfect way of categorizing the literature or the concept.

The intermediate perspective

Translated literally, 'intermediate' means 'coming between two things in time, place, order character etc.' (Oxford Pocket Dictionary, 1999). Intermediate care describes services that are just that – 'intermediate' – and as such provides a very loose concept for care that has been used in many contexts (BGS, 1998), encompassing a wide diversity of practices in a plethora of venues (Newman, 1998). Steiner (1997) noted that intermediate care is generally perceived as encompassing care between secondary and primary care and between health and social care. Vaughan et al. (1999) noted other in-betweens, between nursing and medical care, and between support worker and carer role. Of greatest significance perhaps is the fact that intermediate care spans a range of traditional service organizational boundaries that encompass primary, secondary and social care but that also include the public, private, voluntary and informal sectors (Black and Durrow, 1998; DoH, 2001e).

The literature reveals a range of services and venues that are quite varied according to the political, organizational and cultural perspectives used (Griffiths et al., 2001). They may be regarded more as a function than a discrete set of services (Steiner, 1997, 2001). Intermediate care signifies service(s) closer to the individual's home, as advocated by the Department of Health, be it high- or low-tech (DoH, 2000b). While for some it epitomizes low-tech, holistic and person-centred care (Griffiths et al., 2001), for others it represent high-tech models (Ridley, 1998). In summary, the emphasis is on a 'whole systems' approach involving social inclusion and demanding effective partnership working in an integrated way (DoH, 2001e). The complexity of such service development and delivery cannot be overestimated.

Broad perspectives of intermediate care

Most definitions of intermediate care appear all-encompassing, stimulating many contradictions about what the term means and thus adding to the complexity of defining it (Steiner, 1997; Steiner and Vaughan, 1997). A wide range of definitions has been proposed over the years. One of the most frequently quoted is that by Steiner and Vaughan in 1997, later added to by Vaughan in 1998 and cited below. The emphasis of Steiner's definition (1997) is on the transition from hospital to home and promoting recovery or improvement in health. This distinguishes intermediate care from community health services, which have an emphasis on maintenance or long-term care (Steiner, 1997; Steiner and Vaughan, 1997):

> That range of services designed to facilitate the transition from hospital to home and from medical dependence to functional independence, where the objectives of care are not primarily medical, the patient's discharge destination is anticipated and a clinical outcome of recovery (or restoration of health) is desired. (Steiner, 1997)
>
> Intermediate Care encompasses a range of services aimed at meeting the needs of those who are physiologically stable who could improve the quality of their lives, increase their ability to live independently and minimize their longer term dependence on health and care services through timely, intensive therapeutic input. (Steiner and Vaughan, 1997)
>
> Those people who, through timely therapeutic intervention may be diverted from acute physiological crisis and hence admission to an acute bed. (Vaughan, 1998)

As Steiner (1997) acknowledged, however, her emphasis on the role of intermediate care in improving the transition from hospital to home was a narrow one that excluded services designed to avoid admission to hospital even where these shared the other characteristics of her definition of intermediate care. Vaughan and Lathlean (1999) therefore subsequently extended Steiner's original definition to include 'services which will help to divert admission to an acute care setting through timely therapeutic interventions'. In this context it is the transitional and outcome-orientated elements of the original definition rather than the process of discharge from hospital that are the key features of intermediate care (Vaughan, 1998).

Further definitions have been proposed over subsequent years. The Royal College of Physicians definition (Black et al., 2000) seems to provide considerable scope. Here intermediate care included 'those services that do not require the resources of a general acute hospital, but are beyond the scope of the traditional primary care team'. These could include 'substitutional care' and 'care for people with complex needs' with perhaps the added caveat of 'being closer to home'. These early definitions provided guidance for the development of services during these years, but there was a lack of consensus on the goal of intermediate care, leading to many interpretations of the concept and what constituted the construct. For this purpose a diagram has been used to illustrate the range of models/services within the umbrella of intermediate care, as illustrated in Figure 2.1.

Political perspectives: a year of prolific activity?

Steiner (2001) proposed another new definition, which could encompass the breadth of models having an emphasis on 'transition' (Steiner, 1997), and has

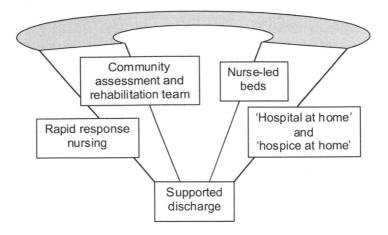

Figure 2.1 The umbrella of intermediate care models/services.

also attempted to offer a framework of models. However, although her work refers to practice, it remains relatively blurred, and perhaps being so broad prevents it from having absolute meaning for those of us not immersed in intermediate care? As Chapter 1 points out, it was not until January 2001 that some more focused guiding principles were released in the form of the *HSC/LAC Intermediate Care Circular* (DoH, 2001e), cited below:

> Intermediate care should be regarded as describing services that meet all the following criteria:
>
> a. Are targeted at people who would otherwise face unnecessarily prolonged hospital stays or inappropriate admission to acute in-patient care, long term residential care, or continuing NHS in-patient care;
> b. Are provided on the basis of a comprehensive assessment, resulting in a structured individual care plan that involves active therapy, treatment or opportunity for recovery;
> c. Have a planned outcome of maximizing independence and typically enabling patient/users to resume living at home;
> d. Arc time limited, normally no longer than six weeks and frequently as little as 1-2 weeks or less; and
> e. Involve cross-professional working, with a single assessment framework, single professional records and shred protocols.

Evidence suggests this definition has tended to form the foundation of developments planned and implemented since this date. For practitioners it provides some commonality and consistency, yet enables local services to be developed in a creative and needs-responsive way. The definition in the

Circular emphasizes the importance of 'Intermediate Care forming an integrated part of a seamless continuum of services linking health promotion, preventative services, primary care, community health services, social care, support for carers and acute hospital care', i.e. a whole-systems approach (DoH, 2001e: 6). It also differs from any previous definition or framework by breaking intermediate care definitions into service models and specific criteria upon which all new intermediate care services should be based. Nevertheless, this prospective approach may not be without its problems.

For example, although there is now a Department of Health definition, it appears to be applicable to a whole range of service models and can serve only as a starting framework. In describing services, the Department of Health stipulate that they must meet all the criteria set. It needs to be asked whether this is possible. Close inspection suggests the Department of Health framework may be flawed. For example, as already discussed, the criteria state six weeks as the stipulated time-frame within which patients should have moved out of intermediate care to their end-point. Evidence suggests that many patients may move into and out of a labyrinth of intermediate care models as their needs fluctuate (Vaughan and Lathlean, 1999). Within the Circular it was not clear from the stated criteria whether the six weeks limit was the total time-frame or limited to one model of care. This ambiguity would appear to have been addressed by the Secretary of State, who has since indicated a more pragmatic approach whereby decisions are left to professional integrity and discretion based on the assessed need of the client for the service.

Despite controversial views expressed by geriatricians (British Geriatrics Society, 1998; Grimley Evans and Tallis, 2001; Martin, 2001), the *National Service Framework for Older People*, also published in March 2001 (DoH, 2001h), includes a key theme on intermediate care. Underlying this is a significant remit to develop intermediate care services to prevent or deflect admission to hospital, promote independence by providing time-limited rehabilitation, and to provide this either at, or as near as possible to, home.

Broad range of models identified from the literature

The number of service models labelled as intermediate care seems to depend upon the focus of the service and the strategic thinking employed by those at the time of implementing the services. For example, intermediate care could be pre-admission screening employed prior to surgery. Alternatively, intermediate care could be interpreted as purely post-acute interventions. Ultimately, it is crucial for service models to be synthesized at an early conceptual stage, thus cementing inextricable links throughout the whole-systems approach. Often the impetus for the service model can be identified from clues within the name: for example, outreach services are usually developed by secondary care to reduce length of stay, whereas community teams are usually developed by primary care to prevent admission. Perhaps even more confusing is the difficulty experienced in trying to gain clarity about the purpose of various intermediate care service models, as it would seem that the objectives and function of service models with the same name can vary depending on their originating purposes – see Table 2.1. These various models will now be examined in more detail, revealing both their complex diversity and their common features.

Table 2.1 The diversity of intended objectives and functions of services with the same name

Intermediate care model	Objective(s)
'Step-up' schemes Community assessment and rehabilitation team GP nursing home beds 'Step-up' schemes	Admission avoidance or Admission prevention
Community assessment and rehabilitation team Rapid-response teams	Rehabilitation at home Rehabilitation in a residential setting Assessment at home Slow-stream rehabilitation
'Hospital at home' Community assessment and rehabilitation team	Supported discharge or Early discharge
Nurse-led units 'Hospital at home' 'Step-down' schemes DVT outreach team Intravenous therapy outreach team	Length of stay reduction
'Hospital at home' Nurse-led units	Early discharge or post-acute care Therapeutic nursing-led care
'Step-up' schemes 'Step-down' schemes	Transitional care Admission prevention for primary care

Rapid-response nursing teams

The literature describing rapid-response teams dates back to 1995 and the development of these teams is increasing (DoH, 2002e). Yet it was only recently that rapid-response teams have been afforded a national definition of their own (DoH, 2001e) as cited:

A service designed to prevent avoidable hospital admissions by providing rapid assessment/diagnosis for patients referred from GPs, A&E, NHS Direct or social services and (if necessary) rapid access on a 24-hour basis to short-term nursing/therapy support and personal care in the patient's own home, together with appropriate contributions from equipment services and/or housing-based support services.

Despite this definition, the remit of rapid response has until recently been vague and has tended to evolve according to 'pressures in the acute sector' (Earl-Slater, 1995). This phenomenon is still supported by the predominantly utilitarian perspective and adaptation of the model through evolution in a practice setting (Lees, 2001). The concept of rapid response may have evolved initially due to a variety of factors, no doubt inextricably linked. This may include poor discharge planning; a need to strengthen district and twilight nursing (Audit Commission, 1992); a reduction in overall bed numbers (British Geriatrics Society, 1998); a need to reduce the length of stay, and a need to reduce admissions to acute hospitals (DoH, 1997); and not least, a need to improve the care of the rising number of older people (Steiner, 2000; Philp, 2001). All this gives the impression of these services acting as a panacea for all ills.

Several teams have been identified from unpublished literature (in the form of service proposals), which illustrate the disparity of names comprising rapid-response nursing services, namely, Rapid Response Integrated Care Services (RRICS), Early Rapid Intervention Teams (ERIT) and Rapid Access Teams (RATs).

Nearly all of the literature cites 'work in progress' (Newman, 1998), adding to the complexity of an absolute definition. For example, as services evolve, their definition may change according to the clinical, organizational and patient focus being addressed. One such definition cited below (Lees, 2001) has changed significantly over the past six months to accommodate the devolution of community services to create a Primary Care Trust lead:

The team will 'rapidly respond' within the hour to assess the patient's needs for intermediate home-based nursing care, to prevent avoidable hospital admission through a single point of access. They collaborate with and refer on to other agencies to institute a care package as required. If the patient is assessed as appropriate, the Rapid Response Team will provide a nursing care package (in addition to any existing services the patient may be receiving) for up to five days.

Those engaged in developing rapid response services are probably aware of the potential diversity of services they can provide (Steiner, 1997). This may have been reinforced through familiarity with characteristics occurring frequently in the literature (Lees, 2001; Earl-Slater, 1995). However, a high degree of ambiguity about what the service provides remains, especially for those less familiar. The critical attributes of 'time', 'access', 'rapid', 'response' and 'action' are the only perspectives that appear common, as they exemplify what is inimitable. The wider intermediate care framework encompasses common themes, inextricably linked yet not unique to rapid response, such as 'prevention', 'transition', 'rehabilitation' and 'time-limited services'. It is evidently not clear whether policy has assisted in shaping and developing the definition of rapid response teams, or whether those teams already established helped to shape policy. Moreover, it could be argued that the policy may have served to inhibit developments. For instance, while the Beds Inquiry (DoH, 2000b) raised the profile of rapid response, it placed a greater emphasis on developing intermediate care beds, potentially detracting from the whole essence of the rapid response concept! At the same time, paradoxically, the national policy definitions (DoH, 2000b, 2001e, h) seem to promote intermediate care, irrespective of the individual model, as the panacea for all health service shortfalls (Vaughan and Lathlean, 1999). Whatever the definition, the two critical attributes seem to be admission prevention and rapid access to services.

'Hospital at home'

Although the literature demonstrates definitions of 'hospital at home' and 'rapid-response teams' that refer to early discharge or admission avoidance, both fit a broader definition of intermediate care (DoH, 2001e). However, not all 'hospital at home' teams are examples of intermediate care (Marks, 1997). For example, in some cases, hospital *from* home, which is the provision of social support, provided by social services (Marks, 1997), is taken to mean 'hospital at home' (Newman, 1998). 'Hospital at home' is the provision of 'hospital-level care in the patient's own home'; in the post-acute phase it can be accessed by the GP direct to prevent admission to the acute or community hospital (Marks, 1997). This model is most appropriate for specific condition groups, such as orthopaedics and elective hip replacements or gynaecology and hysterectomies (Shepperd and Iliffe, 1998c). 'Hospital at home' is co-ordinated to facilitate a care package to support the patient at home, until the point at which the finished consultant episode would have ended had the patient remained in hospital (Earl-Slater, 1995). The patient has equal access to the same level of professional care on a highly individualized basis, and such a model is inextricably linked to community nursing services.

Steiner (1997) specifically excluded 'hospital at home' teams that provided high levels of acute care in patients' homes from her definition, for being 'not consistent' with other aspects of the intermediate care approach. In the UK, 'hospital at home' and rapid response teams have concentrated on lower-technology nursing and therapy interventions that are consistent with an intermediate care approach (Earl-Slater, 1995; Shepperd and Iliffe, 1998c). Alternatively, in the USA, the provision of high-technology care at home has been a feature of 'hospital at home' services (Newman, 1998). The research most commonly suggests that 'hospital at home' services have been established to provide post-acute care for hip replacement and hysterectomy patients (Shepperd and Iliffe, 1998c).

'Hospice at home'

The principle of 'hospice at home' is similar to 'hospital at home', i.e. a hospice-level of care at home, which enables patients to die in their own home surroundings, improves their quality of life and that of their carers, and avoids inappropriate and/or unwanted admission to hospice or hospital. This model is already operational at St Mary's hospice in Birmingham, where there is 'a team of support workers providing care at home, in addition to existing community services, for people in the last stages of their lives, to ensure adequate rest and respite for their lay carers' (Faull, 2000).

Nurse-led wards and post-acute units

Unlike other intermediate care services, this model is generally characterized by the lead professional who has the main responsibility for delivering the service. In this case it is nurses who are regarded as having the lead role with what is called 'nurse-led care' (Steiner, 1997; Griffiths et al., 2001). This contrasts, for example, with community rehabilitation teams, where no individual professional group is identified as having the lead role yet the nurse's contribution to the functioning of the model may be as equal or imperative as it is for a nurse-led setting (Shepperd and Illiffe, 1998c; Earl-Slater, 1995). Conversely, Steiner (2001) does acknowledge that these settings 'may not require nurses to take the lead'. The literature, however, seems to justify the emphasis on the service being nurse-led in relation to nurse-led wards/units, perhaps because the early work and developments focused on a concept of care which challenged the dominance of a medical model and medical control. Because the concept of a more therapeutic/social model care service was not a familiar concept at this time, using the term 'nurse-led' may have been more meaningful in the early evolution of nursing development units (Pearson et al., 1992). These settings are also perhaps the most rigorously researched, accounting for a plethora of research focused on nurse-led wards/post-acute units using randomized controlled trials (Steiner et al., 2001; Griffiths et al., 2001) since 1997.

Most commonly scrutinized features are key outcome measures such as length of stay, functional abilities of patients, costs and readmission rates, comparing this to what would be expected in a traditional post-acute setting (Steiner, 2001). Despite the scrutiny, this model still appears to be relatively loosely defined. Moreover, the definition may be significantly influenced by the particular organizational impetus, such as 'reducing the length of stay' (Steiner, 2001) and the need to provide for post-acute patients requiring low-tech care. Conversely, Vaughan and Lathlean (1999) cite several post-acute units that have specific admission criteria for relatively high-tech nurse-led care such as wound care, nutritional support and multidisciplinary rehabilitation needs. These units employ a high ratio of advanced nurse practitioners, leaving it open to debate whether the nurse-led/post-acute care is 'high- or low-tech' and, moreover, whether it requires senior practitioners (Vaughan, 1998; Wiles et al., 2001). In general it would seem that most post-acute models are seen as 'lower technology settings' for patients who may need rehabilitation after their acute phase is over (Griffiths et al., 2001).

Community assessment and rehabilitation teams

Fourteen different combinations of names for community assessment and rehabilitation teams (CART) were identified from the literature (Steiner, 1997; Newman, 1998; Vaughan and Lathlean, 1999). Three could be differentiated through their focus on rehabilitation in a residential setting, while 11 cited rehabilitation in a patient's home setting as their key remit. It has proved notoriously difficult to distinguish exact 'like for like' comparisons from the literature (Steiner, 1997; BGS, 1998). The names alone have proved to be relatively misleading. For example, depending on the literature, a CART may be an 'intensive home support scheme' (Vaughan and Lathlean, 1999) or an 'intermediate care service' (Newman, 1998), with both being composed of exactly the same components. Moreover, the literature also cites CART under different headings to include multiple functions, namely, early discharge, community rehabilitation and post-acute care (Shepperd and Illiffe, 1998c; Vaughan and Lathlean, 1999).

The concept seems to involve a team of professionals and support workers who can provide rehabilitation for appropriate patients in their own home with the key aim of improving the health of those patients where hospitalization may not be appropriate or necessary (Vaughan and Lathlean, 1999). Such a team aims to improve the rehabilitation outcome by setting goals with the patient, with due consideration to their personal and living circumstances. It is suggested that the community rehabilitation process enhances autonomy, independence and orientation with community reintegration compared to hospital rehabilitation (Steiner, 1997). There are generally two strands of provision, either short-term intensive rehabilitation packages to facilitate early discharge or slow-stream rehabilitation packages for older frail people to prevent admission to hospital or nursing home. It can be used by the acute sector to prevent inappropriate admission to the acute sector *or* where minimization of further functional deterioration is required, thus enabling the patient to continue to live as independently as possible in their own home. Alternatively, it may be used to support an early discharge so as to integrate the older person back to living in his or her own home.

Steiner's work (2001) refers to only CART once, with the most commonly cited model offering rehabilitation either at home or in a residential setting and being referred to as 'supported discharge'. Two further dimensions have been identified, those of 'slow-stream' or 'fast-stream' community rehabilitation (Steiner, 1997; BGS, 1998; Newman, 1998; Vaughan and Lathlean, 1999). In attempting to define CART, the only constant factor would appear to be that it must contain a rehabilitation component, irrespective of the setting and professionals involved (Steiner, 1997; BGS, 1998).

Typically there are four key aspects to the functioning of a CART, as illustrated in Figure 2.2 and highlighted in the shaded boxes: (i) referral; (ii) initial assessment; (iii) setting; (iv) followup. Arguably, however, a reassessment is crucial to such a time-limited service as a CART, but there is also an implicit need for ongoing support and intervention requirements to be identified during the period of time in which the CART service is provided so that transfer of care arrangements can be made in a timely way. Hence these teams have a provider arm inextricably linked to the assessment

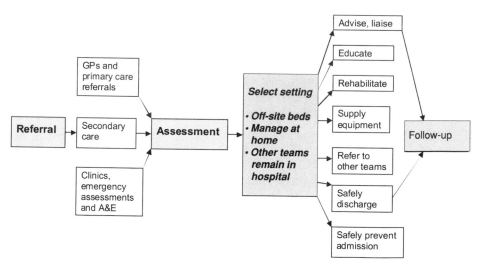

Figure 2.2 Outline care pathway for patients referred to community assessment rehabilitation team.

'Step-up' and 'step-down' schemes

These services are poorly defined in the literature. 'Step-up' tends to be loosely referred to as a safe environment. 'Step-up' schemes are usually developed for patients in community settings whose care needs are stepped up, usually to a point beyond which they would be safe to remain at home. Such schemes perhaps fall outside and beyond the normal provision of health and social care teams (Newman, 1998; Vaughan and Lathlean, 1999). 'Step-up' may take place in a nursing or residential home setting and can be used for a short-term place of safety, convalescence, observation and respite. Comprehensive assessments can be conducted in conjunction with the GP and district nurses visiting to provide additional support to the nursing home.

'Step-up' is distinguishable from 'step-down' by the route of access, which is usually via the patient's GP or primary care team. The term 'step-down' indicates the patient's care needs are no longer deemed to be commensurate with acute or community hospital/intermediate care unit service provision such that their care could be more appropriately delivered in an alternative environment. 'Step-down' provides a safe, well-maintained, sometimes low-intensity, therapeutic environment for the needs of predominantly older adults whose functional rehabilitation potential is perhaps at an end point or has reached optimal potential (Lees and Crouch, 1999), or where patients have complex discharge needs. While patients may still have complex nursing needs, providing some element of rehabilitation and proactive encouragement could avoid the alternative of long-term placement. 'Step-down' allows patients and relatives time to consider the options available to them, especially where pressures upon beds in the acute sector prove excessive. Hence, time spent in such facilities ('step-up' or 'step-down') may be justified by the potential to minimize the unnecessary transfer of patients on to long-term care (Steiner, 1997), and ensures that some elements of rehabilitation are provided.

'Step-down' schemes feature most predominantly in the literature as short-term winter pressure beds (DoH, 2000b) producing extra capacity for the winter (BGS, 1998; Newman, 1998). The latest policy guidance regarding purchasing makes it clear that where a 'step-down' service is provided 'without an element of rehabilitation' it is not advocated as an intermediate service model by the Department of Health (DoH, 2001e, h). The challenge then faced by the Health Service is the provision of care for those older people who have been clearly identified as needing a care home. It could be argued that all such patients should have the opportunity to spend a period of time in a 'step-down' service, since the right environment with a therapeutic approach may allow time for improvement and the opportunity to return home. However, it could also be argued that, for some patients, efforts to enable them to stay at home have been exhausted and a care home remains the only option. For these patients, if a care home placement is not available they may require interim care, where 'interim care' signifies ongoing nursing care without the element of active rehabilitation now associated with intermediate care and 'step-down', as defined by the Department of Health (DoH, 2001e). This interim care would be better provided in a setting other than a busy acute setting. This is an area that has received little attention. Even with the adoption of the Scandinavian model of cross-charging of social services for the care of patients who are waiting for a care home place, it does not address the environment in which this interim care is provided (DoH, 2002f). To date, there seems to have been little attention directed at addressing the care environment of these patients.

High-tech intermediate care

The literature around 'step-down' care usually implies 'to take a step down from hospital' (Steiner, 1997; Newman, 1998). It could equally mean 'to take a step down from an intensive care setting' to an acute medical or surgical ward (Ridley, 1998). The difference in the care considered here is phenomenal, that of a very low-tech setting (Newman, 1998) compared to a very high-tech setting (Ridley, 1998). In reaching a definition, both perspectives of 'step-down' would appear to have one factor in common, that is they are both a by-product of an organizational need to create extra bed capacity by moving patients to another setting (DoH, 2000b).

In the literature reviewed there was little reference to the possibility of high-dependency units falling under the umbrella of intermediate care services (Newman, 1998). In this instance, intermediate care is defined as a high-dependency unit 'providing a level of intermediate care that is between a general ward and intensive care' (Ridley, 1998). Other aspects of this type of intermediate care are less clear; for example, intensive care suffers 'inappropriate admissions' and its intermediate relief, namely high dependency, can act as 'step-up' or 'step-down' between general wards and intensive care (Ridley, 1998). So what is it that distinguishes high-tech intermediate care from other intermediate care facilities? Key defining features, not advocated in the literature but clear nonetheless, are that patients need to remain in hospital beds, they are not medically stable and costs per patient are generally regarded as being higher.

Summary

Early research indicated model definitions and their expected outcomes to be quite distinctive, probably quite isolated from mainstream acute and primary care services (Steiner, 1997). Furthermore, the definitions were rarely transferable to other intermediate care settings. Contrary to any difficulty presently experienced in defining intermediate care, this, if anything, should have made it easier. More recently, the complexity surrounding intermediate care definitions has increased. In part, this may be due to the media attention that winter pressures have received, but it is also due to the new impetus to develop services which interface between primary and secondary care (DoH, 2002f). To summarize, there appear to be four significant dimensions that are evident, irrespective of the intermediate care model: critical attributes, context, patient objectives, and organizational objectives. Figure 2.3, based on Walker and Avant's (1995) framework for conceptual analysis and Rodgers's (1989) evolutionary framework, has been used to illustrate this point.

Conclusion

Practitioners seeking explicit guidance may be frustrated by the consistent stream of contradictions evident in the literature, which can confuse even the most experienced of intermediate-care staff. There are various kinds of intermediate service and they are defined differently, according to the definer's perspective, in terms of their utility, or idealistically or realistically. What is needed is a common approach to defining them that demonstrates their purpose and scope, and provides examples of appropriate patients and

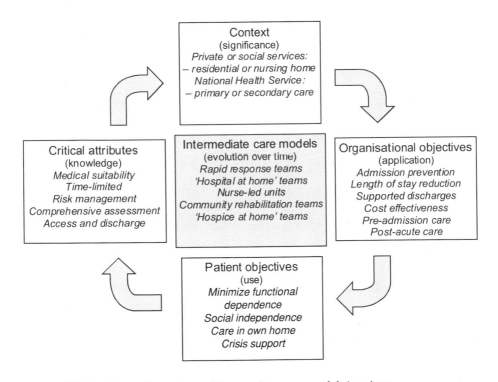

Figure 2.3 Significant dimensions of intermediate care models/services.

relevant condition groups. The caveat, of course, is that both services and definitions are evolving at the same time: there are currently few services delivering intermediate care whose establishment is sufficiently stable to indicate a way forward for longer-term stability. While it is neither appropriate nor desirable to divide services rigidly according to definitions, the confusion is perpetuated by the latest metamorphoses of rapid response and community assessment teams that create phenomenally complex services. Even more alarming are the acronyms adopted. For example, CARRT may mean two completely different things, namely Community Assessment and Rapid Rehabilitation Team, or Community Assessment and Rapid Response Team. Furthermore, teams and services originally distinguishable for their functional role, particularly rehabilitation, may merge under one umbrella. This could undermine effective rehabilitation, but on the other hand it could provide a means of assessing needs and providing the correct service and range of support.

Finally, the prevailing focus seems to be on what intermediate care services *already* achieve rather than on what they *might* achieve. While there is much current good practice to be observed, it is often characterized by limitations and contradictions that hinder the full development of the process of referral, assessment and reassessment.

For some, intermediate care has been viewed as patient focused and for others organization focused. With the former, patient-focused goals have been described as 'recovery', 'maintaining people in their homes' or 'finding suitable alternatives to home' (Steiner, 2001). Organizational objectives, on the other hand, have tended to emphasize shorter lengths of stay, lower costs, improved throughput or more appropriate hospital admissions, while recognizing the opportunities for nurse/therapy-led developments (Griffiths et al., 2001; Steiner, 2001). The latest policy documents refer to a 'seamless' continuum of intermediate care services. Perhaps this needs to be interpreted as a series of stages from which the selection of an appropriate service model can occur. Moreover, comprehensive assessment for entry into and exit out of the models can be considered across the whole system, from acute to primary care, ensuring patient care will not be compromised along any particular pathway.

The history of intermediate care begins with rehabilitation, care of older people and community services. If intermediate care is to be further embraced, history rather than nostalgia should be reflected in intermediate care definitions, to inspire the future rather than relive the past. The potential of intermediate care to meet some of the health and social care needs of older people is explored further in the next chapter.

KEY POINTS

- There is a range of service models or schemes that come under the umbrella of intermediate care.
- Analysis of the range of service models reveals the diversity of the actual services/schemes that exist within these models.
- Some common attributes or themes can be identified as associated with specific service models, but these remain quite wide-ranging and open to interpretation.
- Diversity rather than commonality is perhaps the main feature of intermediate care services/schemes, and this perhaps reflects the ad hoc needs-responsive way that they have developed.
- In the longer term, greater cohesion and consistency might better serve the effective provision of these services/schemes from the perspective of the patient.

CHAPTER 3
Meeting the needs of older people

SIÂN WADE

Introduction

This chapter further analyses the emergence of older people as a significant client group perceived both as using and as having the potential to benefit from intermediate care. In order to ensure that older people do benefit, however, there is a need to explore appropriate ways to address their health and social care needs so that intermediate care services do not become second-rate or replicate the old 'Cinderella services' of the past. A range of care models is explored, with a particular emphasis on ways in which the medical care needs of older people can be met both within intermediate care and within acute and specialist acute services.

Intermediate care for older people – why?

Significant rhetoric has been used to justify the direction of recent policies and developments regarding intermediate care, in both humanistic and financial terms (DoH, 1998b). On analysis of the situation, however, there can be no doubt that an organizational impetus to clear acute beds has put the focus of intermediate care firmly upon the sub-acute care of people who are deemed physiologically stable (Hanford et al., 1999). This impetus, and strategies to avoid or defer acute admissions where possible and prevent long-term institutional care, are perhaps seen as the key motives behind intermediate care. Indeed, as suggested in Chapter 1, intermediate care has been heralded as a solution to many 'bed-blocking' and bed capacity problems of recent years. Such problems have inevitably been seen in terms of older people, whose increased likelihood of multiple pathology and reduced functional reserve make them likely to require longer recovery times (see Chapter 4). The argument is that, once they have become reasonably medically stable, many of these patients would benefit as well, if not better, from rehabilitation and a more therapeutic and social model of care provided within intermediate care settings than from an acute bed.

MacMahon (2001) argues that during the 1980s and 1990s pressures on the health service and a concentration on acute care and patient throughput led to a fragmentation and loss of emphasis on rehabilitation services, with their subsequent demise throughout the health service (Audit Commission, 1992, 1997, 2000; Clinical Standards Advisory Group, 1998; CSP, 2001). The opportunity to adopt the open-ended funding available from the Department of Social Services for long-term care provided a perverse incentive to reduce pressure on acute beds by discharging older people to such care, probably before many had been able to maximize rehabilitation opportunities. Changes in the law and pressures on social services funding with the NHS and Community Care Act (DoH, 1990b) meant this model of care could not be sustained, leading to competition rather than collaboration between Health and Social Services in recent years (Age Concern, 1999a). The re-emphasis of attention on a collaborative and rehabilitative model of care within intermediate care would suggest that the motives behind intermediate care are to provide older people with the opportunity to benefit from rehabilitation in a timely and responsive way, thus increasing their independence and reducing the need for institutional care or costly/intensive home care. The benefits of rehabilitation have been poignantly described by the Royal Commission Report (1998) which suggests that a 1 per cent decrease in age-specific dependency rates would almost halve the costs of long-term care between 1995 and 2051. This could have a major impact on funding issues.

Martin (2001) suggests that older people have been considered as prime candidates for alternative care services such as those encompassed by intermediate care because they are perceived as over-users of acute hospital beds. The assumption is that this will lead to more suitable care. However, in assuming this it is important to ensure that older people are not denied access to specialist acute care, including gerontology as well as appropriate rehabilitation care, or the supportive and caring facilities that are needed to deal with illness, disability and dying. Martin suggests that, if it is otherwise, 'the [new intermediate care] strategy is ageism, albeit "with a softer heart"' (2001: 9). Some of this concern is reflected in the goals and performance indicators outlined within the NHS Plan and modernization agenda (DoH, 2000c, 2002f). First, there is a requirement to reduce the length of stay of older people in acute beds through the use of intermediate care services. Second, there is a demand that the annual increases in acute admission rates for people over 75 years of age rise by less than 2 per cent. As Grimley Evans and Tallis (2001) point out, there is no evidence to suggest that the percentage identified in this latter indicator will match clinical need, and as such the proposal appears to reflect institutionalized ageism, 'betraying' the very aspirations described within the National Service Framework for older people to wipe out ageism and age discrimination (DoH, 2001h). Also, it could be argued, there is limited evidence to suggest that intermediate care is more effective either in cost or outcome (Steiner, 2001). As discussed in Chapter 1, one of the greatest concerns expressed about intermediate care is that older patients may receive a marginalized service and may perceive it as 'a second-rate service', both in terms of access to medical care and to skilled care.

With the focus on older people there seems to be a major concern that 'intermediate care is a new name designed to deal with an old problem – that of older patients staying in acute beds and causing crises during winter time' (Kirby, 2000: 109). There is thus a considerable risk that intermediate care may become a strategy for bed-management and capacity management rather than one for meeting clinical or therapeutic need. The drive to address winter pressures and prevent trolley waits can become an urgent and merciless force in the use of beds. Indeed, personal experience and evidence has shown that, unless used very carefully, the delay in discharge of patients is simply transferred out of acute settings on into intermediate care settings. This prevents further transfers of patients out of acute settings and challenges the smooth flow of patients through service settings, still leading to the inappropriate placement of patients. Alternatively, criteria for admission to intermediate care services are so strict that beds and places are left empty while acute services experience bed management crisis on a daily basis. There is also the risk of a patient being referred to a number of different intermediate care, primary care or private care services, all of which may be reasonably suitable, even if a specific one is deemed the most appropriate. This is simply in the guise of trying to transfer/discharge the patient from an acute bed. Thus the problem is shifted or moved, but not necessarily addressed. This can also lead to fragmented care between providers in acute, community and private care networks. Consequently, instead of diverting care away from long-term care these new developments could end up compounding existing problems and replicating the present and past. Another challenge is that where different providers deliver services, e.g. Acute Trusts or PCTs, there is the risk that active intervention may be withdrawn, with care becoming fragmented once transfer to a new service is imminent. This is most likely to occur in terms of therapy or care management, where resources are limited such that priorities have to be made.

In defining and developing intermediate care services or schemes, therefore, one of the things we need to be most alert to is that such services genuinely contribute to an improved and integrated service with specific outcome measures for those using them. There is probably a need to have criteria for referral to various services, and yet there needs to be the opportunity to use professional integrity when referring and accepting patients. As previously suggested, if these criteria are too strict, services may be under-utilized at a time when they could be utilized more constructively in the best interests of patients. This is where the input of staff with experience and skill in the care of older people is important – it is in fact crucial.

Models that might best serve older people

If older people are going to have their care needs addressed appropriately there is a need to consider very carefully what should be provided in acute hospitals, intermediate care services, and community and primary care. These sectors need to interface effectively both to provide integrated, timely and needs-responsive services and care, and also to ensure a smooth and continuous transition between these services. Intermediate care can provide the opportunity to plan and develop a whole new service to meet the needs of older people – not just an 'add-on'.

Within the acute sector it would seem that care will increasingly focus on specialist care needs and on meeting the needs of older people who are medically unstable or unfit. This would include those services that require access to scarce or skilled staff, equipment, facilities or resources that are best provided centrally unless effective outreach models or technology systems can be developed. While many aspects of a particular care need or care pathway may be provided in primary or intermediate care, referral to more specialist care may be necessary on occasion, although follow-up may occur back within a community setting or service. Medical assessment units are increasingly being developed which should allow access to consultation, diagnostics and investigations without admission. Other models of care that could be developed will be discussed below.

If older people are not to be denied appropriate care, it is essential that current care models ensure their access not only to specialist care in terms of investigations, diagnostics and treatment but also to care delivered by skilled practitioners with knowledge of older people. What is crucial is the need for a comprehensive set of services across the care pathway needs of patients.

Within the acute sector, four principal models of service organization have evolved, as outlined by the Royal College of Physicians (RCP, 2000b), in which the care of older people with medical problems is addressed:

1. age-defined;
2. needs-related (traditional);
3. common admission;
4. integrated (or a hybrid model).

The degree of integration with services for younger adults varies within these models, and according to the RCP no single model has been shown to be more effective. The particular model that has evolved will most likely have been determined by local priorities, the preferences of local consultants and the availability of resources, although a survey of patients showed that an integrated model of care was preferred, especially by older people (Bend and Solomon, 1999). However, both the Health Advisory Service, in *Not Because They Are Old* (HAS, 1998), and Age Concern, in *Turning Your Back On Us* (Age Concern, 1999b) report incidents where older people may have fared better in 'elderly-friendly' acute wards.

With the increasing number of older people in the population and in hospital, the provision of designated direct acute specialist admission wards for older people may become increasingly unrealistic, and thought needs to be given to the best means of using the skills of geriatricians and specialist staff. This must be considered within the context of evolving intermediate care services and schemes and the ways in which they will be supported by specialist gerontological expertise. How and where care is best delivered may need to be rethought. Within the four principal acute models of care identified by the Royal College of Physicians (RCP, 2000b), the first three all have specialist acute wards for older people as well as rehabilitation wards. In the integrated care model, no specific acute ward for older people is evident but they do have specialist rehabilitation settings.

It is not clear how much 24-hour medical support will be provided with new intermediate care rehabilitation services and schemes, and indeed, given their diversity across the country, this is likely to vary quite considerably. Similarly, it is not clear how well developed or intense rehabilitation will be within these services and schemes. However, they increasingly have the potential to provide the rehabilitation needs of the more stable older person, with rapid access to emergency or specialist care as needed (see below), so long as medical and therapy input is consistent and does not become 'patchy'. If this were the case, then it would seem that some changes could occur within the four principal acute models of care outlined by the Royal College of Physicians. Within the integrated care model, the rehabilitation wards may increasingly become more acute/sub-acute, with patients transferring from the integrated medical wards fairly rapidly after only a few days. Rehabilitation would still be provided within these wards so that it could be introduced as soon as the older person were able to begin to benefit – which might already be very much the focus of such wards. A similar shift of emphasis may well occur within the rehabilitation wards described in the RCP's first three models. Here the acute and rehabilitation activities could merge more, to provide acute/sub-acute care and rehabilitation for the more medically unstable older person as intermediate care services develop. This, however, will depend to some extent upon the siting of these settings and the level of medical cover provided, and will vary from Trust to Trust.

The provision of specialist rehabilitation within the acute service, such as that for stroke and orthopaedic rehabilitation, has been variable, some settings having designated wards and others providing the care within acute or general rehabilitation wards. Research shows that these patients do well within a designated rehabilitation setting compared to medical wards, and there are some quite specific and specialized skills required to meet the needs of these patients (Dennis and Langhorne, 1994; Audit Commission, 1995). If developing intermediate care services/schemes can provide this level of rehabilitative skills within focused intermediate care settings, this would be satisfactory provided there is also reasonable access and review by specialist consultants. For patients whose condition is more unstable or unpredictable but who are well enough to leave the acute wards (acute stroke wards in many cases, and orthopaedic/trauma wards), their needs may be best cared for in a sub-acute/rehabilitation setting that provides access to 24-hour medical care and acute facilities. If an adequate level of specialist rehabilitation for these conditions cannot be provided for in intermediate care services/schemes, then it should be provided within the acute service, perhaps best designated as part of the specialist gerontology service (or as part of a shared service between gerontology and neurology or gerontology and orthopaedics).

As stated above, surveys suggest that older people have not always been best served by the acute integrated model of care (HAS, 1998; Age Concern, 1999b). With an ageing population, however, it is inevitable that many older people will be cared for within a range of acute settings and specialities. If expert or specialist gerontological knowledge, care or advice has not been provided in the past, this area must surely be addressed, a proposal supported by the National Service Framework for Older People – Standard 4 (DoH, 2001h).

Within current service provision a geriatrician may not necessarily see all older people, and often only those referred to their care will be seen and receive a comprehensive assessment. Hopefully, the effective development of the Single Assessment Process (DoH, 2001j; see also Chapter 10) will enable those who would benefit to receive this level of assessment. This may initiate referral to a geriatrician or specialist gerontological practitioner, if there is one. It is evident that there has been a lack of staff with the skills and competency to care or contribute to the care of older people across acute settings (HAS, 1998; Age Concern, 1999b). This could perhaps be attributed to the need to equip staff to care for other specialist care interventions, but could equally be attributed to the belief that caring for older people requires only 'basic' care skills and that these can be provided by any health care professional or worker. This, as stated above, has been picked up within the National Service Framework for Older People, with the requirements to undertake a skills analysis of staff in acute care and to ensure that staff are competent to provide care to older people. The development of a competency framework related to the care of older people for all staff in any setting involved in looking after older people would be a natural extension of this work. This would perhaps be best addressed by interested practitioners and educationalists working together to create and validate a national competency framework, so that when staff transfer between jobs, having achieved particular competencies, there is a common understanding of the skills and attributes that they have gained.

The National Service Framework for Older People (DoH, 2001h) also recommends that a centre of excellence in the care of older people should be developed. This could be a natural extension of the specialist sub-acute/rehabilitation settings, as is already the case in some Trusts. There is then the potential for the centre to assist staff from different settings and specialities in developing the skills and attributes needed to care for older people. Different models could be used to address these development needs. Rotations across specialist or general medical/surgical wards, intermediate care services and specialist gerontology sub-acute/rehabilitation settings could be an effective way forward. It would be appropriate to develop teaching programmes with an accompanying competency framework for staff from all professions, to be delivered via such rotations or to staff working within their own settings/services, and funding could be sought from the confederations.

A specialist and skilled multi-professional team based in the specialist centre, as recommended in the National Service Framework, could be set up to provide support and advice to staff on wards without taking over care. This team could also work with staff and discharge co-ordinators or teams in undertaking the assessment of older people who have been identified as needing ongoing rehabilitation or care, to identify the most appropriate service/setting to which they should be referred. This could help to overcome the ad hoc referrals that often occur, especially when there are bed management crises.

Perhaps a key role of this specialist centre and team would be to take a lead in driving forward the strategic agenda for services for older people within a health economy. This would involve working closely with teams and staff across the locality, so promoting a whole-systems approach as discussed in earlier chapters. An essential part of this agenda would involve collaborative partnership working to establish a robust model and programme for the development of staff who care for older people. This would require the development of staff knowledge and attributes across acute, specialist, intermediate and primary care services, and would need to recognize the importance of establishing attractive and responsive career pathways for staff, ensuring effective succession planning (discussed in later chapters).

In the past, health care professionals with a special interest in and knowledge of this field have not necessarily assessed older people who have been transferred to nursing homes for their rehabilitation potential. The introduction of the assessment for the health care element of funding for patients going to nursing homes, and the requirement for health care workers to play a role in this assessment, means these multidisciplinary teams could play a key role. This would ensure not only a skilled assessment of the health care element, but also that all patients going to care homes have been assessed as appropriate for that level of care and that their full potential for rehabilitation has been explored and realized. Utilizing the Single Assessment Process (DoH, 2001h, 2002g) should help here, older patients being more likely to receive a more specialist and comprehensive assessment. Geriatricians would also be part of the membership of the specialist multidisciplinary teams, although how this would be managed would vary. A major benefit for older people would be for geriatricians to have a key role in the assessment of older people for whom major surgery is proposed, and indeed for those for whom it has been decided surgery is not recommended. This would ensure expert advice and assessment was available to specialist consultants and surgeons, who may not have particular knowledge about the ageing process and the consequences of ageing on post-surgical recovery. Hopefully, this would mean that appropriate intervention is offered and that quality of life for the individual is carefully considered and promoted.

Access to specialists at the acute/intermediate care interface

While a social or therapeutic model of care may be desirable once an older person has recovered from ill health and is medically stable, there should still be the opportunity for an older person to be assessed by a consultant geriatrician and/or nurses and therapists with appropriate expertise (Martin, 2001). Equally, if an older person has avoided admission to acute care by the utilization of an intermediate care service/scheme, it is important that a patient who needs or would benefit from specialist care is screened or assessed and is able to access this care if necessary.

The modelling and delivery of gerontological care is still evolving; one way forward in developing services would seem to be a 'hub and spoke' model that involves joint working or strong links between acute and community care. Systems by which patients can be referred, reviewed or discussed at multidisciplinary team meetings within intermediate care settings may be more appropriate than the rather more traditional model of ward rounds, perceived by some as being medically dominated, and would promote the concept of nurse/therapy-led services. Access to medical care and involvement of a skilled multidisciplinary team could be achieved through outreach by consultant geriatricians to teams within the community including intermediate care settings and services, out-patient clinics and care homes (as recommended by the RCP/RCN/BGS 2000; RCN/BGS 2001). To work in teams across these settings would require staff to have appropriate expertise and a shared vision and accountability for the comprehensive delivery of services, and would develop good practice in care for older people. Where and how these teams would work would be variable, depending upon local factors.

The way in which specialist gerontology services are provided within the acute sector may need to change or at least be extended, and there are a number of models that might be considered. One such model involves Rapid Access Clinics (RAC). This service offers GPs a next-day or post-weekend service, whereby within a specified length of time a patient can be referred to and seen by a multi-professional team experienced in the care of older people. The service is probably best provided within an assessment and treatment day unit (perhaps known as a day hospital in some settings). Such a team needs to include a consultant geriatrician, nurse, physiotherapist and occupational therapist and have access to other expertise such as podiatry, speech therapy and dietetics etc., together with diagnostics and investigations. It is also helpful to have direct admitting rights to beds within specialist gerontology wards. This type of service provides the opportunity for a fairly rigorous comprehensive assessment; while some patients do require admission, others are able to access further investigations or treatment via the assessment and intervention unit, while retaining continuity of care from the team and remaining at home. Access to these investigations and treatments may be more rapid than might have been possible as an outpatient. If admission is needed this can be expedited, minimizing the length of hospital stay, and where possible the patient can remain under the care of the RAC geriatrician. Where it is available this service has been received very positively by GPs. Evaluation of one such service has shown that the practitioners involved in providing the service do need to be experienced.

A similar model of care could be established for in-patient care within specialist gerontological services. For example, in addition to referring patients from an acute or integrated care ward within an acute service, referrals could also be made through a rapid access service. Patients could be referred from an intermediate care service or direct from the community for a short stay, during which they gain access to specialists, investigations, skills, diagnostics and treatment. The stay could be overnight or as long as required, followed by patients returning to their home or intermediate care service with ongoing care or support as appropriate. Temporary readmission could be arranged for further treatment and/or follow-up if necessary. Patients could be referred by a GP or any member of the multidisciplinary team; alternatively, a geriatrician working within an outreach programme could refer a patient and then follow up once the patient is transferred back to intermediate care.

With this model, geriatricians would retain their acute remit while incorporating a number of clinics/sessions within the community and intermediate care settings. The community localities would need to be sectorized with regard to the way each geriatrician worked, and possibly for other team members also, so that they would be linked to their own sector. Patients in these settings could remain under the care of their GP but the consultant would provide the service with an overview of patients who caused concern or were identified as benefiting from a consultant or specialist opinion. Alternatively, the patient could be transferred to the acute gerontology service under the direct care of the consultant for a period of time before being referred back to their GP. The consultant could also follow up patients who had been in their acute setting, as discussed. GPs could also be used in more specialist roles, e.g. as associate specialist, while a model of in-reach to the acute setting could be adopted, with other specialist or community practitioners playing a part who may or may not already be involved in a patient's care. Such a service would not replace direct acute/emergency or planned admissions to either integrated care or other specialist care.

Within such models of care the emphasis would be on sound, effective multi- or interdisciplinary working. Such an approach, however, is poorly developed in this field, and will require considerable work in some services/settings (see Chapter 16). There needs to be a greater emphasis on inter-professional education and collaborative working that maintains the uniqueness and value of each profession yet gives rise to the emergence of shared values and working with mutual respect and regard for all team members (UKCC, 2001). Such an environment would give rise to new ways of working that would create further opportunities, such as undertaking action research, or making use of team-members' expertise as a learning resource.

Primary care

There is the potential to develop new preventive, supportive and health promotion services in either intermediate care or primary care. Falls clinics, for example, can be developed in these settings, with many of the required interventions being provided either there or nearby, e.g. exercise classes such as Tai Chi, education and information, home assessments and physical assessments. Older people in need of more specialist intervention can be screened through these clinics and referred on as necessary to various staff members or services, with assessment by a geriatrician in either an intermediate care or an acute setting, e.g. where assessment for the use of a Tilt table is needed.

Mental health

Although policy directives and guidelines have not emphasized it, intermediate care has considerable potential within the field of mental health care. A range of schemes and services has already been established and mental health trusts appear to be quite active in exploring the role of intermediate care within care pathways for older people in need of mental health care (*Nursing Older People*, 2002). Intermediate care seems highly relevant for such patients, especially since admission or relocation can be particularly distressing for those with cognitive impairment problems or depression.

The potential of new models of working

By embracing developments in intermediate care in a proactive and opportunistic way there is the potential to address the holistic care needs of older people right across the health and social care economy, i.e. acute care, intermediate care, primary care, and long-term care. To achieve effective partnership and inter-agency working will require overcoming many current barriers and challenges – no easy task (see Chapter 6). It will also require good leadership and effective co-ordination. The potential benefit of such services, developed as whole systems and supported by skilled care and support, is that, with effective management, they could in some cases reduce the need for acute admissions, and in others ensure that acute admission is timely and needs-responsive. They could also help to ensure a return by an older person to the community as soon as possible, so reducing extended stays in the acute sector, which are so often not in the best interests of older people. This would both better meet the needs of older people and also save many of the bed-days in acute settings that older people are so often criticized for wasting. It will be no easy feat: there needs to be investment or transfer of money to establish services across the economy to provide sufficient capacity and skills to provide such care and support. Furthermore, close partnership working, new ways of working, and a change of culture rarely come easily to practitioners.

Staffing

The achievement of expanded and extended services for older people will inevitably be a challenge, due both to recruitment and retention issues and to limitations of skills and expertise. Geriatricians have increasingly played a significant part within the integrated acute-take of patients within Acute Trusts, and with this goes the subsequent post-take rounds and care. This means that they are giving care to patients of all ages. By having to focus dedicated time in this way, elements of their time have been diverted from addressing the needs of older people. In many areas, the number of geriatricians for the size of the population is well below that recommended by the RCP (2000b), while in others medical care for older people is provided by medical physicians with an interest in older people, or indeed by nurse practitioners.

Various benefits arise from geriatricians having a range of roles. They can be a member of multidisciplinary teams providing support and advice within acute services, they can provide medical care within specialist gerontological wards in an Acute Trust, they can have a role within an integrated medical care service, and can support intermediate care through outreach/hub-and-spoke activities. If geriatricians are to play an effective and active role in all these settings then there is a need for more to be appointed. It is possible to make joint appointments or shared appointments between PCTs and acute services to maintain the range of skills of doctors and meet the Royal College of Physicians requirements. However, there is a national shortage of geriatricians and aspiring Specialist Registrars in this field, which is likely to become worse as greater awareness of their value brings about an increased demand for them (BGS, 2002). The BGS found in a recent survey that not only is the general medicine component of the role felt to be too dominant by trainees, but also the innovations of intermediate care do not appear to be popular. Nevertheless, interest and confidence in engaging in new models of working involving intermediate care could well improve as geriatricians become more engaged in this work and as training opportunities are increased (BGS, 2002). This can succeed only if the demands of other elements of their work, such as acute medicine, are addressed, otherwise making such models of care a reality could be compromised.

There is also a shortage of therapists – currently a considerable shortfall (18 per cent) across the country (DoH, 2002f) – and this shortage is reflected within the field of gerontology and intermediate care (CSP, 2001). Although the NHS Plan (DoH, 2000c) made a clear commitment to increase investment and recruitment of therapists, especially physiotherapists, it will take some time to make up the current shortfall, despite high application rates for training. There are also difficulties with regard to the way physiotherapists prefer to work, e.g. specializing early, which may challenge recruitment to more generalist rehabilitation. At present there is a scenario of 'robbing Peter to pay Paul', i.e. taking staff from one service to resource another, possibly diluting staffing across all services. Thus the concept of seamless care will be even more challenged due to lack of resources. The shortage has been so critical that in some areas the success of new services such as CARTs (Community Assessment Rehabilitation Teams) have been compromised due to the inability to recruit adequately. The same picture is reflected in nursing, where retention is possibly an even greater issue than in other professions (Finlayson et al., 2002). While intermediate care offers a range of opportunities (as discussed in Chapter 1), the general national shortage will directly impact on the aspirations to deliver an integrated and seamless service.

The increased emphasis on developing services for older people and rehabilitation has placed a sudden demand upon recruitment to this field at a time when there is a national shortage of personnel in almost all health care disciplines (Finlayson et al., 2002). Against this backdrop of a national shortage of staff, however, there seems to be limited interest by many in caring for this client group (Akid, 2001). Akid draws attention to a study with nurses, and records a number of quotes from it, suggesting that 'care for older people is nothing more than a "babysitting" service, carried out by nurses "sent to geriatrics because they can't do any harm"'. In another quotation, a nurse describes it 'as a waste of three years of training'. Akid suggests that research shows this field of work often holds little recognition by physicians, summed up by a doctor outside the speciality: 'If the worst comes to the worst you can always work in Geriatrics.' According to Ian Philp, however, care for older people is far from this – it is in fact 'caring ... at the highest level' (Akid, 2001: 13).

The situation does not seem to be helped by the current education systems for pre-registration courses, where there appears to be a lack of emphasis on the skills and complexity of looking after older people (Wade 2000). For doctors, the element related to older people within their pre-registration curriculum may be only a few days, while for nurses and therapists it may vary considerably. Although there seems to be an increasing interest and willingness to provide multi-professional post-registration courses in gerontology, the uptake of places on these specialist courses has generally been low compared to other specialist courses, such as critical care, that have more kudos and status. Thus, while intermediate care may be seen to offer other rewards that attract nurses and other practitioners (Vaughan et al. 1999), care must be taken to prepare and support them adequately and to prevent them becoming disillusioned. How to achieve this is addressed in later chapters.

There has also been a dearth of opportunities for clinical career promotion in the field of gerontology, especially for nurses and professionals allied to medicine. For example, historically in nursing few specialist nurse roles have been available, so that the only pathway for nurses beyond the role of ward sister/manager has been into management or education. Not only has this meant that nurses have left the speciality, but it may also have given the message that care of older people is not perceived as a speciality and not valued in the same way as other services or client groups. With the new importance of providing smoothly co-ordinated care for older people with complex needs across an increasingly diverse range of services, it becomes highly appropriate and desirable to develop a range of specialist posts, particularly roles such as consultant nurse/therapist, specialist nurse and intermediate care co-ordinator (see Chapter 8). The overall objective of such roles, however, must be to promote effective and integrated care by working across the interfaces and boundaries of these services – they must not fragment the care further. This means that the direct responsibility for and co-ordination of the care of any individual older person must be transparently clear, and in most cases remain with the service provider – looking to others for advice, support and reassurance.

For the time being, the dearth of expertise required across all settings is likely to continue, and there is a need for creative approaches and solutions to these problems. Even where these are sought, there is inevitably going to be a shortage of skilled professionals, given the sudden increased demand for them. One of the greatest challenges for at least the next few years will simply be enabling services to function, which is likely to be a major challenge for intermediate care developments in particular. Addressing this issue will need some creative thinking and planning, including 'out of the box thinking'. There are opportunities for new roles such as generic workers and rehabilitation assistants, and the potential of such roles seems to be being explored quite proactively in some areas. Indeed, the National Service Framework for Older People's changing workforce programme group is looking at a range of initiatives related to roles within the care of the older person, as stated by Ian Philp in his Keynote address at the Modernizing Older Peoples' Services Conference (NHS Modernization Agency, 2002). At least one university is planning to introduce a degree for generic workers at level 3 and is exploring the career pathway of these practitioners. While unable to resolve this recruitment and retention crisis, this book does provide suggestions on how to prepare and develop staff and discusses strategies that may help both recruitment and retention.

Conclusion

This chapter has explored some of the motives that lie behind the development of intermediate care and has explored some of the ways in which intermediate care could be developed to support the health and social care needs of older people. The ideas suggested here provide just a flavour of how services for older people could embrace the evolution of intermediate care. Each health economy will have evolved differently and be at different stages of this evolution, delivering services in very different ways. Developments have to be locally responsive, and allow for the fact that one size does not fit all. There is no single right answer or way forward, except that it is imperative that the care needs of older people are proactively addressed and provided for as part of the whole system as intermediate care emerges, so that that there is access for older people to appropriate expertise, care, support and advice across the whole health economy, wherever they live.

So far in this book the specific and unique needs of older people have been referred to but not described. The next section (Part II) provides an overview of the ageing process and how this can affect the older person, in Chapter 4, while Chapter 5 looks at the older person in society and especially within health and social care.

KEY POINTS

- A range of motives lies behind the development of intermediate care.
- It is important to ensure that the holistic needs of older people are not lost within these developments and organizational pressures.
- There is scope for the development for some creative and needs-responsive services for older people if these are thought through and given prominence and priority.
- Issues related to manpower and staff development across all disciplines present a major challenge and need to be addressed creatively and proactively.
- The development of intermediate care offers the opportunity to plan and develop a whole new service for older people, not just an add-on.

PART II

Understanding Ageing and the Older Person in Society and in Health Care

CHAPTER 4

Ageing and the older person

SIÂN WADE

Introduction

Older people are expected to be the main client group to access intermediate care services and schemes (Martin, 2001), and as such intermediate care could be described as becoming synonymous with older people. While other age groups will access and benefit from these services, and indeed require skilled care, it is imperative that the skills and attributes required to care for older people are recognized and provided within intermediate care services/schemes. These skills and attributes need to be identified in order to establish and ensure provision of staff development and education plans.

What is the challenge?

Older people may have extremely complex health and social care needs, making their care both challenging and rewarding, and providing a very positive experience for many staff who choose to work in this field. A wide range of expertise is required to meet the multi-faceted care needs of many older people. In general, older people lead an active, varied and generally full life, with life expectancy increasing consistently during the twentieth century (Bond et al., 1999), due to a general improvement in standards of living and to some extent due to improved health care. For many older people, their contact with health or social care services is minimal and for specific reasons only. Despite this, there are an increasing number of older people who may have more complex needs and these may require considerable input from services, either for a specific period or in the long term. Failure to utilize appropriate skills and attributes to assist older people can lead to deterioration in their health, possibly increasing their dependency and leading to a reduction in their quality of life.

One challenge that is faced is to recognize the status of older people as competent adults with all the attendant rights, while also accepting that some have specific and often specialist needs. These needs may be multiple and could be any combination of physiological, sociological, psychological and environmental needs. There are younger adults who also have this range of care needs, and these will extend into later life. However, due to a range of reasons, older people increasingly develop the need for special consideration should they come into contact with health or social care services.

This chapter looks at some aspects of biological ageing and some of the physiological changes that can occur as an individual ages. While by no means comprehensive, some insight into these is essential for practitioners if they are to be able to provide needs-responsive care to older people. The chapter goes on to touch on some of the attributes and skills required by practitioners in the care of older people that have direct relevance to those staff working in intermediate care services/schemes. Later chapters of the book consider of these in more detail.

The spectrum of care for older people

With the development of the integrated model of care for older people within acute care (RCP, 2000a), there has been an ongoing debate about the strengths and limitations of this model compared to specialist care of older people. In reality, if older people are to access the full range of specialist assessment, diagnostics and treatment to which other patients have access, integrated care will need to continue, and this is the model preferred by older people (Bend and Solomon, 1999). This is further justified by the fact that older people account for a large proportion of patients receiving health care in any acute setting. Many, however, may need specialist gerontological care as well as specialist rehabilitation, with the latter being eroded in many Acute Trusts in recent years (Grimley Evans, 2001; MacMahon, 2001)

During the 1990s the emergence of integrated care within acute settings and the effects of the NHS and Community Care Act (DoH, 1990) were beginning to bed down. The main objective and underlying drive behind this Act was to enable people with less acute care needs to stay in, or as near to, their community and home as possible. Over recent years, as discussed in earlier chapters, there has been a missing element, demonstrated by recent winter crises and bed management problems. From this has emerged intermediate care, aiming, it would seem, to fill a gap and address the full spectrum of care needs – particularly those of older people and rehabilitation.

As suggested, older people will be cared for across the full spectrum and continuum of care settings. This requires practitioners who are informed and skilled in the care of older people across all settings, and justifies the importance of ensuring that the needs of older people are understood, acknowledged and promoted by practitioners in all these settings. To some extent this is backed up in the National Service Framework for Older People both in relation to Standard 1 and Standard 4. Within Standard 1, 'Rooting out age-discrimination', there is a recommendation that 'health and social organizations should provide additional training and support for staff at all levels to build their knowledge base and foster more positive attitudes towards older people' (DoH, 2001h: 21). Within Standard 4, 'General hospital care', there is a requirement for older people to receive appropriate care (52–58), for a skills profile to have been completed for all the staff (60) and for staff to be competent in the care of older people. Strangely enough, this standard applies only to staff in a general hospital, and not to staff in any other setting. If older people are to receive effective care throughout all these services and if performance indicators are to be achieved (NHS Exec, 2000a), this standard must surely be brought to apply to all staff.

Understanding the complexity

In claiming that older people have specialist needs, it is necessary to explain why this is the case. This is particularly important for nurses who are present over a 24-hour day and therefore often in the position to observe changes and to deal with problems as they arise. By being more articulate about the complexity of care in this field, they can perhaps provide more clarity about the requisite skills and attributes to other colleagues, including student nurses, many of whom have difficulty in identifying the care of older people as being any more than 'basic care' (Akid, 2001).

The care needs of older people may range across the spectrum of physical, social, psychological, environmental and financial issues. Where these needs develop in later life they may result from the effects of earlier lifestyles and living standards along with societal attitudes and policies as discussed in Chapter 5. Biological ageing, however, is very likely to have some influence on the experience of later life. For this reason, an overview of biological ageing and some of the related physiological changes is presented here, exploring how it might affect the health of the older person. This is intended to provide some understanding of why older people may have both specialist gerontological care needs and also need access to the spectrum of other specialist and general health care needs, and why this is just as important for staff in intermediate care services as for staff in other settings.

Normal ageing and age-related pathology

There is much debate and theorizing about the ageing process, but nevertheless it is acknowledged that everyone does age. Ageing is not a disease, it is a normal part of the human lifespan and is known as primary ageing. This must be distinguished from abnormal processes which cause pathology, disability and disease, and which are described as secondary ageing. Primary ageing is a continuous process which starts at conception and ends with death. Strehler (1977) identified four criteria which distinguish primary ageing from other biological processes:

1. Universality: it happens to every member of the population, e.g. normal and inevitable skin changes vs skin cancer; normal eye changes versus diabetic cataracts.
2. Intrinsic: the processes must come from within, not from external sources or lifestyle factors such as smoking, diet, environmental or occupational hazards.
3. Progressive: the changes must occur gradually over time. Ageing is a progressive and inevitable process whose effects are cumulative, not an acute event.
4. Deleterious: the changes have a deleterious effect, and have an affect on the ability to cope with the environment – the final result being death.

There is a range of theories proposed to account for primary ageing (Medina, 1996; Woodrow, 2002). It is clear, however, that ageing does not occur as a uniform process across all systems, e.g. maximum oxygen uptake in the lungs and maximum strength of muscle contraction declines with age, while other systems do not appear to deteriorate to any great extent (Herbert, 1992). Nor is the rate of progress of ageing consistent between individuals, meaning that chronological age is a poor indicator of biological ageing. The effects of secondary ageing will depend upon a range of factors, some of which at least are likely to be associated with lifestyle and exposure to assaults and stressors on the body. Thus there is increased diversity in what is 'normal' ageing and this variability makes predicting ageing changes almost impossible. When assessing someone's health status, therefore, it is their biological age that is important, not their chronological age.

The consequences of primary ageing and pathology are to challenge and compromise physiological systems in their functioning. The systems in our body have a functional reserve and this assists the individual to maintain homeostasis. With primary ageing, functional reserve is compromised and reduced, hence the viability of each system is challenged (Figure 4.1). This leads to reduced efficacy of most systems in the older person, some of which are outlined in Table 4.1.

When older people are subjected to physiological stress, therefore, they are more likely to experience a decreased capacity to cope and adapt, challenging the ability of the body to retain or return to homeostasis, and

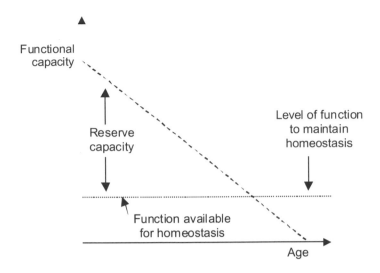

Figure 4.1 Homeostasis and functional reserve. System failure occurs only when function is depleted and homeostasis can no longer be maintained or restored. This may be after years of continual functional capacity.

Table 4.1 Changes in systems that can challenge the functional ability and reserve of the older person and which can increase their vulnerability to stressors

- Reduced immune resistance and increased risk of auto-immune disease
- Reduced perception of visceral sensation leading to reduced perception of pain
- Conduction of nerve velocity is reduced by 15%
- Reduced elasticity of collagen leading to reduced elasticity of muscles such that
  - ➢ Lung capacity is reduced by 50%
  - ➢ Resting cardiac output is reduced by 30%
  - ➢ Muscle strength is reduced, especially thigh muscles to enable individual to stand up
  - ➢ Reduced elasticity of the skin
- Renal blood and perfusion is reduced by 50% therefore renal filtration and excretion of waste products is compromised
- Speed of return to normal blood pH is slowed by 80%
- Blood vessel walls thicken (atheroma/atherosclerosis) challenging blood perfusion

meaning that recovery may often take longer (see Table 4.2). However, within the body, systems work in an interrelated way, working to compensate for each other. This is often referred to as 'cancelling out'; the effect of this for older people should not be underestimated, and it can help to overcome the assault from stressors.

Table 4.2 Effects of physiological stressors on ageing systems

When subjected to physiological stress, older people are more likely to:

- Have difficulty controlling core body temperature – leading to increased risk of hypothermia/hyperthermia (Watson, 1995)
- Fail to maintain fluid balance leading to increased risk of dehydration
- Experience hypotension and consequently dizziness and falls (Robertson, 1990)
- Have lowered inflammatory or fever response
- Fail to always perceive acute pain
- Display signs of confusion

Since the rate at which ageing occurs varies widely with each individual, chronological age cannot be used as a predictor of biological ageing. However, while it is not inevitable, older people are more prone to developing features or symptoms that lead to illness and disability. Their patterns of disease and illness often differ from those of younger people, as they tend to suffer from multiple pathology and often present with atypical features, as outlined in Table 4.3. These tend to relate to four key presenting features related to mobility and instability problems, confusional states and incontinence when the older person is ill (RCP, 2000a). Brocklehurst (1978) described these as the four 'geriatric giants':

1. mental confusion
2. falls or instability
3. incontinence
4. immobility.

These can be regarded as the classical presenting features of many older people when they are unwell; they should ring an alarm bell with

Table 4.3 Presenting signs and symptoms of pneumonia at different ages

Patient 1: 40 years old	Patient 2: 80 years old
Productive cough	Confusion
Fever and rigours	Dizziness and fall
Pleuritic chest pain	Incontinence
Elevated white blood cell count	Inability to perform normal self-care

Source: adapted from Dunbar (1996).

practitioners that something is amiss and that further investigations need to be instigated. Superimposed upon these physiological challenges may be an array of sociological, psychological, cultural and environmental factors, all of which have an impact upon older people, their later life, their health and well-being. There is also a greater likelihood for the older person to experience a combination of mental health needs and physical disease (RCP, 2000b). Older people usually take longer to recover from acute illness, due primarily to the effects of primary and secondary ageing and compromised functional reserve, as illustrated in Figure 4. 1. Terms like 'off legs' or 'acopia' which seem to have increasingly crept into practitioners' language have no place in the care of the older person. There will be reasons for the older person having mobility problems or not coping that require investigation, and may well have an underlying physiological basis.

Physiological assessment of older people

While assessment is central to any caring situation (Schaefer, 1974; Moore, 1996), the physiological assessment of older people is particularly important and difficult. The physical assessment of the older person is significant since not only do older people present with multiple pathologies but also they often present with symptoms that are unusual, atypical and unique to the older person (Exton-Smith, 1985; Herbert, 1992, Dunbar, 1996). There is a need to have knowledge of ageing and of the older person in order to make an accurate assessment (Herbert, 1992), especially as presenting psychological, social or environmental needs may be directly related to a physical illness that may be overcome, at least partially, if identified and treated. It is only through this knowledge that those symptoms closely associated with illness in later life become meaningful and contribute to accurate diagnosis and intervention. Table 4.3 depicts the kind of predicament that may be experienced in the diagnosis of pneumonia (Dunbar, 1996).

Case study 4.1 illustrates the challenge of diagnosing a myocardial infarct, since older people do not present with classical symptoms of a myocardial infarct. They are often likely to present with:

- general malaise – reduced self-caring, physical, social and psychological malaise/depression;
- breathlessness;
- vague weakness;
- confusion/disorientation (in over 20 per cent of people over 85).

According to Cocchi et al. (1988) normal features of diagnosis such as typical history, ECG changes, and elevated cardiac enzyme levels occur in only 24 per cent of patients over 85 years of age.

Case study 4.1

Mr B, an 87-year-old, was admitted to an acute medical ward late on a Sunday evening. There was no clear diagnosis and no infection was apparent. A UTI was suspected, however, and it was felt necessary to observe him. He was very disorientated, incontinent, had great difficulty co-ordinating his actions, was unstable on his feet and appeared somewhat breathless. As the night progressed Mr B became restless, and somehow managed to reach the patient next to his bed, where he began interfering with the IV infusions. The nursing staff returned him to bed, but he continued to be agitated. This led them to become irritated and they accused Mr B of being a nuisance and an inappropriate admission. In the morning, the sense of his inappropriateness was emphasized by his being allocated a bank nurse to care for him. Fortunately she was experienced in working with older people, and was anxious to know if he had been seen yet by a doctor, as she was concerned about his symptoms. She suggested he could have had an MI, and called the on-call doctor, who was unimpressed. Eventually he arrived late morning, and as a result of further examination and investigations it was established that Mr B had indeed experienced an MI. Diagnosis could have been delayed or unrecognized, with Mr B labelled as a 'bed-blocker', had the staff nurse not been informed and proactive.

Older people often have a reduced perception of visceral sensation and their immune response may be compromised so they may present differently. In one study, only 20 per cent of older people with appendicitis presented with the typical presenting features of nausea, fever, lower right quadrant pain and a raised white blood cell count. Symptoms and diagnostic test results of the remaining 80 per cent failed to result in an initial definite diagnosis, and more than 50 per cent of deaths associated with appendicitis are among older people, leading to an increased mortality rate in elders (Lyder and Molony, 1999)

Interpreting laboratory results and physiological measurements

Some physiological measurement readings may indicate abnormality for the younger person, while they may be regarded as normal for the older person. For example, there is an expectation that the normal blood pressure will rise with age (Jolly, 1991; Hurst, 2002). Also, while it should be normal practice to take the blood pressure using the person's left arm whenever possible, to ensure consistency, it is particularly important to use the same arm each time when taking the BP of an older person, as research has shown inter-arm differences that can be significant. Atheromatous disease or the presence of emboli or thrombi are most likely to cause these differences (Fotherby et al., 1993).

Laboratory results and values for older people often do not fall within normal ranges – see Tables 4.4 and 4.5 (Somerfield, 1999). This makes interpretation difficult (Herbert, 1992; Dunbar, 1996). Alternatively, the results or findings obtained may not easily contribute to a current diagnosis, since abnormal findings may arise due to concurrent pathology (Cawley, 1983). Thus it may be difficult to differentiate between physiological signs associated with ageing, early signs of pathological changes and disease, such as in cancer (Cunningham, 1996), and the side effects or interactions of drugs due to prescribing or poor compliance with a complicated medication regime (Hudson and Boyter, 1997). Add to this the unstable homeostasis and reduced functional reserve of an older person, together with the speed and degree at which a condition can deteriorate, and it is evident that assessment of an older person's needs presents a considerable challenge (Levkoff et al., 1988; Herbert, 1992; Dunbar, 1996).

It is not hard to see that practitioners may feel as if they are 'working in the dark' sometimes. However, skill and knowledge of older people usually

Table 4.4 Some laboratory results that do not usually alter significantly with age

Haemoglobin

Erythrocytes

Coagulation tests

Thyroid function tests

Cortisol

Bilirubin

HDL (although wider range of values)

Potassium

pH

Source: adapted from Somerfield (1999).

Table 4.5 Some laboratory values that alter with age

Decrease	Increase
Leukocytes	ESR
Serum iron	Alkaline phosphotase
Testosterone	Serum urea
Albumin	Serum creatinine

Source: adapted from Somerfield (1999).

means that the experienced nurse or practitioner is very subtly able to assess and identify their changing needs. These changes require continuous assessment and reassessment and the ability to decide if medical or other referral and intervention is required (Herbert, 1992; Dunbar, 1996), taking account of social, psychological and environmental needs while focusing on the wishes of the older person. This leads on to the importance of undertaking a holistic assessment and focusing on person-centred care (see Chapter 14). Access to a review by a geriatrician or experienced specialist registrar in the field will also keep the team alert and is significant if the medical needs of patients are to be effectively met and their care not marginalized.

Pharmacotherapy and the older person

When considering the care needs of older people, especially those with multiple pathology, the place of pharmacotherapy, the use of medications in the treatment of illness, cannot go unrecognized within intermediate care services and schemes.

Pharmacotherapy can be very effective and important in the care of older people. With correct medication management, tremendous improvements in health and well-being can be achieved in their care and in their quality of life. For some older people, effective medication enables them to continue to live independently. However, poor prescribing or misuse of medications can lead to considerable physical and psychological impairment and can even lead to death (Col et al., 1990; Ewing, 2002). The key benefits associated with effective medication are in the appropriate diagnosis of illness, correct prescribing of drugs and vigilant monitoring of intended and unintended effects of the prescribed treatment (Watson, 2001).

Older people account for about 18 per cent of the population but receive nearly half of all prescribed drugs (RPS, 1997; Hudson and Boyter, 1997). Special care and attention are required when prescribing medications for older people for a number of reasons, particularly because of some of the physiological changes that accompany ageing. In addition to these changes, those drugs used to treat a range of different conditions may each have their own side effects and may possibly interact with other drugs already being taken. Taking multiple drug regimes is known as polypharmacy, often taken to be four or more medications (Watson, 2001), and this is closely associated with older people due to treatment for multiple pathologies. Older people may also experience difficulty in complying with their prescribed medications, and they are at greater risk when buying over-the-counter drugs (OTCs), because of interactions with drugs already prescribed.

Thus pharmacotherapy for the older person is a very complex area of care. While it cannot be adequately addressed within a book of this kind, some aspects of pharmacotherapy are discussed below, since it is likely to have a key place within intermediate care settings and schemes. This is of particular significance since practitioners often work in isolation and will often not have easy access to medical support.

Physiological changes and their effects

Ageing may result in physiological changes which may influence the activity of drugs (Table 4.6). This may lead to altered *pharmacokinetics* – the way in which the body affects the drug with time – and altered *pharmacodynamics* – the way in which the drug affects the body (Kelly, 1995; Ewing, 2002). Very often the effect of these changes leads to the altered *bio-availability* of the drug, i.e. the rate and extent to which it is absorbed from a given pharmaceutical preparation and becomes available at its site of action (O.L. Wade, 1996; Downie et al., 1999). This can lead to an increase in the *half-life*, which in effect leads to the prolonged activity of the drug within the body due to an increase in plasma concentration (Figure 4.2). It can also lead to an increased risk of toxicity as described below. It is important to keep in mind that these changes cannot be attributed to chronological age, but to the effects of ageing, and therefore it is difficult to predict the response by any one individual. What it does mean is that caution is needed when prescribing for an older person.

Table 4.6 Age-related changes in the gastrointestinal tract, liver and kidneys which may have an effect on drug activity

---

- Reduced gastric secretion
- Decreased gastrointestinal motility
- Reduced total surface area of absorption
- Reduced splanchic blood flow
- Reduced liver size
- Reduced liver blood flow
- Reduced glomerula filtration
- Reduced renal tubular function

Source: Shetty and Woodhouse (1994).

Pharmacokinetics

With regard to altered pharmacokinetics, there are a number of possible effects related to ageing.

Absorption

While there may be changes related to the structure and function of the gastrointestinal tract with ageing, their effect on the absorption of drugs is probably of limited significance.

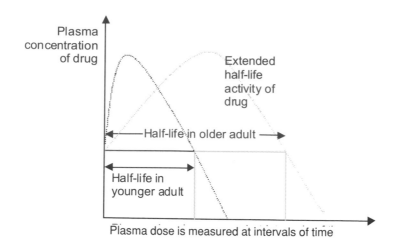

Figure 4.2 Extended half-life resulting from altered pharmacokinetics and pharmacodynamics.

Metabolism

Within the liver there may be a reduction in the liver enzyme activity so that the rate at which drugs that are normally metabolized within the liver by first-past effect may be reduced, leading to the subsequent enhanced or sustained activity of the drug. Impaired first-past metabolism has been demonstrated for several drugs with older people, including chlormethiazole, labetalol, nifedipine, nitrates and others (Shetty and Woodhouse, 1994).

Distribution

There may be age-related physiological changes that affect the way drugs are distributed within the body (Table 4.7). This may be due to increases in body fat, which can have an impact on the expected activity of both fat- and water-soluble drugs. There may be an increased volume of distribution of lipophilic drugs, while there is a reduction in the distribution of water-soluble agents (Macphee and Brodie, 1992). There may also be a reduction in the volume of serum plasma due to ageing or due to illnesses often associated with the older person. Since these drugs are bound to plasma proteins there is the potential that their clinical effect will be enhanced. Also, since with multiple pathology there is likely to be greater prescribing, there is greater likelihood of more than one of these prescribed drugs being bound to plasma protein, which can lead to competition for the available plasma binding sites. The effect of this is that there will be greater availability of the non-bound and therefore active drug element, which can lead to a prolonged half-life (Macphee and Brodie, 1992; Hudson et al., 1997). The challenge of this is really going to be applicable only in acute administration of drugs during the early stages of illness, while the dose of the drug is being stabilized and the plasma concentration of free drug is determined by drug clearance.

Table 4.7 Age-related changes in body composition

- Reduced lean body mass
- Reduced total body water
- Increased total body fat
- Lower serum albumin
- Alpha[1]-acid glycoprotein unchanged or slightly raised

Source: Shetty and Woodhouse (1994).

Renal clearance

Perhaps the most important and predictable alteration in pharmacokinetics associated with age is the reduction in elimination of drugs excreted by the kidney. This is due to a decline in glomerular filtration – 50 per cent between the ages of 50 years and 90 years (Macphee and Brodie, 1992). This in effect means that the drug remains in circulation in the body and continues to be active, leading again to an enhanced or sustained effect for the same dose, i.e. increased half-life. This is particularly important where drugs have a narrow therapeutic range/index since it can lead to a build-up of the drug and increased risk of toxicity, as occurs with digoxin and gentamicin (Figure 4.3). This calls for the prescribing of a reduced dose and careful monitoring of levels over time. Since digoxin is a drug that many older people are maintained on while in the community, it is important to look out for the effects of toxicity and also even to ask for a review where the dose appears quite high. Staff in intermediate care are well placed to request such a review if contact is made through one of these services.

Hepatic clearance

Blood flow through the liver declines between the ages of 40 and 80 years (Macphee and Brodie, 1992), as does the liver size, affinity and activity of the enzymes, and the uptake of hepatocytes. This can lead to a reduced rate of clearance of some hepatically eliminated drugs – the second-past effect – and sustained activity due to a prolonged half-life.

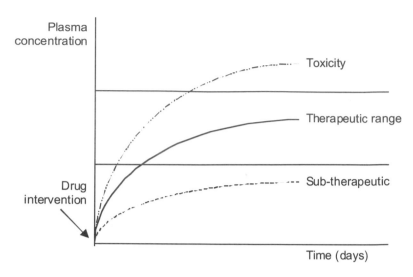

Figure 4.3 Therapeutic range.

Altered pharmacodynamics

With ageing, the way the drug affects the body may alter, often increasing the
sensitivity and reaction to it. For example, as discussed earlier, homeostatic
reserve may be reduced with ageing, which with some drugs leads to an
altered orthostatic circulatory response. This can lead to hypotension and an
increased likelihood of falling, as with some antihypertensive drugs, drugs
that decrease the sympathetic outflow from the central nervous system, and
anti-Parkinsonian drugs. Postural control may also be compromised by some
drugs as the individual ages, leading to an increased likelihood of postural
sway, as for example with some hypnotics and tranquillizers.

Some drugs seem to affect the thermoregulatory systems of the older
person, increasing the risk of hypothermia, which older people are less likely
to recognize. Tricyclic antidepressants, opioids, benzodiazepines and
phenothiazides are all implicated. With ageing, there may be neurochemical
changes within the central nervous system so that certain drugs may
predispose to confusion. This frequently occurs with hypnotics, anticholinergics, H2-antagonists and β-adrenoreceptor blockers. Similarly, with
ageing there may be reduced gastrointestinal motility, so predisposing to
constipation, and this effect may be promoted by some drugs such as
tricyclics, anticholinergics and antihistimines. Anticholinergic drugs may
cause urinary retention in older men, especially those with prostatic
hypertrophy and bladder instability. Urethral dysfunction is more prevalent in
older women, and diuretics, especially loop diuretics, also predispose to

incontinence (Shetty and Woodhouse, 1994). It is also apparent that ageing may be associated with the response of some cell receptors, which may affect enzyme activation or alter the response of target tissues. This is quite a complex process but it is important to be aware of this when considering the ageing individual.

Because of the effects that ageing can have on the activity of drugs and the unpredictability of this with older people (since these changes cannot be directly associated with chronological age), great care should be given when selecting doses to be prescribed, especially where giving a loading dose. In particular, great caution should be taken when prescribing anxiolytics, anti-depressants and sedatives. Each older person should be treated individually, and the response of the older person should be monitored carefully, acknowledging that the build-up of the drug may be slow with a delay in the real effect. For the nurse/practitioner a key role is to be alert to the kind of doses being prescribed and, if concern is felt, the prescription should be reviewed with the doctor. Case study 4.2 describes the kind of scenario that can occur in clinical areas, especially on busy acute wards, if tolerance is not or cannot be adopted. As can be seen, the consequences of requesting additional medication to be prescribed when a situation seems to be unmanageable can have unfortunate consequences for the older person.

Case study 4.2

Mr A, an anxious and agitated man, was admitted to a medical ward for investigations. His condition meant that he may have been more agitated than usual and a small dose of sedative had been prescribed for him at night. It was after midnight and Mr A had still not settled. In fact, he had got up from his bed and was wandering around the ward fiddling with other patients' belongings, and tampering with drips and equipment. The ward was poorly staffed and the staff nurse somewhat stressed. Eventually when Mr A caused an intravenous drip counter alarm to go off for the third time the staff nurse phoned the on-call houseman to come and prescribe a further sedative. The houseman obliged and soon Mr A was heavily asleep. The next morning at breakfast he was still heavily asleep and still asleep at lunchtime. When the senior staff nurse came on duty on a late shift, she was quite concerned to find Mr A still drowsy and contacted his own doctor. The issue was discussed and it was agreed that in future the initial medication would be given at 8 p.m. to allow time for it to take affect and promote sleep at a reasonable time. In the meantime, Mr A had missed his breakfast and lunch and had been subjected to the many risks of extended bed rest.

Compliance and concordance

Pharmacotherapy can be very important and effective, but one of the challenges faced with increased prescribing and resulting polypharmacy is the ability of older people to take their medications. Traditionally there has been an expectation that when medications are prescribed, patients will take them and simply 'comply'. Non-compliance or failure to take medications and the consequences of this has been well documented for many years (Shulman, 1985; Marinker, 1997; Playle and Keeley, 1998; Shepherd, 1998). There may be a range of reasons why patients, especially older people, do not take their medications as prescribed, some of which are outlined in Table 4.8.

Table 4.8 Actions that may account for older people complying poorly with their prescribed medications

Physical difficulties	• Poor dexterity • Poor eyesight to read labels
Memory problems	• Made worse by complex regimes
Cognitive difficulties	
Unclear or ambiguous instruction on labels	• Take 4 times a day. (But when? There is the risk of taking them closely together?) • Instil eyedrops. (But how, and how much?) • Apply sparingly. (What is sparingly?) • Take as directed by doctor/nurse. (But these cannot be remembered or were not clear.)
Inadequate explanations about the medication by the health care professional	
Concerns about side effects, especially if unpleasant	
Medication does not appear to be doing anything and could also cause side-effects	
Poor knowledge of care and storage of medicines	• Mixing different tablets in same bottle so that those taken may be incorrect • Inappropriate storage, e.g. glycerol trinitrate needs to be in a dark bottle • Sharing tablets with a friend who appears to have the same problem so as to avoid troubling the doctor • Purchasing over-the-counter medications and taking these with prescribed medications
Poor understanding of how hypnotics work and over-relying on them	

The term 'compliance' is no longer helpful and has been replaced by the term 'therapeutic alliance' (Heath and Webster, 1999).

There are a number of ways in which the ability to take medications as prescribed can be enhanced, outlined in Table 4.9. If patients are in-patients within a ward, especially within intermediate care environments, where the drug regimen is likely to have been reasonably stabilized, there is the potential to implement a self-medication programme (Bird and Cottrell, 1990). This needs to be managed and monitored carefully so that the patient is carefully assessed in his or her capabilities and potential to take the medications. While this process can be time-consuming it is an ideal way to identify any problems, and to find ways of overcoming them for when the individual goes home. It is also likely to improve the likelihood of patients taking their prescribed medications correctly, as hopefully these problems will have been addressed. This concept fits well with the concept of rehabilitation within intermediate care.

Table 4.9 Managing polypharmacy and helping older people to take their medications in a reasonable way

Minimize drug treatment	• Ensure drug is still necessary • Consider risks and benefits • Review whole drug regimens
Optimize compliance	• Avoid complex regimens, and simplify these, e.g. once daily regimens or slow release • Review packaging: ensure medications can be accessed by the individual and bottles are easy to open • Ensure labels can be clearly read and are unambiguous • Consider dosage form and consider pre-packed or monitored dose formats, but be aware of rights of individual
Teach about medications wherever possible	• Name and reason for taking • Instructions on how to take safely • Possible side effects (considered so as not to cause unnecessary alarm) • Time and dose to take • Education about condition • Maintain a personal record of an individual's medications (which can be shown to a doctor or nurse or when buying OTCs) • Advise on how to care and store medications • Advise and ask for help and advice when purchasing over-the-counter medications; show the personal record of medications so a pharmacist can check possible side effects and interactions

Although efforts have been made to improve compliance, there is little evidence of sustained success (McGavock, 1996), and it is evident that for many people not taking medications is a conscious decision and indeed could be regarded as intelligent non-compliance. In the past there has been an implication that non-compliance, as an intentional act, was deviant behaviour. Increasingly over the past few years, however, the medical profession has come to accept 'that non-compliance might be no more deviant a behaviour than compliance, and that this has often had serious effects' (Marinker, 1997: 747). They have recognized that the behaviour of a patient will be related to their own health beliefs – which may be in conflict with those of the doctor, and that where there is an internal locus of control patients will exert their own behaviour – hence the more recent adoption of the term 'therapeutic alliance'. This has led the medical profession to acknowledge the importance of 'concordance', where the doctor/practitioner discusses with the patient the diagnosis and proposed treatment, providing information and explanation. They also need to discuss the consequences for the patient of choices he or she may make with regard to taking medications or otherwise (Marinker, 1997; RPS, 1997). This can be regarded as a form of negotiation, and in some cases the practitioner may have to acknowledge the need to prescribe a different treatment or dose than might have been originally envisaged, if this is likely to lead the patient to take this newly negotiated prescription. This means that monitoring the patient's response to prescribed medication can hopefully be more reliable, in the fairly dependable knowledge that the patient is taking what he or she claims.

The use of monitored dosing systems, etc. is seen by many as the solution to non-compliance. Individuals need to be assessed for their ability to use the system, and for their cognitive ability and memory to use it. It is also important to consider if they can choose whether or not to take their tablets as presented. Where the responsibility has been given to others, e.g. nurses in care homes, or relatives or carers, either to give medicine or remind patients, patients' control may be removed or compromised. They may not be able to make choices about which medications to take or not, and this takes away their rights and autonomy. This needs to be considered when using measures such as monitored dosing systems.

Nurse and extended prescribing

There is considerable scope for nurses and other professionals who have prescribing rights to have a role within intermediate care settings. While it may be some considerable time, if at all, before major prescribing can be undertaken with older people (for this is some of the most complex of prescribing) there is considerable potential with regard to some prescribing. Prescribing from a limited formulary certainly makes sense (McHale, 2002), and being excluded from this has been very restricting for nurses within settings such as community hospitals and nurse-led units or services in the past. Dependent prescribing also has considerable potential for staff in these settings/services, while the opportunity to prescribe from the extended formulary and to become a supplementary prescriber provides many opportunities. It is probable that some staff will not wish to adopt this kind of role. Appropriate education and assessment is required, of course, and must be offered and available (DoH, 2002a), but the opportunities open to practitioners with prescribing rights in these settings/schemes could be very beneficial to older people.

With advances in modern pharmacology and pharmacotherapy, it is not surprising that prescribing for older people has become even more complex. This is made even more challenging for those prescribing due to the increasing size of the older population (Hudson and Boyter, 1997). In 1997 the Royal College of Physicians set up a working party which made recommendations to health professionals on principles for prescribing for older people (RCP, 1997). Indeed the whole issue of medications with regard to older people is addressed within Section 9 of the *National Service Framework for Older People*. Section 9, while not one of the specified Standards, provides clear guidance on actions and measures that need to be met (DoH, 2001h).

Communicating with older people

Interpersonal skills and communication are central in the successful care of an individual (Altshul, 1972; Wade, 1992). The Kellog International Committee suggested that 'the ability to communicate is frequently a deciding factor in determining a person's autonomy, independence, and overall well-being and happiness' (Salomon, 1986). Older people in particular may find that their abilities to communicate effectively are compromised, and this may present quite a challenge to those providing care. Age-related changes and pathology may affect hearing ability, comprehension and the ability to talk or articulate wishes. The natural ageing process tends to mean that older people think more slowly and take a more considered approach to their responses, although normally the intelligence and ability of older people to learn is not compromised (Cunningham and Brookbank, 1988). Furthermore, being polite and making small talk before entering into serious and personal conversation is often seen as courtesy and good manners by the contemporary older generation. While not inevitable, hearing and sight are often compromised and it is important that the practitioner is able to recognize and assess any problems appropriately so that the older person is able to access specialist advice and make informed decisions about any aids that might help.

The prevalence of hearing impairment among the general population is 37 per cent in the age-band 61–70 years and 60 per cent between 71 and 80 years. Much of this is age-related, although its pathological basis is unclear (Tolson and Nolan, 2000). In a study of hospitalized patients it was estimated that 80 per cent of dependent older patients between 71 and 80 would benefit from a hearing aid; this rose to 99 per cent in those over 81 (Tolson and Stevens, 1997). Older people are often reluctant to admit to a hearing problem, and yet it can have a significant impact on their ability to communicate, can cause family tensions (Cowie et al., 1987) and can affect intimate relationships (Hetu et al., 1993) – thus the importance of effective assessment and referral for more specialist assessment (Tolson and Nolan, 2000). Should older people have aids, it is important that staff are familiar with their use, care and potential problems, since it is evident that this knowledge is often lacking (Tolson, 1991). Within rehabilitation and intermediate care environments the importance of using a hearing aid effectively will be particularly important if the older person is to maximize the benefits of rehabilitation. Attention also needs to be given to environmental noise, especially background music, which can interfere considerably with a hearing aid's effectiveness.

It is important to make sure that glasses are worn if they are needed; not only are they important for seeing, but they can indirectly affect someone's ability to hear and communicate. Wearing properly fitted dentures is likewise important for speaking and general communication and comfort. Those with speech or comprehension problems, such as may occur after a stroke, may experience great difficulty in communicating their wishes and needs, with the risk of isolation and considerable frustration. It is important that staff know and understand what is happening and what such patients need, and are equipped with the skills to maximize effective communication.

Those who have the misfortune to have some form of cognitive impairment may be quite severely compromised in their ability to understand and communicate effectively. This can be very challenging for those caring for the older person in any environment, particularly in busy, noisy, acute settings, and it supports the need for slower stream care settings, which are more appropriate to the needs of older people. Unfortunately, the skill required to give appropriate care may go unrecognized by those who are uninformed, or it may appear as 'invisible care' and be misinterpreted (Case study 4.3).

Case study 4.3

It seemed a very busy morning on Ward X, an acute assessment ward caring for older people. Mrs W, who had dementia and had been admitted three days previously with an acute chest infection, seemed very agitated and unsettled.

S/N B was aware of the demands on herself, the other two trained nurses and three care assistants. By 10 a.m. Mrs W seemed increasingly agitated. This was not helped by the tensions and pressures evident upon the staff. S/N approached Mrs W calmly, suggesting they 'take a walk into the garden'. Mrs W willingly accepted and they spent some five minutes sitting by the fountain.

Mrs W was then keen to return to the safety of the ward. S/N B collected a cup of tea for each of them, and sat talking with Mrs W while she settled her back on the ward. At this point a manager came in and was surprised to see the S/N sitting 'chatting' when the ward was supposedly so busy. A few minutes later the S/N left Mrs W contentedly by her bed. She was able to return to attend to her other duties undisturbed, giving her full attention and concentration.

Some weeks later when there was a demand to reduce staff the manager remembered the morning she had seen the S/N sitting chatting. She suggested this ward could afford some reduction in their establishment, since staff seemed to be able to sit and chat, and the ward seemed well organized. Within six months of this change, the ward had recorded a substantial increase in incidents involving aggressive outbursts by patients together with an increase in incidents and complaints. In addition, a number of committed and skilled staff had handed in their notice, and the vacancies remained unfilled. The 'skilled invisible work' had been unrecognized and all were now paying the cost.

It may appear that staff are 'doing very little' and that care seems very straightforward and simple in a care setting, especially for patients with mental health care needs such as dementia. This may give the impression of the setting being 'well-staffed'! The temptation for managers is to reduce the skilled staff and resources, but in fact it is the very expertise of the staff that creates and establishes such a calm and tranquil therapeutic caring environment. This implicit expertise can be difficult to articulate and justify, especially when managers are under pressure to cut costs. The consequences can lead to cutbacks and the creation of a problematic caring environment, as illustrated in the case study, where the S/N demonstrated great skill, which it appears impacted on other staff and the organization of the ward. Once cutbacks have been made, however, staff will have left, and the care of patients will have been compromised.

Communication and multi- and interdisciplinary care

The multiple needs of older people mean, as Thomas (1995) and Castledine (1994) argue, that it is rare for a single profession to meet the often complex health and social care needs of the older individual. Areskog (1988: 252) asserts that this requires the preparation of the minds and attitudes of those who teach and those who care. To ensure effective collaborative working and continuity of care between different professionals requires competent skilled working and communication. This becomes easier when those involved are working towards the same goals, with mutual agreement about what is to be achieved, and when the skills and attributes of each member are valued and respected. As Sellick argues, this is 'not easily achieved or maintained' (1985: 35); it is discussed in more depth in Chapter 16. Similarly, relatives and carers needs to be approached sensitively to ensure their needs and concerns are met, and that they are involved appropriately according to their wishes. Any change in an older person's condition will need to be communicated through sensitive discussion with both the family and the older person to establish an appropriate level of intervention, while trying to respect the wishes of the older person.

Rehabilitation and risk-taking

When an older person becomes ill or is required to reduce their level of mobility in any way, it is very possible that they will require some level of rehabilitation. Young (1996: 313) identifies rehabilitation as being 'concerned with lessening the impact of disabling conditions'. The importance of preventing deterioration or complications together with maintaining or improving functional abilities and quality of life is paramount in the effective care of older people (Squires and Hastings, 2002). It is important to recognize that continuing rehabilitation has a central role in every type of setting, and especially in intermediate care services. It is not just the domain of therapists and the therapy department but very much an ongoing activity that involves participation by all of those involved in the care of an older person.

However, initiating and maintaining the activity and promoting the independence of an older person will inevitably create potential risks, and at a time of increasing fear of litigation this can be very challenging for staff. Risk assessment with planned intervention and prevention for the older person is therefore of great importance in all settings, and is explored again in Chapter 16. Effective management of interventions will create confidence and needs continual monitoring. Careful and reasoned discussion with the patient will enable mutually agreed goals and activities to be set, and sensitive discussion of any possible risks will reduce anxiety and fear. This may be difficult, especially if there is cognitive impairment, and demands clear and careful explanation and information.

It is essential, therefore, that staff providing care are proactive as opposed to reactive. Relatives need to be involved in discussion of risks so that they can overcome their concern for possible consequences. Staff need to be aware of the importance of their role as listeners, so that risks can be mutually acknowledged and accepted. For example, relatives or carers may be anxious that a cognitively impaired patient who is wandering will fall; they may believe the patient should be restrained. Such concern is understandable, so it is essential at an early stage to discuss the pros and cons of allowing the person to wander versus the risks and dangers of restraint. Such action may help to prevent complaints at a later date should an injury occur, and it helps relatives feel acknowledged and respected.

The process of co-ordinating and planning a successful transfer or discharge from care settings is often a highly complex activity when the older person has considerable needs (Nazarko, 1997). Because of their altered situation, an older person may no longer be able to live independently in the community without the help of others. It is often the nurse who co-ordinates such discharges, and who feels responsible for their smooth running. Considerable skill and experience is necessary to achieve this. The breakdown of one small aspect of discharge arrangements for a vulnerable older person may cause chaos, leaving the nurse feeling the 'finger is pointed at them'. In view of the importance of effective transfer and discharge of care in relation to older people, the topic is examined in more detail in Chapter 18.

The challenge of working in isolated settings or services

Working in isolated settings and services can be very challenging when caring for older people. Decisions must be made that may have a major impact upon the future lifestyle of the older person. These may relate to the level and extent of medical intervention to be offered, to consideration of individual wishes and choices of the older person, to discharge plans or referral, and to the use of a range of different services as found in intermediate care.

Decisions about medical intervention may be influenced by the availability of resources. Alternatively, they may be influenced by expectations of likely outcomes, by preferences of doctors, by attitudes of those involved in care, by wishes of relatives or carers, and by those of the older person themselves. Such decisions are often very difficult. They may be swayed by power and by bias and may lead to competing demands and wishes, all of which require discussion and negotiation.

While making decisions in an acute setting may be difficult, the nurses and staff working in the comparatively isolated environment of an intermediate care setting, care home or patient's own home may find themselves feeling very vulnerable, alone and exposed when making some decisions. They may have to make a complex decision there and then, without the support of another trained nurse, doctor or senior colleague (McMurray, 1990). Personal experience suggest that the level of vulnerability experienced by staff in isolated settings often seems to go unrecognized or is at least underestimated. For example, there is much skill involved in deciding whether or not to call a busy doctor, especially at night or when the doctor is 'on take' or 'on call'. Once the decision to call the doctor is made then it is necessary to be able to explain and justify the reason for calling. Because older people tend to present with unusual or unclear symptoms, it may be difficult to convince the doctor, especially if he or she is busy or tired, has limited expertise of caring for older people, or is not interested in their care needs (Dunbar, 1996). The nurse requires quite exceptional skill to communicate such a request, and may feel accountable for the decision but may to some extent lack the responsibility.

Those familiar with working in community or small intermediate care settings will recognize that the experience of requesting a GP to come in urgently is often daunting. Somehow it is easier to influence a GP to attend when in a patient's own home setting. It seems that the bricks and mortar of a ward or hospital or care home building suggest that the patient is safer or not in so much need of intervention. Even persuading the GP to visit, or to act upon the assessed needs of the older person, such as referral of the patient to another specialist (perhaps because they are making no progress or deteriorating), may be very challenging, and should not be underestimated – as illustrated in Case study 4.4.

Case study 4.4

A senior staff nurse in a community hospital came on duty on a late shift. She noted an older lady (Mrs M) in the side room, in bed, appearing very dishevelled and almost falling out of the bed. She went into the room and tried to assist her into a more comfortable position, but the lady seemed unable to co-operate in a meaningful way. At report the S/N asked what was wrong with Mrs M, and was told the GP suspected a UTI. The S/N had considerable experience and was convinced that this was an incorrect diagnosis from the way the lady presented. While she could not put her finger on it, she suspected something like a spatial lesion, especially as the lady had no previous history of confusion. She phoned the GP who refused to come in, as she had visited the day before and would be in the next day. When seen again by the GP the S/N suggested a referral to the Consultant

Geriatrician. This idea was rejected. A week later, Mrs M was referred to the Geriatrician and was immediately transferred to the acute sector, where the S/N later heard she had died. She could never establish what was wrong with Mrs M, and subsequently always felt guilty that she had not been more persuasive when talking to the GP.

Some nurses transferring from the acute sector to take up a post in an intermediate care setting or service may experience difficulty when faced with the reality of how isolated they feel and the need to make decisions independently and without support. While it is frequently acknowledged that practitioners do often work in isolation or with a low skill mix of staff in community-based environments (RCN, 1992; RCN, 1996; UKCC, 1997) the implications for these staff and the experience they require need to be recognized. Coping with isolation and independence is one of the challenges of working in these kinds of environment; it is a skill and attribute that should be acknowledged and admired, and for which staff should be prepared.

Having no doctor on site or easily accessible also means that nurses in these settings/services need to be proactive in ensuring that care can continue without the intervention, signature or say-so of the doctor. The need to pre-empt the rewriting of a script, prescribing medication p.r.n., or prescribing a syringe driver should it be required out of hours, falls very much to the nurse, even though it is primarily the doctor's responsibility. Nurse prescribing may go some way to help nurses, and indeed other professionals working in intermediate care services, as already discussed, but they may experience limitations due to the complexity of prescribing for older people, and staff will also need to receive the mandatory training (DoH, 2002a).

The undertaking of extended roles is also necessary in these isolated environments. While not unique to nursing in these settings, it needs to be acknowledged that the veins of older people are very fragile and collapse easily when it comes to venepuncture. Similarly, it can be particularly challenging when undertaking apparently simple procedures such as X-rays or ECGs with little support from others, for older people may be anxious, have cognitive difficulties or major mobility problems. These abilities again require knowledge, skills and attributes that need to be acknowledged and recognized.

Managing changed life circumstances and transition

While holistic, comprehensive and individual assessment is important for all those receiving care, for the older person there may be specific aspects that need careful and considered regard that arise as a result of the effects of ageing and their care needs. Individuals may have to face the realization that they may not recover from an illness or disability and that it could be progressive, leading to changes in lifestyle, ability, independence and other losses. Losing control of life and facing the inevitability that life is nearing an end may be distressing. Older people often have extensive and complex life histories. Erikson (1980) describes a number of developmental stages that a person passes through during life. He suggests that each stage may be only partially resolved at that time of life. As a result, unresolved issues may present at subsequent stages, particularly in later life when other life goals are threatened. This may influence the way older people deal with their situation and their presenting behaviour, and may complicate recovery or the adaptation of older people to their current situation when faced with ill health. For the nurse assessing and trying to help the older patient, there is a need to develop a relationship of some trust and to develop an awareness and understanding of the patient's background.

This area of care is probably of particular significance for staff in specialized settings caring primarily for older people. It may be that the older person in any setting will be unable to make progress until they are helped to work through these psychological and sociological issues. It is likely that in an acute hospital setting there is little opportunity to address these needs, and this may account for the fact that older people often fare badly in these settings once the acute phase of their illness has passed (HAS, 1998). This is a justification for slower-stream and longer-stay settings such as specialist units and intermediate care settings/services; staffing is often more stable, and care can be given on an ongoing basis, allowing time to assess and form relationships (S.E. O'Connor, 1996). This allows the nurse to help the older person actively work through and adapt to the transitions they are undergoing. The older person may be enabled to return home more successfully or transfer to a care home with greater psychological well-being (Morgan et al., 1997).

Once back at home, great skill may also be needed in helping the older person to adapt to a changed way of life, perhaps with personal space being constantly invaded by those coming in to help and assist. The impact of this is discussed by Begley in Chapter 12. Such work is equally important in a care home context where it is likely that a frail older person is finding his or her life and future very much changed and challenged. Considerable help and understanding may be needed to make this transition and to help older people experience a satisfactory quality of life in their new home (Morgan et al., 1997). Because of its significance for staff in services such as intermediate care, the concept of transitions is examined in more detail in Chapter 15.

For those giving end-of-life care for older people, adequate knowledge and skills required to offer effective palliative care are of particular importance. While death is not the main focus of caring for older people, it is still of significance. Hospice care seems to attract great attention, but recognizing the necessity for the same kind of care, together with expertise in palliative and end-of-life care of older people in all environments, sometimes seems to be forgotten and neglected. Only 5 per cent of those dying each year are cared for in a hospice (Bennett and Ebrahim, 1995). It is only in recent years that the need has been recognized to share the knowledge and skills developed in hospices and that steps have been taken to influence standards across other health care environments and professionals (Bennett and Ebrahim 1995). Unfortunately, palliative care does not seem to bed in with intermediate care service developments as defined by the HSC/LAC Circular (DoH, 2001e), although it is highlighted in the *National Service Framework for Older People* (DoH, 2001h). It is therefore imperative that attention is given to how this service is to be appropriately provided within the health and social care economy.

Organizational management and professional/personal development in isolated settings

Registered nurses and staff in more isolated settings have traditionally tended to work primarily with unregistered staff. While these staff have much to offer and are greatly valued, they have not always had much training or education in health care, and have not been able or allowed to undertake certain activities. While this is being increasingly addressed with NVQs or equivalent educational opportunities, the requirements of the Care Standards Act (DoH, 2000a) and the *National Service Framework for Older People* (DoH, 2001h), there is some way to go. Registered nurses and staff in these areas therefore need skills in delegation, supervision and prioritizing, so that unregistered staff can give effective care and feel respected while the registered nurse remains responsible and accountable.

It is ironic that the need for time and skill is so evident in meeting the needs of older people effectively. Sadly, the importance of this has been continuously ignored, and there has been a failure to prove that competent, professional nursing and care is beneficial and cost-effective (Pembrey, 1983). When such evidence has been demonstrated it has been disregarded (University of York, 1992). Specialist settings caring for older people are often poorly staffed and made up of a low skill mix. This seems to emerge from an historical context when the expertise to care effectively for older people was not recognized. To some extent it would seem that the need for these skills has still not been made evident, and this is reflected in the way that settings which care specifically for older people are staffed (Buchan and Ball, 1991). The environments themselves may offer little help, for hospital units discarded by others have often been cheaply upgraded to accommodate older people, and tend to be sited peripherally, isolating them from mainstream services (see Chapter 5).

Early successful intermediate care services tended to develop with a rich skill mix and establishment (Vaughan et al., 1999). The part played by such staffing in their success should not be underestimated nor forgotten, for to do so and to err on the side of saving money could dilute the effectiveness of these services and create a new 'Cinderella service'. Because the care of older people can be challenging, demanding and emotionally draining, staff who work in these settings need support and supervision. Similarly, education for all staff working in these settings is important if quality of care is to be enhanced. Thus, preparation and development needs to be carefully considered and planned and is considered as in the last section.

Conclusion

It is evident that the effective care of older people requires extensive knowledge, skill, experience and expertise. The needs of older people extend over a broad spectrum of care needs, including physiological, psychosocial, cultural and environmental. It is rare for an older person to have only a single need identified; they are more likely to present with a complex, interrelated set of needs that require careful, considered and often complicated intervention, drawing upon the skills of many, but often co-ordinated and overseen by the nurse. With the current national shortage of registered practitioners, together with the historical difficulties in attracting staff to care for older people, the future could seem dismal. This reaffirms the need for the effective care of older people to be recognized as skilled, for gerontological education to be encouraged, and indeed mandatory in some areas, for this to be easily available, and for care assistants to be appropriately prepared. It confirms the need to make every effort to promote this speciality of care and ensure it is addressed in developing intermediate care services.

KEY POINTS

- Caring for older people requires as much skill as any other speciality: it is both challenging and demanding, but also rewarding.
- Assessment is often complicated: observations, recordings and readings may fall outside normally expected ranges, and presenting features may also often be altered; this can be further compounded by a range of communication difficulties often experienced by older people.
- Due to the effects of primary and secondary ageing and the increasing likelihood of multiple pathology, older people are more likely to need an extended period of rehabilitation and may need help with making life-changing transitions, which call for skilled, collaborative, multidisciplinary working.
- Prescribing for older people can be difficult, due to the likelihood of multiple pathologies and changes with age in the way drugs are processed

within the body; staff working within intermediate care can play an important role in promoting good practice.

- These changes also put older people at risk of complications and side-effects: skill and attention are therefore needed in assessing and adopting preventive measures and trying to minimize risk.
- Staff caring for older people often work in isolated situations or settings; they require well-developed decision-making and problem-solving skills to ensure their patients gain access to all their care needs, and it is therefore important that personal and professional development and support is provided.

CHAPTER 5

The older person within health care

SIÂN WADE

Introduction

This chapter provides an understanding of how the social standing of older people has emerged over recent decades. While respected and valued in many quarters, there is the potential for many older people to be treated in an ageist way and for discriminatory practice to influence their care and treatment. This chapter explores how ageism may be reflected in practice, highlighting the importance of treating older people as individuals. Raising awareness of ageism and what is meant by age discrimination is important for practitioners involved in the care of older people. Not only can they address it in their own practice, but they can influence others by articulating and providing support for the rights and needs of older people as individuals.

Background

Butler (1975) defines ageism as 'systematic stereotyping and discrimination against people, simply because of their age'. Ageist attitudes and ageism have been found to pervade the health and social care community across the whole spectrum of care (HAS, 1998). Intermediate care has been heralded as the way forward in addressing many of the ills of the health and social care services, in particular those experienced by older people. In particular, it has been identified as providing opportunities for staff to take on new roles and responsibilities, providing a challenge and greater clinical autonomy (Vaughan et al., 1999). While early intermediate care services/schemes may offer optimism and status for staff and service users, there is an inherent risk that this image could shift as time passes, leading to problems related to ageism and ageist practice, as seems to have occurred in many other services (HAS, 1998). This is particularly likely to happen as the novelty of this kind of service wears off and staffing becomes problematic, or if the skills and expertise required by staff are not available and not developed. Recruitment of staff to this area of care rarely requires evidence of a special interest in older people or any such specialist experience or personal development in this field. Intermediate care is required after all to meet the needs of a wide range of care and specialities; arguably, it will benefit from a wide range of previous experience. Experience shows, however, that the skills required to look after older people are not evident in many other practice areas and will probably not be brought to intermediate care services/schemes (HAS, 1998; Age Concern, 1999b). Because of the novelty of intermediate care, there is the underlying risk of forgetting that the key client group is older people and that staff require specialist skills, as do staff in any practice area.

It is evident that one of the greatest challenges for health and social care staff is to recognize just this, that caring for older people does require specialist skills and expertise, and then to realize that they themselves may lack these (see Chapter 4). Similarly, it may be difficult for staff to understand that their own practice may be ageist. This is particularly important since staff in intermediate care services so often work in isolated, autonomous positions and need to be able to appreciate the care skills required and to know when to refer on to more specialist expertise. To appreciate this requires a level of inherent skill that needs to be addressed as staff are appointed to positions within developing services. While work related to Standard 1 in the *National Service Framework for Older People –* 'Rooting out Age Discrimination' – may help this, it will still be important to prepare staff adequately to appreciate and understand the factors that underlie and contribute to ageism, ageist practice and age discrimination (DoH, 2001h). Hence the need to address this issue within a book on intermediate care.

From its inception, intermediate care has been in a good position to address these issues, as it has been perceived positively and has gained status as a new range of services with many opportunities for staff to promote high-quality care. This needs to be sustained and built upon, and will be assisted if staffing skill mix is maintained and staff are adequately equipped to work in isolated roles and autonomous positions. There is an inherent risk that intermediate care services could go the way of other services in terms of the status and expertise involved in caring for older people. This could emerge through the need to staff services where resources are lacking and where there is a failure to address staff development needs. These could be compromised if decisions are made to reduce skill mix due to lack of qualified staff and the need to save money.

The emergence of ageism

Understanding theories of ageing is helpful in appreciating the way that society views older people and ageing, and to some extent helps to explain behaviour towards older people. Theories are the basis on which ideas about specific concepts develop. They provide frameworks for understandings, hypotheses, speculations, values, etc. that influence and form the basis of many activities in our personal and professional lives. Actions do not arise from an ideological vacuum, they emerge from beliefs and values; these, along with our knowledge, form the mainspring of behaviour and provide the reasons why we think and do things. In professional practice, theories may have a particular impact: the judgments we have to make are based upon our current knowledge base and values, etc. and to justify our judgments and decisions requires that these be made explicit .

Theories about humans, unlike scientific theories, are not objective and value-free. At all levels in the human sciences, theories are based on certain fundamental assumptions or values that have to be made explicit (Howe, 1987). Furthermore, different theories lead policy makers and professionals in quite different directions in terms of what, if anything, needs to be done. This can be depicted as shown in Figure 5.1.

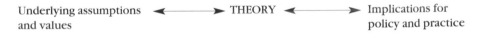

Underlying assumptions ◄————► THEORY ◄————► Implications for
and values   policy and practice

Figure 5.1 How different theories lead policy makers in different directions.

In gerontology, theories to propound or explain later life have emerged at a macro-level, whereby generalizations are made and applied to all older people; superimposed upon these are more micro-level theories related to knowledge, e.g. about race, gender, mental health, family dynamics, etc. Gerontological theories have been divided into three main types: biological, psychological and sociological (Victor, 1994; Medina, 1996; Bond et al., 1999).

Biological theories, particularly older ones, have tended to depict ageing as a negative process, e.g. programmed ageing and ageing due to random damage (Medina, 1996). Strehler (1977), as outlined in Chapter 4, also presented a rather pessimistic view of primary ageing, describing it as a process with four key features:

1. universal and inevitable
2. intrinsic
3. progressive
4. deleterious.

While these features are true, there is little recognition of biological ageing as a developmental process wherein individuals may adapt or be helped to accommodate to their changing circumstances so that they may enjoy a high quality of life, as indeed they so often do (Bond et al., 1999; Hughes, 1995).

Psychological theories have also tended to depict a negative perspective. Early theories focused on studies that later proved to have been inappropriately performed and failed to reflect accurately the general experiences and capabilities of older people. They depicted older people in a negative light, as being slow to learn and remember, etc. Early theories of human development were notable for taking little account of the development and experiences of older people. Not until the work of Erikson in 1965 was the ageing process depicted as a time of maturity and acceptance of earlier life experience. Such work emphasizes the increasingly unique individuality of older people, whose later lives are the culmination of an ever-widening diversity of life experiences.

A number of academics have tried to provide explanations on the basis of sociological theories. The Concise Oxford Dictionary defines sociology as 'the science of the development and nature and laws of human society', although it is in reality much more complex than this. One of the early sociologists was Durkheim, founder of the concept of structural functionalism (Cox, 1983). Functionalists are interested in the structure of societies and how changes in one part of society may set up chain reactions leading to changes elsewhere. Functionalism tends to attribute most of the problems of older people to the natural consequences of physical decline, mental fragility or individual failure. The onus is then on individuals to adapt and adjust to their ageing selves, instead of society and institutions of the state trying to assist older people to function more easily in later life. Society may actually be seen to contribute actively to dependency in old age, in that it legitimizes the exclusion of older people from the labour market and from significant alternative roles, and promotes acceptance of low incomes and pensions. The power of this tradition cannot be overestimated (Phillipson, 1998), and could be said to legitimize ageism in practice. Various other theories took a similar line. Disengagement theory (Cummings and Henry, 1961) provided a convenient explanation to account for why older people should be allowed to withdraw from society. Role theory depicted negative perceptions towards older people. While activity theory did endeavour to redress the balance, in general such early theories helped to legitimize the marginalization of and discrimination against older people and the nature of care practice – practice that has almost certainly contributed to negative perceptions of later life by much of society (Phillipson, 1998). What these theories and the emerging concepts seem to have done, however, was to initiate an exploration of the relationship between the changing needs of an individual and those of the social system (Passuth and Bengston, 1996).

The social construction of old age

The political economy perspective, as put forward by Estes (1979) has been a major contributor to the argument that old age has been socially constructed. The political economy perspective is not concerned with old age as a biological or social problem. Rather, it is interested in old age as a problem for societies because it is characterized by major inequalities in the distribution of power, income and property.

By the 1970s there was growing awareness that the experience of old age was influenced by social problems and conditions. Phillipson (1982) identified how these were shaped by the social relations and institutions characteristic of a capitalist society. With the fiscal crisis in the 1980s and early 1990s older people became perceived as the main beneficiaries of public expenditure. They began to be seen as a burden on the economy, and with the predicted demographic changes and declining ratio of younger people to older people, this was seen as creating an intolerable pressure on public expenditure (Phillipson, 1998).

One particular argument considers whether the logic of capitalism as an economic and social system is reconcilable with meeting the needs of older people. Phillipson (1982) makes four observations in relation to this:

1. When capitalism is in crisis – as in the 1930s, and again in the 1990s – it attempts to solve its problems through cuts in the living standards of working people.
2. Capitalism seems to have a distinct set of priorities, which almost always tend to relegate social and individual needs behind the search for profits.
3. Because of the cyclical nature of capitalist economies, older people often find themselves caught between their own need for better services and the steady decline of facilities within their neighbourhoods.
4. In capitalist economies there are distinct inequalities in the distribution of income and wealth. This results in considerable problems for groups such as poor and disadvantaged older people.

Modernization theory

Modernization theory, which emerged during the 1950s, has also contributed to our perceptions of older people. It proposed an explanation of what happens to older people when a society makes advances towards becoming a 'modern society'. Modernization theorists view development as an evolutionary process going through various stages and transforming all societies from traditional to modern. Each successive stage is not only different from, but superior to, the one preceding it. Development is a cumulative process where there is no turning back. In other words, modernization implies that these changes are in the technological, economic, political and social systems of developing countries, so that they become increasingly like Western European and North American countries.

Using the concepts of modernization theory, Cowgill and Holmes (1972) made a series of studies of ageing in 14 societies at various stages of modernization, ranging from pre-literate societies such as the Sidam, Igbo and Bantu peoples of Africa to the highly Westernized societies of Austria, Norway and the USA. As a result of these studies, Cowgill and Holmes (1972; Cowgill 1974) advanced a modernization theory of ageing, which states that the societal process of modernization leads to a progressive decline in the status of old people:

> Modernization is declared to be associated with later onset of old age, increased use of chronological criteria, increased longevity, an ageing population ... lower status of the aged, decline in leadership roles of the aged, decline in power and influence of the aged ... (Cowgill 1974)

A constant theme in modernization theory is that in pre-industrial societies older people have extensive kinship networks that provide the older person with valued roles, respect and economic security. As a country moves towards modernization, these family support mechanisms tend to break up and the nuclear family becomes the norm, with the state providing for the economic and social needs of older people. The underlying assumption in this theory is that the status of older people in pre-industrial society was high.

Cowgill (1974) states that four significant changes occur with industrialization to alter the status of older people:

1. high technology
2. economic technology
3. urbanization
4. literacy and mass education.

There are, however, a number of criticisms of modernization theory:

- It is not clear what is meant by the term 'high-status'. This term is not defined explicitly and it might be argued that this is only one factor that must be considered for understanding older people from a cross-cultural perspective.
- The contemporary world is so intertwined that changes in the areas adjoining rural areas of the third world countries can have an important effect on the status of older people in these areas.

- The viewpoint assumes a high status for older people in traditional societies – this is almost certainly a misleading over-generalization. Certainly there is research that shows the perils facing older people in small, face-to-face tribal societies (Victor, 1994).
- Shanus (1979) and Bengston et al. (1990) would challenge the claim that extensive and supportive kinships were in existence in traditional societies.

Perceptions of old age

Two perceptions of older people, both influenced to some extent by facts and by theory, have dominated the formation of public policy, particularly in the reduction of public expenditure and provision for older people. One is that there is a rising tide of dependent older people, whose lack of productivity and increasing need for income maintenance and care have created a social problem of enormous proportions. It is believed that the resource implications of this will need to be borne by the section of the population which is younger and economically active, and, crucially, steadily shrinking (this assumes that ageing is synonymous with disability and dependency). On the other hand, there is the notion of the Woopie (Well Off Older Person), based on the assumption that most older people are in a situation of secure finance, good health, pleasant material conditions and lifestyle (Falkingham and Victor, 1991). This may well be the case for white middle-class professionals. This group, however, is only a minority, and unrepresentative of the older population as a whole.

What emerges is that someone's experience of life as an older person is very much influenced by the accumulation of circumstances, attributes and experiences they have acquired throughout life. On the one hand, older people will have commonalities related to their cohort and the particular society of which they have been a part – with its particular images, attitudes, provision and policies towards life, retirement and old age. On the other hand, it is important to acknowledge the diversity that exists between older people and the extent to which other sources of individual life experience will have influenced later life. These may be related to factors such as class, gender and race that will have shaped earlier life circumstances and carry on into later life. In old age, they are likely to be compounded to create each individual's particular experience of life at this stage. Despite this diversity, older people still tend to be grouped together as one homogeneous group and often seem to experience discrimination. There are four particular dimensions where this is evident.

Income

There is a view that older people enter a golden age due to the relative income position of their pension compared to certain other groups, e.g.

single mothers, the decline in the proportion claiming income support (although actual numbers have stayed stable) and the emergence of Woopies, as mentioned above. There is evidence of age discrimination within the state income and benefit system. This seems to endorse the idea that older people should expect to be impoverished and disabled, and should not expect the same assistance as younger people to whom these misfortunes may befall. For example, non-means-tested disability benefits are denied older people unless the claimant has submitted the first claim before reaching pensionable age. Becoming disabled after this age apparently deems one ineligible, presumably on the assumption that pensioners must expect to become disabled, a view many older people themselves hold.

Housing

Older people proportionately live in poorer housing conditions with poorer or fewer amenities, and twice as many live in privately rented unfurnished accommodation (Wheeler, 1986). A range of reasons may account for this. Some may lack adequate finances, and if they remain in their family home or their lifelong home, this along with lack of wherewithal or access to help and assistance may mean the house is run down and poorly maintained (Bond, 1999).

Health

Older people experience more acute and chronic ill health, due to both the normal ageing process and to lifelong inequalities (Arber and Ginn, 1991). There is also evidence, however, to suggest that older people are not taken as seriously or treated as rapidly or thoroughly as younger people (Arrol, 2001). It is not uncommon for an older person to be expected to 'Grin and bear it', or to be told 'What can you expect at your age?' or 'It's your age'. The health care received in the contemporary political climate may be even more adversely affected by health economies and rationing and the shift towards a market system of delivery of health care services over the past decade or so (HAS, 2000; Age Concern, 1999b). Recognition of this is evident within the National Service Framework for Older People along with the milestones identified.

Social attitudes

Ageism and other forms of discrimination against older people as a group can exist only where there is a general attitude that lacks concern or demonstrates negative views about older people. The social construction of ageing within Britain tends to give rise to a number of stereotypical images of older people including the 'rocking-chair' image, the 'awkward old woman' image, and the 'dirty old man' image. While there is a cursory recognition of the importance of celebrating old age and long life, and there may be reference to older people as being wise and revered, there is no doubt that in reality older people, as a group, experience social discrimination. This is evident in the inequalities addressed above, reflected in the National Service Framework for Older People, particularly within the two early standards, 'Rooting out Ageism' and 'Person-centred Care' (DoH, 2001h).

Ageism in the making

Despite the common images of old age, there is great diversity between older people. As a group, however, they do seem to fare worse in relation to a wide variety of indicators compared with other social groups (Hughes, 1995). It is clear that they experience considerable social and economic inequalities compared with the rest of the population and subgroups. Thus it is legitimate to assume that a wide variety of social policies are also based, implicitly or otherwise, on a set of assumptions or attitudes that, first, allow such inequality to be generated and, second, permit it to continue unchallenged.

We are not born to old age, as are most other minority or subgroups. Old age is a potentially universal characteristic, for we all, if we live, enter into old age. Yet old age, as Hughes (1995) suggests, seems to define a different kind of 'minority group', being treated as if it were a differentiating variable, conferring a fixed social identity on those within the group and disconnecting old age from other age-related life phases and experiences that precede it. Thus age is interpreted as a basic source of biological variation between people and over the course of life. It seems, however, that older people are defined both biologically and in other ways as different from other people.

It is not hard to see how these emerging images could become internalized by society and policy makers, even where they have not been fully justified or substantiated. The result of this is that policies, directives and sometimes Acts of Parliament may have been created that are often based upon unsubstantiated ideas, theories and ageist attitudes as well as upon other unfounded information. Not only do attitudes towards older people emerge from early personal socialization founded on inherent beliefs and values, but also from the socially constructed views that are dependent on society's values.

For example, the imposition of a fixed retirement age has had the effect of forcing older people to withdraw from economic activity, contributing to the view that older people are socially and politically redundant and reinforcing their marginalization. Hughes (1995) argues that not only do social attitudes towards old age develop in response to the historical legacy and cultural traditions of a particular society (our early primary socialization), but also from the structure of a society, in particular its economic structure and the relationship between the economic, social and political systems.

Furthermore, Hughes suggests that the existence of old people may touch deeply atavistic fears about death: their appearance may bring to mind images of wizards, witches and mystics, presenting us with aspects of our own mortality and bodily changes that we may try to deny. Hughes argues that ageism may be a related social response – designed to protect the 'not so old' from dwelling too long on painful, unpalatable but inalienable aspects of their futures. 'Old people' are always other people, never oneself, however old one may be, suggests Hughes.

Images of old age and older people seem then to derive from an array of prevailing political, economic and social attitudes as well as from historical developments (Townsend, 1962; Estes, 1979; Phillipson and Walker, 1986). Biological, psychological and sociological theories have all tended to portray later life in a negative light, perceived it as a time of physical and mental decline marked by social withdrawal and increasing self-preoccupation. These changes have been accounted for as part of the normal ageing process and so attributed to the individual. These images have become established and then continually reinforced by icons (in drama, advertising, literature), by powerful commentators (politicians, actors, teachers, nurses), through family life, and through primary socialization (Bytheway, 1995).

This ageist iconography of old age has seeped into people's lives through several routes, three of which are described by Hughes (1995):

1. policies which marginalize older people;
2. personal values as expressed by others through conversation, behaviour etc.;
3. personal experience – older people themselves and their own self-perpetuating views of being older.

The features of ageism outlined here help to explain the context within which health and social care services for older people have become established, and give rise to an interesting discourse about how older people are cared for and how their care is perceived within health and social care.

The biomedicalization of old age and the 'ageing enterprise'

Estes (1979) examined the issues of social construction of old age in more detail by actually looking at the way older people have been marginalized as a perceived dependent group within health and social care. He coined the term 'the ageing enterprise' and attributed this to the 'biomedicalization of ageing'. Estes argued that this resulted in the development of a service industry of agencies, providers and planners who reaffirmed the 'outgroup' status of older people in order to maintain their own professional jobs –

nurses, social workers, geriatricians. He also believed that it attracted people who wished to make money and see it as a business, a criticism that has been directed towards the private independent sector (although hardly profitable presently). This could be argued to marginalize further the specialized care and services provided for older people, in addition to their perceived lack of glamour. On the other hand, it could be argued that it has prevented older people becoming entrapped within a medical model of care, which is another issue of concern.

Policy solutions have tended to focus on integrating and socializing older people to adapt to their status rather than engaging in efforts to fundamentally alter social and economic conditions in order to incorporate the needs and abilities of older people. However, within the proposals outlined in the *National Service Framework for Older People* (DoH 2001h) and *Intermediate Care Guidance* (DoH, 2001e), there is the potential to create a set of specialist services within intermediate care that retain a more therapeutic and social model of care but ensure equitable access to appropriate services and expertise based on need. This could be the making of services for older people, but it could equally become a 'new Cinderella service'.

Ageism in health care

While ageism and age discrimination appear to be rife within society, it is also very evident within the health and social care community. Over the decades, a litany of reports and publications has condemned the quality of health and social care experienced by older people (Townsend, 1962; Rowntree Report, 1980; Means and Smith, 1985). Although various strategies have been implemented in response to these, the concerns still remain, as evidenced by recent reports including the UKCC Continuing Care policy paper (UKCC, 1997), the Health Advisory Service Report (HAS, 1998), *Turning Your Back on Us* (Age Concern, 1999b) and the Royal Commission into the Long Term Care of Older People (DoH, 1999c; DoH, 2001c). A range of factors contribute to the continued failure to improve the health care situation for older people, many of which are listed in the HAS Report (1998). Underlying these, and indeed fuelling them, is the persistence of ageist attitudes, and age-based discrimination regarding access to resources. This is probably reinforced by the history of negative perceptions of this area of care and by the failure to make specialist education a prerequisite for nursing staff and other practitioners working in this area (UKCC, 1997).

Ageism in context

Ageism pervades almost every walk of life, health and social care workers included, where according to the HAS Report it 'permeated even the highest levels of organizations' (1998: 67). Evidence suggests that nurses, who are the key workforce over the 24-hour period, and who will play a predominant part within intermediate care services, are as guilty as others in demonstrating negative attitudes towards older patients (Slevin, 1991; UKCC, 1997). Like other health professionals, they often show little interest in working with this age group. This seems to be particularly true of students and newly qualified nurses (Penner et al., 1983; Snape, 1986; HAS, 1998). Treharne (1990) found that attitudes of student nurses became more negative towards older people following placement on an 'elderly care' ward. Sheffler (1995) attributed this to the negative attitudes that were found among the qualified nursing staff and other disciplines working in these placement areas. There are many well-meaning, motivated staff who demonstrate significant commitment in working hard to maintain and improve the standards of care received by older people; their work, however, is hampered by such ageist attitudes and their influence (HAS, 1998).

Slevin (1991) argues that older people are blamed for their condition by the wider social group, similar to the way that other 'out-groups' are victimized (Ryan, 1971). Nurses and health care workers may themselves adopt these views. Those working in non-specialized settings with older people in their care may also play an active part in contributing to the development of ageist views, exemplified by such comments as 'They shouldn't be here' irrespective of the individual's equal right to care. This view in particular is picked up in one of the key sections of the National Service Framework (DoH, 2001h), which focuses on equity of access by all based on individual needs, not age.

Within the medical profession there has been insufficient recognition of the value of addressing the educational needs of caring for older people (assessment, diagnosis and treatment) at both undergraduate and postgraduate level (Morris et al., 2000). Physiotherapists tend to specialize in functional activities, which may not focus on the holistic needs of the older person. They may, therefore, prefer not to participate in the more general holistic rehabilitation so often required by older people, especially within intermediate care services. Occupational therapists, it might be argued, are the most appropriately prepared to look after this client group and others with compromised independence.

The status of technical skills

Ageist attitudes within health care may be connected to the perceived value of caring for older people contrasted with the value so often placed on highly technical activities which seem to engender a high-status image of nursing and health care. Davis (1968) described how student nurses internalized a body of professional attitudes and behaviour; little seems to have changed as evidenced by Stevens and Crouch (1995). This has tended to encourage a narrow, disease-orientated, biomedical model approach to care, which values high technology and devalues essential therapeutic patient care involving a range of psychosocial and environmental factors. The specific yet complex skills required for such care have almost been dismissed as inferior, and indeed as unnecessary and not requiring expertise. When older people require technical intervention, the need for care in the acute sector seems to be recognized as justifiable and is valued, at least to some extent. Once acute medical treatment and intervention is no longer required, however, care needs to change, and compete with those more acute highly technical care needs of others. An acute setting is no longer necessary, nor is it suitable for these changing care needs. The skills and expertise required to meet the care needs of older people alter, but because the 'glamour' associated with technical care subsides this expertise is perceived as inferior, at least by those preoccupied by a medical model of care. It is this view that gives rise to the longer-term concerns related to staff working in intermediate care.

Birchall and Waters (1996) suggest that ageist attitudes lead to a lack of attention to the changing needs of older people in more acute settings, contributing to their increased dependency and subsequent delays in discharge or transfer when in hospital. It is often older people who are moved around wards when there is a bed crisis. This can cause considerable distress and disorientation to the older person, possibly leading to regression. It may also help to give the impression that their care needs are less important than other patients'. These difficulties provide a good argument to invest funding in the development of other settings or services so that they better meet the care needs of older people (Royal Commission, DoH, 1999c; NHS Plan, DoH, 2000c; Intermediate Care Circular, DoH, 2001e). It is also important to have patient tracking systems in place that can confirm that patients are in the right place, at the right time, with the right skills to meet their needs (see Chapter 18).

The image of caring for older people

Although the glamour of technical skills and high-status nursing has done little to promote the expertise of caring for older people, neither has the historical image of caring for this client group in specialized settings. Long-term care has been associated with the workhouse and the asylum, where recipients of care occupied a marginalized and stigmatized position in society. In Goffman's analysis of the 'total institution' he described how the institution controlled the behaviour of both 'inmates' and staff, with highly stylized and ritualistic behaviour patterns emerging. These were justified in terms of meeting the aims and functions of the institution (Goffman, 1961). Unfortunately, this image of care in some settings may still remain and to some extent is borne out by more recent studies such as those by Salmon (1993) and Armstrong-Esther et al. (1994).

More recently, Norman (1997) has built upon this image by citing reports of the low morale and demoralization among staff in care homes. He believes this arises from a number of contributory factors, identified by Levi et al. (1983) as quantitative overload, qualitative underload, lack of control and lack of social support. Staff have heavy caseloads and carry out care that is mainly physical and routinized, often performed as 'tasks'. In contrast with person-centred therapeutic care, this kind of caregiving can lead to feelings of tedium and lack of stimulation, where staff feel they have little or no control over the care they give. This, together with the unglamorous image of this kind of care in both acute and other settings, can lead to feelings of isolation and being undervalued, and may create an 'inferiority complex' for staff (Wade, 2001). It is not beyond the realms of possibility that intermediate care could develop such an image if attention is not given to providing person-centred care and to supporting staff effectively.

Negative perspectives may also be perpetuated by employing a low skill mix of staff to care for older people in specialized areas. Hill et al. (1987) found that as the dependency of the patients in a setting rose, so the number of registered and learner nurses fell. A survey of nursing homes and some NHS settings would no doubt reflect this picture today. The contemporary shortage of nurses adds to the difficulty of recruitment in this area and leads to the easier solution of employing unregistered staff. In acute settings likewise, it is often unregistered staff who are allocated to care for older people. While these staff are often good and well-meaning and may give more continuity of care than would occur with bank or agency staff, the acceptance of an unregistered worker caring for a highly dependent older person does little to dispel the view that such work is unskilled (King, 1995). Instead, as King argues, this area of care is complex, demanding and sophisticated and must be nurtured and valued.

This situation is perpetuated by management acceptance of low staffing levels and skill mix provision for this client group, especially when faced with staffing difficulties. Staff working in these settings may feel powerless to question this situation, especially when challenged by the burden of work, the lack of peer support from other qualified staff, and the often isolated setting. This lack of control and support are comparable to the factors identified by Levi et al. (1983) that contribute to low moral. The ability to determine quality of care can be associated with the sense of ownership felt by staff and their ability to influence and make decisions. A sense of powerlessness helps to account for the reluctance (or, indeed, resistance) of staff to change practice, despite any external pressures and obvious benefits. Furthermore, multiple layers of management in some organizations may create a 'depth and distance' (Frey, 1990), which can jeopardize changes in practice since 'the greater the distance a proposal must travel, the greater the likelihood it will meet with resistance'. Further obstacles include the remoteness of management or their reluctance to seek views, along with the frequent changes of senior staff which may be found within the NHS and care homes. These factors serve to underline the importance of addressing the skill mix and expertise of staff in intermediate care settings.

Perceptions of what constitutes skilled nursing care are controversial. It seems nurse education has failed to convey the expertise required where caring activities predominate. Stevens and Crouch (1995) argue this contrasts with the espoused 'essence' of nursing, which is perceived to be holistic therapeutic care. They suggest that one reason for this is that the principles of therapeutic care and expertise are usually illustrated using examples from highly technical areas such as intensive care units. They cite eminent nursing theorists such as Orem (1980), Newman (1979) and Watson (1988), who tend to use examples related to rather technical aspects of care. Similarly, when Benner (1984) tries to illustrate the continuum from novice to expert, and talks of intuition, she again often refers to highly technical areas of care. Stevens and Crouch argue that by implication the message conveyed is that these situations are the most professionally demanding. Elzinga (1990: 157) suggests that the caring stance 'is now grafted onto a scientific core with the help of a philosophical discourse and the incorporation of humanistic studies'. Furthermore, Stevens and Crouch (1995: 239) assert that, in Bourdieu's terms:

> 'the pedagogic work' undertaken to embed student nurses in their appropriate 'habitus' defines technological/scientific expertise as the most significant 'symbolic capital' of the profession.

Stevens and Crouch go on to suggest that medicine, regarded as the top profession in health care, has been characterized as the achievement of competence, knowledge and monopoly over clinical and technical tasks and the application of that knowledge. It is therefore, they argue, not surprising that nurses who aspire to professional status regard such technical skills as desirable. They go on to suggest that these activities are regarded as needing such attributes as expertise, defined responsibilities and, most especially, autonomy and independent control.

If, as Stevens and Crouch suggest, these latter attributes are seen as desirable for professionalism, then this could be seen to bode well for more nurse-led environments such as intermediate care settings. Patient care in these settings is very much nurse led, and the delivery of good, effective care calls for skilled decision-making and problem-solving skills requiring autonomy, independent control and responsibility, often within exposed and vulnerable situations (UKCC, 1997; Vaughan et al., 1999). In addition, expert interpersonal skills together with effective interdisciplinary and collaborative working are essential (Philipose et al., 1991).

These skills and attributes need to be emphasized as a valuable aspect of giving high-quality person-centred care to older people. They will, however, not develop if, as in some settings, there are inadequate support systems and a lack of opportunity for ongoing professional development (King, 1995; UKCC, 1997). In isolated or unsupported environments, the lack of such helping strategies may result in the nurse struggling to obtain resources and being forced to lower standards. This may lead to poor practice being delivered with a relatively inadequate knowledge of the complex needs of older people (Beckingham and DuGas, 1993). It may be these unsupported areas where care becomes compromised that contribute to the poor reputation of some institutions caring for older people and the general low status and stereotyping of the speciality of caring for older people (Knowles and Sarver, 1985). This further emphasizes the need to provide comprehensive support mechanisms for staff working in intermediate care settings.

Strategies to combat ageism

Having discussed ageism and its context, and the problems of ensuring high-quality care for older people, it is appropriate now to identify some strategies that may help to address developmental needs and combat ageism. A key concern has been the failure of professional education to address the care needs of older people or to convey the expertise required for their care. This is true of both nursing (Stevens and Crouch, 1995) and medicine (Morris et al., 2000). The multi-faceted nature of the problem means that a number of strategies need to be considered.

Early surveys have suggested that increased knowledge in gerontology should help to foster positive attitudes among nurses (Campbell, 1971; Heller and Walsh, 1976) and should be carefully addressed within nursing curricula. Eddy (1986) argues, however, that other variables have a significant influence, such as environment and attitudes of others, as identified by Nolan et al. (2001). This same issue applies to doctors and is recognized by the RCP (2000b) in its recommendations for the education needs of medical students. The RCP advocates attachments to firms specializing in this field, in the belief that students will gain opportunities to 'develop core clinical skills, and to learn a holistic approach to the practice of medicine' (p. 19). Education related to the care of older people also needs to be present in both pre- and post-registration-level curricula for all professional disciplines. Staff who care for older people, in whatever setting, should be actively involved in continuing professional development and education. All courses should have a gerontological focus seeded across their curricula (with the exclusion perhaps of obstetrics and paediatrics – although it could be argued there should be a small curricular element even here). Furthermore, the requirement of a specialist educational course for staff working predominantly with older people (as in other specialist areas) may help to raise awareness that caring for older people does require skill and expertise. Specialist registrars in geriatric medicine should be required to aim for accreditation in general internal medicine and specialist gerontology, while continuing personal development for all physicians should encompass training in internal and geriatric medicine as well as in sub-specialities.

The practice fields of training for trainee doctors will also need to encompass intermediate care services so that confidence and competence within the area is developed. This can happen only once consultants have a remit to support intermediate care services. Enhanced practice in working with older people will perhaps best be achieved through multi-professional education and development (Philipose et al., 1991), as recommended in *Making a Difference* (DoH, 1999c). This is supported by Thomas (1995) and Castledine (1994), who argue that it is rare for a single profession to meet the often complex health and social care needs of the older individual.

Wallace (1992) advocates that nurse educators must focus on *care* (the therapeutic approach) rather than *cure*, promoting the value and interest of this. The approach to teaching should be on a health–illness continuum, focused on enabling older people to maximize independence and self-determination, and recognizing the variety of settings in which older people are cared for. Medicine likewise needs to value the complexity of caring for older people, recognizing the challenges of assessment, diagnosis and treatment of illness that often presents differently in the older person. Equally, the holistic care needs of this client group should be addressed, not neglected in favour of a biomedical model (RCP, 2000a). Another increasingly relevant approach is the recognition that most patients in care are older. Thus for most health care professionals their curricula would be better based around the central theme that the average patient is older. This whole area will need to be addressed within Standard 4 of the National Service Framework for Older People (DoH, 2001h). However, this standard focuses on a skills analysis and competency framework for staff in District General Hospitals. That staff in these settings have been selected for special attention may arise from an historical failure to appreciate that the key client group they care for are older people, and also because critical reports such as the HAS Report (1998) and the Age Concern Report (1999b) focused on these setting. It would perhaps be most appropriate, however, to address the education and development needs of staff in all settings and services that care for older people, across all disciplines and professions.

Preparation of unregistered caring staff

There is a growing dependence upon unregistered care staff in all settings, and it is paramount that their educational and development needs are addressed seriously. With the current shortage of registered nurses, care assistants will continue to provide the greater part of hands-on care to older people. They need appropriate practice-based in-house training such as NVQs and other educational and development strategies, with appropriately educated qualified staff to act as assessors. The creation of generic workers and rehabilitation assistants with a recognized programme of preparation is another responsive approach for unqualified staff. There is an urgent need, however, to clarify the roles of these workers, especially that of rehabilitation assistants. All these developments need to feed into more advanced educational opportunities so that staff can progress and move forward in their practice and responsibilities, and if they so wish and are able, enter education schemes to become appropriately qualified practitioners (Apps, 1997; DoH, 1999a).

Teaching needs to be provided by appropriately qualified staff with a committed interest in older people, who keep in touch with practice and the reality (King, 1995). In medicine, it is more usual for geriatricians to play a key role in the education of medical students in their speciality. However, the lack of status of this speciality evidently rubs off on to students, impeding for many the commitment to specialize in this area.

Practice settings

Sheffler (1995) demonstrated that both hospital and nursing home placements, if suitable, lead to improved attitudes. Fox and Wold (1996) also described the emergence of some very positive and rewarding outcomes, particularly in relation to attitude change among nursing students, when they were placed in settings conducive to caring for older people. These findings are backed up by the more recent work of Nolan et al. (2001). It is therefore critical that appropriate settings or philosophies of care (where care is provided in the home) are available for staff to be able to undertake their care appropriately and for students to experience competent person-centred care of older people with clinical staff who are equipped to teach. This provides a strong argument to ensure all care teams and settings are suitable, both from the ethical view point of equitable care for all older people, but also because of the current difficulty experienced in finding adequate placements for students at all.

With the emergence of intermediate care services, opportunities should arise for staff to take on more specialist roles as in nurse/therapy-led services. If real leadership, inspiration and encouragement can be developed at this level then students may well be encouraged to return to these areas (DoH, 1999c, 2001h). Good leadership is important, as is the level of commitment at a strategic executive level. An absence of expertise at a senior level may give the impression that the speciality is not deemed important or significant, so contributing to a general sense of staff feeling devalued. The appointment of specialist nurses/roles, e.g. consultant nurses, gerontological specialist nurses and nurse practitioners, should help to raise the profile of the field of care and contribute to staff development, so increasing the confidence of staff to care for this client group across all settings (see Chapter 8).

The discussion so far has explored ways of improving the way staff in recognized roles are prepared to care for older people. To some extent this may simply be 'tinkering with the edges'. The roles of doctors, nurses, social workers, physiotherapists and occupational therapists as they are currently known may perhaps be outdated for the needs of contemporary health and social care provision. It may be time for a fundamental review of the roles of those providing health and social care. Such an approach would indeed be radical: it would have major practical and logistical implications in terms of what it is we do need and how this could be introduced within the context of current roles. Consideration would also need to be given to professional registration and indeed career pathways and progression, but as stated in Chapter 3, programmes are already being introduced, and developments are under way. Much thought and planning would be necessary to prepare for the possible consequences and repercussions, the implications of which may be unpredictable.

Conclusion

This chapter has examined the concept of ageism and age discrimination. It has perhaps given a rather gloomy impression of the care provided to many older people in contemporary health and social care settings, and painted a rather pessimistic picture of the possible development of intermediate care services. None of this is inevitable; it can be avoided. It does provide a warning, however, to those involved in developing and providing intermediate care services, of the real dangers of inherent ageism, and highlights the need to pay attention to staff preparation and development. The advantages for such services is that many very aptly address the needs of older people, and in so doing promote the need and importance of person-centred care. This should to some extent protect against ageism at a time when there is greater recognition, emphasis and respect for older people.

The first two parts of this book have addressed the concept and context of intermediate care in relation to older people, and have provided an overview of ageing and older people within heath and social care. The next part moves on to look in more detail at the practicalities of planning and developing intermediate care services within the context of health and social care policy and drivers. In the final part, the focus shifts to preparing for the delivery of intermediate care services/schemes and focuses in particular on staff, exploring in some depth some of their development needs.

KEY POINTS

- There is continued concern about the quality of care received by some older people in health care settings, with ageism and age discrimination possibly playing a fundamental role in perpetuating low standards.
- A number of factors have been identified that contribute to ageism and age discrimination.
- Senior management and administrators are in a key position to guide and influence the factors that can resolve this continued concern.
- Education plays a significant part in challenging ageism, which needs to be addressed at pre-registration, post-registration and care assistant levels.
- Those responsible for providing education need to have appropriate postgraduate gerontological education and demonstrate positive attitudes.
- Relevant settings, environments and teams need to be provided with support and ongoing staff development to promote positive attitudes towards the care of older people and provide positive learning environments.

PART III

Planning, Developing, Monitoring and Evaluating New Intermediate Care Services

CHAPTER 6

Planning and preparing for intermediate care

JON GLASBY

Introduction

So far in this book, attention has been given to exploring the concept of intermediate care and models of care within the context of providing a whole systems service for older people with health and social care needs. Ageing and uniqueness of the older person has been examined along with the social context within which older people access services. In this part, the more practical aspects of planning and setting up intermediate care services will begin to be explored. In this chapter the experience of the logistics and complexities, along with the opportunities, of setting up a new intermediate care services are shared and examined.

Setting the scene

Although intermediate care is often seen as a panacea for resolving the various pressures experienced by health and social services, operationalizing the concept is more difficult than many agencies may first realize. Precisely because it is 'intermediate', intermediate care spans a range of traditional service boundaries encompassing primary, secondary and social care, as well as the public, private, voluntary and informal sectors. This inevitably means that the person or people responsible for developing an intermediate care strategy will have to work with and overcome a range of competing agendas, organizational tensions and different approaches. Perhaps more significantly, the resultant strategy will have to draw on money from a range of different budgets, and asking for money has an awkward habit of 'putting people's backs up'. When things are going well, it can really seem as if everyone is rising above their positions as representatives of a particular organizational stance and pulling in the same direction for the common good. When difficulties arise, however, such apparent collaboration can quickly disintegrate into mutual suspicion, a refusal to give ground, and cost shunting, making it all but impossible to reach a satisfactory compromise and to achieve a shared vision of the way forward. This situation is not aided by a number of practical difficulties and 'teething problems' that often arise when a new concept or service is being planned. As a result, senior managers and planners can find themselves distracted from the task of achieving a collective inter-agency approach by unresolved technical issues such as registration and inspection, guidelines for constructing new buildings and question marks over whether the anticipated funds for the project have really materialized.

Against this background, this chapter draws on personal experience of developing an intermediate care business plan, highlighting the practical difficulties that can develop and that need to be overcome if a new service is to be successfully introduced. After setting out the context within which the business plan was commissioned and produced, attention turns to the tensions that can be generated by inter-agency working and specific issues that emerged as the plan progressed. Finally, a framework is suggested that may help others seeking to develop intermediate care services to produce the shared ownership necessary to deal with some of these complexities and achieve mutually beneficial outcomes for users/carers and all the individual agencies involved.

Background

In 1999, a West Midlands Primary Care Group (PCG) commissioned a firm of external consultants to carry out a feasibility study with a view to establishing a new intermediate care facility. Working with a steering group made up of local health and social care representatives, the consultants drew up a provisional staff profile, estimated the number of beds/domiciliary places required and began to consider some of the financial implications of establishing a new service. As part of the brief, the consultants also worked with a range of stakeholders from local health and social care agencies and from the voluntary sector in order to consider the overall model that the proposed service should adopt. In the event, the feasibility study produced a number of options for local practitioners and managers to consider:

- two hospital-based intermediate care facilities;
- one hospital-based and one nursing home-based intermediate care facility;
- two nursing home-based intermediate care facilities;
- a single nursing home-based intermediate care facility in a central location;
- a single, purpose-built joint health and social care facility.

Each option was then evaluated according to a series of criteria drawn up by the consultants and key stakeholders. By far the most favoured option was for a single, purpose-built intermediate care facility for the PCG, and this model was subsequently recommended to and accepted by the PCG Board.

In 2000, the PCG in question was named as a pilot site for NHS LIFT, a new form of public–private partnership announced in the government's NHS Plan (DoH, 2000c) and designed to provide the capital and expertise necessary to improve primary care buildings. While LIFT is very much in its infancy at the time of writing, the scheme essentially involves local agencies working with a private sector partner to identify and build new primary care premises, with the health service leasing such premises from the local LIFT partnership. To capitalize on this new opportunity, the PCG decided to take forward its plans for intermediate care much more rapidly than it had previously planned, commissioning an independent researcher to draw up a business plan for the proposed intermediate care facility.

Specifically, the brief was to:

- identify and agree with partners the existing services that will be redirected into intermediate care, and the timescales for this;
- work with local managers to develop an agreed staff profile;
- ensure detailed financial costings are produced for the capital and revenue costs of the service;
- identify potential sites and providers;
- produce a plan for consulting on the business plan and communicating to staff.

Inter-agency working

Securing effective collaboration between different health and social care organizations has long been recognized as problematic and has proved remarkably resistant to official attempts at reform (Glasby and Littlechild, 2000b). Although bringing down the 'Berlin Wall' that exists between health and social care is currently a key government priority (House of Commons Debates, 1997), the evidence suggests that differences and tensions both within and between health and social care remain difficult to overcome, (Henwood et al. (1997), Horne (1998), Hudson (2000)). In recent years, the key obstacles to joint working have been summarized in research conducted by the Nuffield Institute for Health (see Figure 6.1).

Almost by definition, those charged with delivering the government's targets for intermediate care will have to address and overcome such barriers if their work is to be effective. Although the inter-agency and cross-cutting nature of intermediate care is one of its great strengths as a concept, it is also

- **Structural** (fragmentation of service responsibilities across agency boundaries, within and between sectors)
- **Procedural** (differences in planning horizons and cycles; differences in budgetary cycles and procedures; differences in information systems and protocols regarding confidentiality and access)
- **Financial** (differences in funding mechanisms and bases; differences in the stocks and flows of financial resources)
- **Professional** (professional self-interest and autonomy and inter-professional competition for domains; competitive ideologies and values; threats to job security; conflicting views about clients/ consumers interests and roles)
- **Status and legitimacy** (organizational self-interest and autonomy and inter-organizational competition for domains; differences in legitimacy between elected and appointed agencies)

Source: Hudson et al. (1997: 11).

Figure 6.1 Barriers to inter-agency collaboration.

one of the factors that make successful intermediate care difficult to achieve. As a result, developing new intermediate care services will require a concerted effort on behalf of all participating agencies to look above and beyond their own individual agendas, reach workable compromises and collaborate to achieve positive outcomes for users and carers.

In seeking to draw up an intermediate care business plan, the PCG worked with a range of practitioners from different professional backgrounds and employed by a range of different agencies, as outlined in Figure 6.2. This raised a number of practical difficulties as the project progressed, which had not always been anticipated from the beginning:

Participating agencies	Participating practitioners
PCG	GPs
Health authority	Public health workers
Local authority	Social workers
An acute/community health trust	Nurses
Independent sector	Occupational therapists
Other PCGs in same health authority	Physiotherapists
PCGs in nearby health authority	Speech and language therapists
Neighbouring local authority	Dieticians
Nearby acute hospital	Chiropodists
Nearby community health trust	Consultant geriatricians

Figure 6.2 Key stakeholders involved in planning and commissioning a new intermediate care service.

Different values: Different participants were from different professional backgrounds, had undergone different types of training and had developed different personal and professional values. Whereas some agencies tended to emphasize the importance of professional power, others stressed the need to promote choice and autonomy for users and carers. While some professionals prioritized security and stability, others called for greater risk-taking. Perhaps the best example of a potential clash of different value systems came with regard to interpretation and translation services. The area concerned was very multicultural, and the provision of culturally sensitive services was felt to be important by most participating agencies and individuals. However, opinions varied as to the extent to which professionally trained interpreters and translators would be needed in the proposed intermediate care facility. Although some stakeholders from a health background felt that it would be acceptable for family members to interpret on behalf of individual patients or for members of staff from ethnic minorities to take on this role, participants with a social services training believed this to be inappropriate, exploiting staff and giving people from ethnic minorities a second-class service. Of course, this was far from an insurmountable problem, but does illustrate the different assumptions and approaches that different workers bring with them to the negotiating table.

Organizational agendas: In any partnership, individual participants are likely to have their own priorities, preferences and ideas about how a given project should proceed. These are not always articulated explicitly, but can complicate the task of reaching a compromise and create mutual suspicion among participating organizations. With regard to the intermediate care business plan, some GPs were concerned to have the proposed facility as close to their surgeries as possible to minimize their travelling time, and sometimes objected to locations that were more accessible for the PCG as a whole on the grounds that they were too far away from their individual practice. In contrast, the acute health trust was concerned about a local community hospital some miles away that was already in use but felt to be under-utilized and which it wished to use for the proposed intermediate care facility. This was rejected by other participants who preferred a more community-based approach to intermediate care, but kept surfacing at various stages in the negotiations as the acute trust continued to push its preferred option. Finally, the social services department was eager for the new service to be based in one of its residential homes which it was struggling to refurbish to meet new care standards, hoping to lever in funding from NHS LIFT to renovate a dilapidated building that might otherwise need to close. Despite this, the department was prepared to make the building available only on the grounds that it was chosen to provide the new service – an approach which might not have secured best value for money and an ultimatum which other partners found difficult to accept.

The lack of co-terminosity: Inter-agency working is frequently blighted by the lack of co-terminosity between the various agencies that are trying to work more closely together. This can take a number of forms. Whereas NHS services tend to be based on the GP with which a patient is registered, the local authority and sometimes the voluntary sector is based on strict geographical boundaries. Thus, a patient from a particular PCG may fall under a number of different social services departments depending on where they live, while a local authority may need to work with a range of PCGs who have patients in the local area. At the same time, GPs may choose to send their patients to a number of different acute hospitals, whose typical catchment areas may sometimes overlap. In this case, the PCG was keen to share its learning with nearby PCGs in the same health authority and had traditionally been served by two separate acute hospital trusts. While the majority of PCG patients lived in one local authority, a substantial minority lived across the border in a neighbouring authority. There was also a possibility of a joint approach to intermediate care in conjunction with a nearby PCG in a neighbouring health authority. This was problematic for the PCG, since it had to work with a range of different partners and since negotiations were inevitably complex. It was also problematic for the local authority and for the voluntary sector, who wished to adopt an authority-wide approach to intermediate care and were frustrated by the failure of local PCGs to develop a co-ordinated strategy.

Organizational upheaval: All these negotiations took place at the same time as a large-scale process of organizational change within the NHS and local authorities. As partners met to discuss intermediate care, they were also having to cope with a range of internal problems and demands which could not help but distract them from the task in hand. Thus, the PCG was in the process of becoming a Primary Care Trust (PCT) and there were plans for it to merge with other local PCTs at a later stage to form a Care Trust – a new form of agency that provides both health and social care commissions. The acute/community health trust was about to merge with a nearby hospital trust and was discussing how best to transfer its community staff and a number of buildings to the newly formed PCT. At the same time, the health authority was about to be abolished in anticipation of new strategic health authorities recently announced by the government. The social services department was facing something of a financial crisis and was also in the process of an internal reorganization. A nearby social services department serving a number of PCG patients was also struggling with a significant projected overspend and had recently received a very negative report from government inspectors. Since most criticism had been reserved for the children and families service, moreover, the department was understandably concentrating its attention on this aspect of its work and did not seem to be prioritizing intermediate care.

Faced with these barriers to progress, the intermediate care business plan was very much a case of 'the art of the possible' – achieving the best possible result that could be obtained in the time and with the resources available. This meant a series of planning meetings, compromises and crisis talks, as well as a host of informal contacts and discussions with key personnel outside of formal meetings. Although a satisfactory result was eventually obtained which seemed to please all key stakeholders as for as possible, this was neither quick nor easy, and required considerable time, patience and management input.

Additional difficulties

In addition to the complexities which joint working can create, the intermediate care business plan also had to overcome a number of practical problems which arose during the course of the project. In many cases, these were the result of unforeseen issues which began to emerge once local agencies started to operationalize the concept of intermediate care set out in government guidance (DoH, 2001e, 2001h). Intermediate care is a relatively recent concept, and government targets require swift action from a range of health and social care agencies. With any new initiative there is bound to be a number of practical difficulties that gradually emerge (particularly in a situation such as this where there are very tight timescales and where front-line organizations feel under pressure to deliver a central agenda). The following is a brief account of some of the key issues that arose during the intermediate care business plan in question.

Registration and inspection

The intermediate care business plan was developed in the second half of 2001 as the government was consulting on new arrangements for registering and inspecting health and social care facilities (DoH, 2001b, 2001d, 2001g). The arrangements were complex, and made it very difficult for the PCG to think through and take full account of the registration and inspection issues that may arise once the proposed facility was operational. To take but one example, the PCG wished to establish a service that provided a combination of in-patient beds and a domiciliary team to support people in their own homes, and was prepared to consider a range of different providers to run the new service. However, input from the local registration and inspection unit suggested that this might be complicated. Whereas an independent sector provider or a social services department would need to be registered and inspected under the Care Standards Act 2000 (DoH, 2001a), a facility run by an NHS organization would not fall under the remit of this legislation. If registration was required, the service may need to be registered both as a provider of in-patient accommodation and as a domiciliary agency. It would also need to be registered for every different type of service user who would use it (older people, people with physical disabilities, people with learning difficulties etc.). In addition, there was confusion as to how the in-patient beds would be classified under the new system. With no category for intermediate care, the beds would either be designated as a nursing home or as an independent hospital (with the local registration and inspection unit wondering whether the latter may be the most accurate description of the proposed service). Whatever decision was reached, registration and inspection could have considerable administrative and financial implications for the new service, and it seems strange that no national decision had been taken prior to the launch of intermediate care about how such services should be monitored.

Technical specifications

NHS Estates produce a large number of technical publications which set out guidelines for constructing new NHS buildings. These cover topics ranging from in-patient accommodation to mortuaries, and from rehabilitation services to cancer care, setting out the type and size of rooms required, the facilities that may be needed for particular services, and allowances for circulation, utilities, telecommunications and so on (see, for example, NHS Estates, 2000). Unfortunately, there was no guidance for intermediate care at the time of writing, and the PCG had to work closely with a consultant surveyor and NHS Estates in order to establish the technical specifications of the proposed building, adopting something of a 'pick-and-mix' approach from a number of existing guides.

Financial confusion

Although the government had announced 'an extra £900 million' to be spent on intermediate care by 2003–04 (DoH, 2000c: 71), there was considerable confusion locally as to how much money had been received, how much was actually available and where the 'extra' money had gone. In the event, input from finance staff suggested that the 'new' money had not been specifically set aside for intermediate care, but had simply been incorporated into the annual budget. Due to inflation and previous overspends, most of the money had already been accounted for and there was no new investment available for a new intermediate care service. As a result, the business plan had to identify existing projects that could be incorporated into the proposed intermediate care facility, redirecting existing resources into the new service. Hardly surprisingly, this created significant tensions among local agencies and meant that the project was under considerable financial pressure before it had even begun. It was also difficult to explain this situation to front-line workers and to users/carers, reconciling government announcements of additional funding with the cash-strapped reality.

Delivering within tight timescales

Due to perceived government pressure and due to the opportunities provided by NHS LIFT, the PCG was keen to develop and implement its intermediate care business plan as soon as possible and set extremely tight timescales for completion. This had a range of implications for the project, and meant that much of the work was extremely pressured. It also meant that the researcher had to rely heavily on the goodwill of individuals from outside agencies in order to provide requested information and/or support in a very short (and sometimes unreasonably so) space of time. Clearly, this could create tensions in light of the difficulties of inter-agency working described above, and some agencies simply refused to co-operate within the PCG's timescales, making the project all the more complex.

Consultation

One area where time constraints were particularly problematic was the need to consult with service users/carers and front-line staff – something that the PCG wished to do but which could have been problematic within the PCG's timescales. Involving people in decisions about service changes takes time, and there is little point 'consulting' if the agency concerned is not able to listen to the answers it receives or act upon them. This is frequently a source of tension for users and carers, who feel that most consultation is merely tokenistic, going through the motions of involvement without genuinely seeking the views of local people, and is discussed further by Thewlis in Chapter 7. This can quickly lead to disillusionment, with users and carers quite rightly feeling that there is little point wasting their time in consultation exercises that simply confirm what the management has already decided (see Age Concern, 2000; Barnes, 1997; Barnes and Walker, 1996 for further discussion and details of consultation/involvement). To avoid these pitfalls in this particular project, a twofold approach was recommended which included a very rapid consultation with key user/carer representatives together with much longer-term research that sought to consider the priorities of users/carers, what they value about current services, what they would like to see changed, how they like to be treated by service providers, and so on. A similar process was also recommended for front-line staff, once again combining a 'quick and dirty' consultation with longer-term research to address issues such as the strengths and weaknesses of current services, attitudes to intermediate care and possible implications for other agencies.

NHS LIFT

Although technically a separate issue, the inclusion of the PCG in an NHS LIFT pilot raised additional difficulties that had not originally been foreseen. During the project, a range of questions quickly emerged which the central government sometimes struggled to answer with any degree of conviction and which made planning the new intermediate care facility all the more complex: How much should the PCG allow for 'rent' payable to the local NHS LIFT for new premises? Should allowances be made for VAT or will this be recoverable (as is the case with some other areas of primary care)? How should GPs deal with issues of negative equity?

A framework for intermediate care

Building on first-hand experience of research and consultancy work with a range of health and social care agencies, the following model may help those seeking to develop intermediate care to secure greater inter-agency collaboration and may give local partnerships a solid foundation from which to tackle some of the practical difficulties and tensions described above.

Generating shared ownership of intermediate care and developing a practical, relevant and workable service depends on five key components:

- *A values-based approach* that seeks to identify the principles on which participating services are operating. Agreeing shared values is an essential preliminary before addressing the organizational dilemmas and tensions that significant change and joint working can generate. If agencies are clear about what they are trying to achieve and why, they will be able to base any future decision on the extent to which it fits the group's shared values and will have an explicit set of criteria with which to evaluate future action.
- *An empowering approach* that recognizes and values the contribution of all stakeholders, from users and carers to front-line staff and from first-level managers to senior officers. Ensuring that all key stakeholders have an opportunity to contribute to the strategy will increase the chance of its success and will aid future dissemination and evaluation. Often, input

from users/carers and front-line staff in particular can be crucial in ensuring that the resultant service is appropriate and really meets the needs it was established to address. Involving people who do not usually get consulted about service changes can also encourage them to feel valued and involved in the project. Ultimately, the success of a new service depends not on the building that houses it or the policies that govern it, but on the people who use and run it.

- A *multidisciplinary approach* that values the skills of practitioners from different professional backgrounds and acknowledges the need for a holistic approach to intermediate care. Health and social care services are ultimately interdependent and a successful strategy must rest on shared ownership and a recognition that 'joined-up solutions' are needed for 'joined-up problems'.

- A *pluralistic approach*: With any significant change in service provision, different agencies will have different priorities and expectations. As a result, it is important to examine the perspectives of all participating agencies and ensure that the strategy is mutually beneficial to key stakeholders. This is likely to facilitate greater co-operation and shared ownership of the strategy.

- A *realistic approach* that costs proposed service developments to ensure that they are feasible within available financial and other resources. This will ensure that any new service is adequately funded and may minimize potentially damaging arguments between partner agencies over the contributions each is making to intermediate care.

Having decided the *principles* by which intermediate care services will be developed, planners and policy makers need to consider the *process* that will be adopted in order to devise and implement the proposed service. Once again, the following model has been developed from first-hand research experience in health and social care, and is also consistent with government guidance for intermediate care (DoH, 2001e, 2001h). Key aspects include:

- The formation of a multi-professional and multi-agency *steering group* to guide and inform the development of an intermediate care strategy. This should include representatives of all key stakeholders, including users, carers, primary care, secondary care, social services, medicine, nursing, occupational therapy, physiotherapy, speech and language, the independent sector and housing.

- A *literature review* to identify and learn from good practice elsewhere. This will ensure that the intermediate care service is based on a sound evidence base and that it is consistent with clinical audit and clinical governance.

- A *scoping exercise* to map existing health and social care services. Often, different agencies already run a range of services that could be incorporated into a new intermediate care strategy, and planners need to avoid 'reinventing the wheel', learning from and utilizing what is already out there.

- A *needs analysis* to identify gaps in existing provision and areas where new services will need to be developed. This should include the collection of quantitative data regarding acute admissions, A&E attendances, bed occupancy rates and residential placements. This information would ensure an evidence-based approach to the intermediate care strategy and would provide base-line data for subsequent evaluations. The use of a clinical review instrument would also be a useful means of estimating the prevalence of patients inappropriately located in hospital and the scope for alternative service provision such as intermediate care. (Clinical review instruments are standardized lists of criteria, often relating to a patient's medical condition and the type and intensity of service provided. If a specified number of criteria are met, the patient is deemed to be appropriately located in hospital.) At the same time, however, the needs analysis should also incorporate more qualitative research to identify the priorities of users, carers and front-line workers. Possible approaches include a stakeholder conference or the use of semi-structured interviews that enable participants to set their own agendas and discuss their experiences and opinions in a frank and open manner (for further details of research methodologies regarding issues such as inappropriate hospital admissions, see Glasby and Littlechild, 2000a, 2001; Littlechild and Glasby, 2000).

- Following the scoping exercise and the needs analysis, *care pathways* and protocols for accessing intermediate care will need to be developed for the major conditions leading to acute admissions and long-stay residential placements, although, as discussed in Chapter 9, it needs to be kept in mind that these have their limitation due to the complexity of the needs of many frail older people who may present with multiple problems. In line with recent government policies such as the *National Service Framework for Older People*, (DoH, 2001h), users will need to receive a single multidisciplinary assessment and a single care plan, as discussed in more detail in Chapter 10. Procedures will also need to be developed regarding information sharing, training and information technology.

- Throughout, the strategy should be underpinned by the *dissemination* of information regarding access to intermediate care and good practice to users, carers, front-line workers and participating agencies. Possible avenues for dissemination include the production of accessible information and the staging of a stakeholder conference, as well as the publication of articles in professional and academic journals.

In the longer-term, a new intermediate care service will also require ongoing evaluation (see Chapter 11) and reappraisal to identify outcomes for users and carers, areas for improvement and the implications of intermediate care for other agencies.

Conclusion

Although it has a number of potential advantages, intermediate care is not necessarily an easy option and can be complex to develop. Designing new approaches that span the boundaries of traditional health and social services requires considerable planning and effort in order to overcome different professional values, different organizational agendas, boundaries that are non-coterminous and other competing priorities. Even once these barriers have been overcome, there is scope for a range of unforeseen practical issues to develop and complicate the process yet further. While the experience of planning an intermediate care setting has been explored here, similar challenges can be expected with the development of any new partnership arrangements or services. What needs to be central to planners' minds and thinking is that any proposed intermediate care service will need to be based on multidisciplinary working and on shared values, together with a firm commitment to empowerment and to holistic care – themes that are picked up again in this book. If an initial plan is to be successfully translated into reality, moreover, it will need to seek the active involvement of key stakeholders – including users/carers and front-line staff – in order to ensure shared and mutually beneficial outcomes. Of course, such an approach is unlikely to be the perfect recipe for success, but it will at least provide a firm foundation from which local partners can work to overcome the obstacles they face and to develop a common vision of the way forward. In the next chapter one approach that has been established to involve older people and carers in services and developments, such as those related to intermediate care, is described and discussed.

KEY POINTS

- Despite both the expressed desire and rhetoric surrounding the promotion of inter-agency collaborative working within intermediate care, a range of barriers challenge these aspirations.
- The very strength behind the concept and the inter-agency and cross-cutting nature of intermediate care is also the very weakness in its achievement.
- To achieve new or revised intermediate care services will require a concerted effort on behalf of all participating agencies to look above and beyond their own individual agendas, reach workable compromises and collaborate to achieve positive outcomes for users and carers.

- Collaborative working also gives rise to a range of practical barriers in the operationalizing of an intermediate care service.
- To achieve secure inter-agency collaboration and give local partnerships a solid foundation from which to tackle some of the practical difficulties and tensions faced, the adoption of a framework of five key components may be the best way forward – fundamentally this means a sharing of values and meeting of ways.

CHAPTER 7

Hearing the voices of older people

Penny Thewlis

Introduction

This chapter looks at both the why and the how of involving older people in planning and evaluating services and, in particular, intermediate care services. It describes one model that offers older people in Oxfordshire an organized opportunity for *having a say* - and *making a difference* - on a wide range of issues of importance to them. The importance of this is summed up in the following quote:

> There's no point coming to all these meetings if they are just going to be talking shops. We need to know that we are making a difference to the way things are for older people. (Oxfordshire Panel member)

Background

The emphasis on improving opportunities for public involvement began with the previous government and has gained momentum under the current administration. All public services are being enjoined to involve service users and local communities in their work. The National Service Framework for Older People (DoH, 2001h) and the HCS/LAC Intermediate care guidance (DoH, 2001e) are no exceptions. The latter makes several references to involvement, including the following statement:

> In planning the best balance of intermediate care services locally, the NHS and councils should consult and take into account the views of patients/users and carers on current patterns of service delivery and on the potential impact of developing new intermediate care services. (HSC 2001/01: LAC; DoH, 2001e)

This renewed emphasis on involvement is good news for those who have been engaged in involvement work over the years. However, actually making a reality out of the rhetoric continues to pose problems. Involvement work is complex, not least because, if it is to be effective, it requires some shifting of the power balance. Resources are required if meaningful involvement is to be supported, and these remain woefully inadequate.

The involvement of older people has not always kept pace with developments among the wider public. Carter and Beresford (2000) emphasize that older people have frequently been marginalized and overlooked in participation initiatives. Too little attention has been paid to developing the means to include them, not helped by the low expectations older generations have often had. Carter and Beresford (2000) argue that this situation has been compounded by the fact that many older people face additional obstacles to participation, such as low income, lack of access to transport, disability, and the reduced confidence that can go with these. The consequence of these factors is that the voices and views of older people have often been excluded.

Recognizing this, the present government has encouraged the development of particular initiatives to improve involvement opportunities for older people. The Better Government for Older People Programme launched in 1998 aimed: 'to promote the better coordination and responsiveness of public services and ... the recognition across Government that for too long older people's interests had been overlooked or undervalued' (BGOP, 2000). These developments have unquestionably moved the agenda forward.

Why involve older people in planning intermediate care services?

> Older people themselves know best what is needed to improve the quality of their own lives and the nature and the quality of the services they need. There is no substitute for first hand experience. (HOPe, Help the Aged (2000)

Older people are the main users of intermediate care services. For a long time they have actively supported the principles of intermediate care – including care closer to home and an increased emphasis on rehabilitation and preventive care, providing an opportunity to 'get back on their feet again' and stay at home for longer. It is clear when working with and talking to older people that they *want* to be involved. The Better Government for Older People initiative demonstrates that older people want to be 'participants not recipients'. Clarke and Dyer (1998) identified the importance to the health and well-being of older people of feeling what they describe as a 'sense of self as a competent member of the adult community'. This, they suggest, is too easily lost as people begin to need more help.

A study undertaken recently in Oxfordshire bears out these findings. For many of the older people involved in the study, this 'sense of self as a competent member of the adult community' was tied up with being an active participant and a giver in some aspects of life, to balance being a recipient in others, as the following quotations show:

> Please have a cup of tea. I don't have a chance to make one for a visitor very often. Most people don't have the time to stay.
>
> I know what has helped me. I'd like to be able to pass that on in some way to help others. Yes, I'd really like that.
>
> I've had a lot of help from people and I wanted to give something back.
> (Thewlis, 2001)

Older people are not a homogeneous group. Their views on what life is like for them and the sort of support they need will be influenced by their individual circumstances and outlook as well as by the nature of the communities in which they live. These views can be discovered only by involving older people direct. Furthermore, there is a growing body of opinion that services developed with the involvement of older people are more responsive to their needs. This has to be a very good reason for involving them.

How to involve older people

There are many different models or approaches by which older people can be involved. Very little, however, has been done to evaluate which models are most effective. Carter and Beresford (2000) have identified a range of different but overlapping approaches or models of involvement, as outlined in Table 7.1.

Carter and Beresford (2000) conclude that each and all of the approaches have their own strengths and weaknesses, and that their effectiveness varies according to the circumstances or the purpose for which they are being used. They also identify 'two helpful distinctions ... between different philosophical approaches to involvement: "consumerist" and "democratic" approaches; and different sources for involvement: "agency-led" and "user/older people-led" initiatives,' which again have their own strengths and weaknesses.

Little is known about how older people themselves *prefer* to be involved, though enough is known to assert that a 'one size fits all' approach is unlikely to suit everyone. This means that a range of opportunities for involvement needs to be offered. Riseborough (1996) identifies that some older people prefer

Table 7.1 Approaches or strategies that can be used to involve older people

- Advocacy and information
- Forums
- User panels
- Consultation
- User/pensioners' groups
- User-led services
- Direct payments
- Networks
- Campaigning
- Direct action
- Initiatives in other countries

involvement rather than 'participation (which appears to restrict the issues) or consultation (which is simply confusing)'. Carter and Beresford (2000) suggest that 'consultation' is probably the form of involvement that most service users, citizens and their organizations like least and are most suspicious about. There is a view that where Public Consultation is offered, decisions have already been made, and the process is simply an empty formality. Involvement at an *early stage* is welcomed, 'before everything gets set in concrete and while we can have a bit of impact' (Oxfordshire Panel member).

One model for involving older people has emerged in Oxfordshire where Age Concern has developed an *Involving Older People Programme* for the county. The programme is based around a network of Older People's Panels and Forums, which were established to provide organized opportunities for older people to have a say and make a difference. The function of Age Concern is to listen to and act on the views of older people, and to provide support for the process.

Carter and Beresford (2000) emphasize the importance of providing support, describing how 'it makes it possible for people to counter the obstacles and discrimination which they face'. They outline a number of features that are incorporated within support, and that prove important if the views and concerns of older people are to be heard:

- support for personal development: to increase people's confidence, assertiveness and expectations;
- support to develop skills: to participate fully and effectively and on their own terms;
- practical support: including information, advocacy, transport, payment and expenses;

- support for equal opportunities: to ensure equal access, regardless of age, 'race', gender, sexuality, disability and communication differences;
- support to get together and work in groups.

These features provide the blueprint for the support Age Concern provides for the involvement network in Oxfordshire which is built around the following.

Age Concern Forums

These are held in the five local authority districts of Oxfordshire twice a year. They are large open forums - open to all older people, their carers and people who work with and for older people. Invitations are distributed widely, along with posters and local media coverage, to encourage as many people as possible to come along, with transport offered. Attendance figures fluctuate, but there is an average attendance of around 200 older people across all the Forums. The aims of the Forums are twofold: most importantly they aim to enable older people, as citizens, to raise any points of interest of importance to them locally, such as issues relating to services, the environment or society as a whole. They also offer an opportunity for service providers to give information about their services and new developments. All the points raised at Forums are noted and circulated to all of those who attend and to those in a position to do something about the issues raised. The points are then taken up by the Panels in their work programmes, and feedback on progress is a routine part of the next forum.

Five local older people's Panels

These meet every six weeks, again in the five local authority districts of the county. There are over 100 members who regularly attend Panel meetings, ranging in age from 50 years to 90+ years. The majority of the membership is female (75 women to 33 men), reflecting to some extent the demography of this age group, but otherwise members come from a very broad spread of interests and backgrounds. The Panels use points raised at local Forum meetings to set their agenda. A good example of how such an issue is picked up relates to community safety. This was raised at one of the Forums, where several older people talked about their experiences and fears of crime, and the effect this had on their quality of life. They also described the difficulties they had experienced in trying to contact the police, and as a result they had concluded that their local police force did not perceive their concerns as a priority. The Local Panel took up this issue and arranged a meeting with representatives of the police and the District Council and this did result in some change. It was also the starting point for an ongoing dialogue. The Panels tackle a wide range of issues of concern to older people, including housing, community hospital developments, preventive services, trading standards, gardening, implementing the NSF standards locally, transport and grandparenting. They have developed links with their local district councils, with PCTs, with MPs and with others in a position to influence change.

The Health and Social Care Panel

This panel meets monthly and has a countywide remit and membership. It brings together 26 older people from all the other Panels together with three older people representing the Community Health Council. It reports back to the local Panels regularly. The Health and Social Care Panel is the most recently established Panel, started because of the sheer size of the health and social care agenda. This increased markedly following the publication of the National Service Framework for Older People (DoH, 2001h) and threatened to overwhelm the local Panels. Panels members recognized the need for a voice and involvement at a time when change was likely to be affected, but were concerned that the agenda might bias or jeopardize their more local activities and priorities. They also recognized the need for a more strategic forum. The Panel grew from an ad hoc group of representatives with an interest in health and social care issues, drawn from all the local Panels, who came together initially to meet Professor Ian Philp, the then newly appointed National Director for Older People who was on a fact-finding visit to Oxfordshire.

How the Health and Social Care Panel works

A style or way of working for the Panel is beginning to emerge. It does not always follow a neat pattern as is the case for so many things human, but when it is working well it should be roughly cyclical (see Figure 7.1, page 122).

1. Information

> We need to make sure that we dig behind the smooth flow of the official line. (Panel Member)

Information about how health and social care services work, about new service developments and about what is happening within the health and social care economy is always the first stage of any work for the Panel. The Panel was quick to identify the need to voice informed opinion – 'we need to make sure we know what we're talking about if people are going to listen to us'. The importance of information from a broad range of perspectives was also identified:

- the professional perspective (both at management and grass roots level) – visitors to the Panel will often come to talk or explain about their services, plans or initiatives;

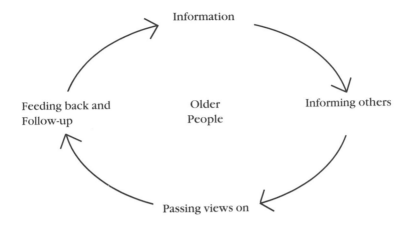

Figure 7.1 How the Health and Social Care Panel works.

- the independent expert's perspective (e.g. Pauline Thompson from Age Concern England joined a Panel meeting on charging for community care, and helped to prepare members for a subsequent meeting with representatives from the Local Authority Treasurer's Department); and most importantly
- the perspective of older people using services.

Reading and discussing policy and planning documents is obviously another important way of keeping abreast of developments. Some members are more comfortable with this than others – increasingly, good teamwork means that not everyone needs to read a document: they trust others to extract and communicate the key points.

2. Informing others and seeking their views

> We have to get out there and really use our networks to ensure that more older people know what's going on. We must listen to what they have to say. (Panel member)

The Panel cannot make claims to be representative of older people, but it can help to ensure that other older people are informed about proposals for change in health and social care services and have an opportunity to have their voices heard. It does this by passing information on through networks and groups of older people, and talking and listening informally to individual older people. Surveys targeted at older people whose voices are seldom heard also have an important role to play in this, and more will said about a couple of examples of this kind of approach later.

3. Passing views on to those with authority to *make a difference*

> We need to make sure that our messages are getting through to the right people.
> (Panel member)

Collating views and finding creative ways of passing them on to those in a position to do something about them is a key activity. The Panel has learnt, from work done by older people elsewhere, the importance of engaging at senior manager level. Patmore et al. (1999) demonstrated that older people believe they can be most influential by involving senior managers, who need 'direct, eyewitness education in older people's everyday realities to be able to influence and act on policy'. Barnes and Bennett-Emslie (1997) usefully showed that managers appear to be less influenced by the views of older people if they are passed on through an intermediary, such as a project worker. Blunden (1998) backed this up with findings that showed that senior managers appeared to be most influenced by direct contact with older people.

4. Feedback and follow-up

> There's a lot of listening goes on but you don't always feel you've been heard.
> (Panel member)

All Panels have regular stocktaking/review sessions, but tracking progress, and therefore evaluating whether the Panels are 'making a difference' is by no means easy, and this is borne out by the literature on involvement. Feedback to the Panel on process has been very good – professionals attending Panel meetings have said that they found them very helpful and many have reflected back to the Panel the points that they have taken away and indicated the processes they will use to take the points forward. However, progress in implementing change is slow – where views expressed by Panel members bear fruit, it may be three years before that fruit is visible. Keeping track over this sort of timescale as personnel move on and priorities change is really challenging.

As indicated, the aim of all the Panels is to give older people a voice and to really make a difference. One of the earliest tasks of the Panel was to draw up what they described as *Principles of Engagement* to try to influence the quality of the Panel's interactions with policy makers and service providers, and maximize their opportunities to make a difference. When the Panel meets, it often has at least one professional or speaker from the local health or social care community. In order to help these visitors or speakers, the Principles are sent to them in advance so that they have some understanding and insight into how the Panel functions and works.

The Principles are outlined in Table 7.2.

Table 7.2 Principles of Engagement for members of the Older Persons' Health and Social Care Panel

---

The Panel welcomes engagement with statutory, voluntary and independent health and social care organizations.

Panel members are an extremely rich resource: they can contribute most effectively and make best use of their knowledge, skills and experience if the following few simple principles of engagement are observed.

Information
Jargon-free information about proposals enables the Panel to consider them properly and to talk to other older people about them. Clarity about the questions to which you need the Panel to consider answers is important. Clarity about what will happen next and what happens as a result of the Panel's involvement is also important.

Time
Adequate time to consider and consult others about issues is vital – the length of time needed will obviously vary with the issue and the amount of other work underway, and is best negotiated.

Setting the agenda
The Panel is happy to respond to requests for input on issues identified by you as being of importance, but must also be able to set the agenda according to their own priorities.

Meet the Panels on their own territory
Wherever possible and practicable, the Panel will welcome your attendance at one of their meetings since this guarantees that all Panel members have an opportunity to contribute to discussions.

The attendance of one or two Panel members at 'one-off' meetings otherwise made up of professionals is not best practice unless there is adequate information and ample time to consider issues and consult in advance.

Diversity
Panel members come from rich and diverse backgrounds, and through their networks are in touch with many more older people in different circumstances. Diversity of views is therefore to be expected and valued: consensus should not be expected.

Feedback
Feedback about progress and what has happened as a result of the Panel's involvement is essential – Panel members are realistic and recognize that it will not always be possible to act in line with their views, but this does not obviate the need for feedback.

Panel members often provide representation on a range of health or social care working groups, forums and Boards, so that they can both influence decisions and feed back progress to their own Panels. This has included regular attendance and involvement in forums and groups looking at the intermediate care agenda.

Since its inception a range of themes have been covered by the Panel, and these have included:

- an overview of the National Service Framework;
- medicines management, single assessment;
- the planning of a new hospital for older people in Oxford;
- charging for community care;
- cross-charging;
- county council funding;
- therapy services for stroke;
- Essence of care benchmarking;
- modern matrons;
- input to Oxford Brookes School of Nursing courses.

Many of these cut across the intermediate care agenda within the county.

Making a difference to intermediate care services

As suggested, Local Panels have all developed links with their local PCTs around the intermediate care agenda, looking particularly at the work of local community hospitals. They have also looked at what might be termed the broader intermediate care agenda, which includes housing and housing support, transport and preventive services – all part of the bigger picture of intermediate care. However, Panels have all experienced problems when trying to relate one component of support to another, provided by a different agency. The Better Government for Older People initiative recognized 'compartmentalization' as a problem for involvement work – the issues raised by older people require 'co-ordinated responses from a whole range of actors' Thornton (2000) – and this is by no means always easy to achieve.

The Health and Social Care Panel takes the lead on countywide initiatives, and members are very conscious that, in relation to intermediate care, one of the major challenges they face is finding ways of ensuring that people with experience of intermediate care services can voice their views. One piece of work in particular is worthy of mention, aiming as it does to enable older people using Day Hospital services at one of the local hospitals to 'have a say' and inform the planning of new and intermediate care services. A small subgroup of five Panel members has undertaken a study of the views of Day Hospital patients. The group has planned the study, designed the semi-structured interview schedule, following discussion with Day Hospital staff, carried out the interviews and analysed the results. The final draft of the report was presented to the full Panel for their agreement and the finished report widely circulated. Panel members will feed back findings to patients at the Day Hospital in the form of a newsletter. They are also due to make a presentation to the County Older People's Programme Board and are feeding results into various working groups of which they are members. The effectiveness of this method of working has yet to be evaluated by the Panel (the work is newly completed), but what is already known is that the voices of 20 frail older service users has influenced the thinking of Panel members, and fed into service planning.

Challenges

The Panels face a number of constantly changing challenges as they continue to develop, but two that are unlikely to change are as follows.

Who sets the agenda?

> We have to be careful that we are not just being reactive. (Panel member)

The Panels have been very clear that they must set their own agenda, but as they become more widely known they are increasingly in demand. On the one hand, this is good news, but it can distort the agenda, and Panels have expressed the frustration of feeling reactive rather than proactive. This frustration is balanced by the recognition that getting views into the system at the right time is more likely to be influential. The healthy tension that results has been modulated by advice from Carter and Beresford (2000), who suggest that 'the first question about any invitation to get involved is what is the cost benefit analysis?' They suggest that 'what this means for people is looking for answers to the following questions:

- what are we really likely to get out of this?
- what will it actually cost us (in energy, time, skill and money)?
- could we get more doing it differently?
- should we be putting our efforts into other things?'

Fun

> The meetings have to be enjoyable to compensate for some of the frustrations. (Panel member)

The need to provide practical support to facilitate involvement has been discussed here and is well documented, particularly by Cormie and Warren (2001). But less is written about the need to make involvement fun. Thornton (2000) emphasizes this aspect 'Many conventional methods of getting people's views are dull and unrewarding for those who take part.' Humour is one tool for making meetings enjoyable – and it is my firm belief that it has an important part to play in involvement work. In collaboration with Oxford

Brookes University, one of the Panels is about to undertake a rurally based project using photography to document older people's lives. Creativity and fun are at the very heart of this project: its focus will be on issues that are raised by older people themselves and how these can influence policy and practice development. It would be surprising if there are no messages in this work for those developing intermediate care services.

Conclusion

This chapter has described one approach whereby older people can be involved in the planning, running and evaluation of public services, particularly in intermediate care. While it is evidently both complex and challenging to establish effective mechanisms for hearing the voices of older people, the results can be both effective and rewarding, and can promote partnership working within a health and social care economy.

KEY POINTS

- The importance of including older people in the planning and running of public services has taken increasing precedence, such that it is high on the agenda of relevant organizations.
- A range of approaches can be adopted to involve older people, and their effectiveness will vary according to circumstances or need.
- One approach that has been adopted with some success is the development of Panels of Older People who are charged with:
  - finding out information;
  - disseminating this to other older people;
  - passing on the views of older people to those in authority;
  - feeding back progress of proposed action to older people.
- There are always challenges to overcome with such initiatives. These include:
  - trying to keep control of the agenda;
  - trying to make sure the activities are fun for those older people involved.

CHAPTER 8

New roles to support services for older people

LIZ LEES AND SIÂN WADE

Introduction

With the planning and development of intermediate care services/schemes and possible developments in the way that care is provided for older people, there is potential, as previously suggested, to introduce a range of new roles. This chapter focuses on the potential of three roles within intermediate care and services for older people. The discussion will try to demonstrate how the creation and development of these roles may go some way to help to integrate, co-ordinate and consolidate the care that older people receive as new models of care and services emerge. Each role can also contribute to the planning, development, monitoring and evaluation of services, to the ongoing development of these services and, most importantly, to the preparation and development of staff within these services. Underlying their work, a fundamental element needs to centre on quality of care issues and initiatives and the improvements in standards of care by providing strong and effective leadership.

Background

A range of reports and national audits in the late 1990s demonstrated the inadequacy of rehabilitation for older people and also how the fragmentation of care of older people was leading to inefficiencies across the system (Clinical Standards Advisory Group, 1998; Audit Commission, 1992, 1997, 2000). The imperative to 'join up' and integrate services in a coherent fashion, under the strategic direction and umbrella of promoting independence and autonomy, has therefore emerged as an important and recurring theme, with intermediate care perhaps being seen as the vehicle by which this can best be achieved. As discussed in Chapter 3, there is considerable potential for developing a range of new roles related to the care of older people and intermediate care, and these roles would be ideal to facilitate this. Thus a key underpinning remit of these roles would need to be upon promoting co-ordinated, integrated and seamless care, which, as suggested in Chapter 3, must enhance the experience for the older person – not fragment it. This will require close working between service providers, with clarity and transparency as to who holds overall responsibility for any one individual older person. In order to fulfil this remit, post-holders in these positions will need to be able to work effectively across services and boundaries so as to promote effective inter-agency collaborative working where a common understanding is reached together with mutual respect.

Among the roles that have a potential to make a difference for older people within intermediate care are the role of the intermediate care co-ordinator, the specialist gerontological nurse, and the consultant nurse/therapist. Each of these three roles will be considered briefly in this chapter, although they by no means represent the full potential of future roles that might play a part.

Intermediate care co-ordinator

Within the HSC/LAC Intermediate Care guidance, there was a clear recommendation that an intermediate care co-ordinator should be appointed within 'at least every Health Authority' (HSC/LAC, DoH, 2001e: 8). Intermediate care co-ordinators have been identified as being responsible for delivering nationally stipulated intermediate care milestones (Intermediate Care Local Authority Circular, January 2001, DoH, 2001e), as part of the National Service Framework for Older People (DoH, 2001h) and NHS Plan (DoH, 2000c). These post holders, however, are also ideally placed to assist with, and facilitate developments to promote, integrated service delivery. For this reason, intermediate care coordinators need to be positioned not only at the interface of health and social care, but also at the interface of primary and secondary care services. At both a national and local level, the role is considered high profile and is perceived as 'breaking new ground'. As with all new roles, intermediate care co-ordinators could be said to be 'entering into unknown territory'.

The concept

While the policy guidance in the intermediate care circular (HSC/LAC, DoH, January 2001e) clearly validated the introduction of this role called 'intermediate care co-ordinator', there was much less clarity about what constituted the role. While some key principles were identified, as outlined in Table 8.1, how this was to be achieved was less clear, and therefore individual job descriptions and specifications were left to the discretion of the employing agencies. For this reason, roles have tended to emerge in a variety of different ways. Similarly, there was no guidance on the professional background from which these post holders should originate. This again has been left to prospective employers, with some specifying a social work background, others a health care background, and yet others either one of these. Because of the broad remit, a management qualification or management experience has often been specified in addition to a health or social care qualification. In reality there is no right or wrong background, and post holders have been drawn from a diverse range of backgrounds, perhaps reflecting the nature of the posts. This has included discharge liaison sisters, occupational therapy managers, district nurses and social work managers.

The reality

In some ways it is not surprising to find that recruitment to these posts has not always been easy. This occurred in Birmingham, where posts had to be advertised on several occasions. This may well have been attributable to the broad, uncertain and evolving remit of the post. Furthermore, there was no recommended pay-scale or facility to monitor this, so that salaries offered for the emerging posts seem to have varied considerably and do not appear always to have been related to the level of complexity of the post held. In addition, national evidence also suggests that some people are already working in similar posts, carrying out an intermediate care co-ordination function as an existing part of their role, while their title and pay may not have equated to this. The fact that the role could also be described as a political 'hot

Table 8.1 Key functions of the intermediate care co-ordinator role

- Co-ordination of services at an operational level
- Co-ordinating multi-agency, multi-team care (seamless care), across community health services, social care, housing and the acute sector
- Service development of established intermediate care services
- Development of new services between health with social services
- Securing agreement on the scope of, and finance for, new projects and developments (unified/pooled budgets)
- Managing a multidisciplinary team, multi-agency team of staff
- Collaborative working between health and social services and all agencies
- Interfacing between primary and secondary care to prevent inappropriate admissions and improve the flow of emergency admissions
- Developing care pathways and protocols for access to services
- Ensuring robust working relationships

potato', with the government anxious to be seen to deliver on its election promises and looking to the intermediate care co-ordinator to fulfil this promise, could be seen by some to have created too much of an onus on the post holder. Thus while in principle the concept of the intermediate care co-ordinator seems an excellent idea, where cohesive working practices should be promoted so as to help translate policy into practice, from its conceptual beginnings it has not been without its difficulties.

Perspectives of the role

Two key elements seem to emerge as fundamental to the role. One is at a strategic level where an overview of the what, where and why of the services required for a locality is needed. The other is at an operational level, looking at the 'how' of services, along with their day-to-day management, to best ensure a high-quality and efficient programme of care for patients (see Table 8.1). Whether the post holder performs all these functions, some are delegated, or some are within the remit of another person's role, often depends upon the complexity of the organization, its size and other unique factors.

Challenges of the post

Inevitably with such a wide-ranging role, challenges have emerged. These challenges seem to have focused on professional, organizational and financial boundary issues, all inextricably linked, but which need to be synchronized if intermediate care is to expedite according to milestones. The exploration of professional boundaries alone could be considered to occur in four distinct phases. These include: 1. operating within the post holders' own professional capacity 2. exploring the role of other professionals 3. engaging and interfacing with other professionals, and 4. expanding out of the 'safe zone' of the individual post holder, albeit on the peripheries, to challenge culture and elicit the change required. In addition, each professional and voluntary organization has its own professional or ideological culture, perspectives and responsibilities, along with distinct funding mechanisms, procedural mechanisms and issues of status and legitimacy. All these make effective inter-agency working seem like a 'minefield', as discussed by Glasby in Chapter 6. This is quite apart from the lack of co-terminosity of service providers and the need to work across geographical and organizational boundaries such as Primary Care Trusts and Social Services' area wards. In addition, since the inception of Primary Care Trusts, they have been bombarded with a plethora of 'must do's' while at the same time trying to develop and emerge organizationally (Banks-Smith et al., 2001).

The development and delivery of intermediate care services has been seen to be a pivotal role of the co-ordinator. At the same time, however, these post are essential to 'drive' other policy initiatives, such as improving the flow of emergency admissions (DoH, 2001f; DoH, 2002c – Modernization Agenda) and an active engagement with the implementation of the Single Assessment Process (NSF, standard, 2, DoH, 2001h). What is more, depending on which organization employs these intermediate care co-ordinators, they may also be required to assist in meeting their specific organizational targets, for example in secondary care in meeting the requirement to reduce lengths of stay and to progress discharges.

The way forward

To achieve effective inter-agency working requires a wide range of attributes and skills, which no one individual is likely to have. It is therefore almost inevitable that these post holders will need considerable investment in their training and leadership for individual personal development. It also seems evident that there is a need for clear support from within the post holder's organization to help to clarify the role and keep the post holder focused. Similarly, some form of external support, such as a formal facilitated network, would allow for exchange of ideas and concerns and help to reach some consistency to the role.

The need to be seen 'to deliver' by the government has led to tight timescales for progressing intermediate care work and other related developments. Yet the very need to take time to reach effective partnership working, let alone overcome obvious barriers, places enormous pressures on the post holders. These mitigating pressures, although all interlinked issues, are further compounded as locally some posts have been time-limited to two years. This potentially inhibits the vital individual development of individual post holders as well as their proficiency in a range of skills, as the role evolves. Furthermore, the longer-term recruitment and retention strategy leaves a little to be desired, as valuable expertise developed by these post-holders may be 'lost' forever after the fixed-term contract expires! It would therefore seem that the longevity of the intermediate care co-ordinator role is paramount if they are to remain key figures, instrumental to the implementation and co-ordination thereafter, of intermediate care and their interface with social service providers. As discussed at intervals throughout this book, the failure to allow something to become established and evaluated fully has been one of the downfalls of intermediate care and early service developments. This should not be allowed to happen here.

Specialist nurses

The concept and perspectives of the role

The potential for developing specialist gerontological nurses to work alongside other professionals within multidisciplinary teams so as to promote the effective care of older people has considerable potential. The specialist nurse is specified here because at present there are limited specialist gerontological nurse posts compared with other client/condition specialities nationally. It is not intended here to suggest that other team members do not have an important role or the potential to develop new, more needs-responsive roles. Nurses may at times, however, be in the best position to assess an older person and begin to identify their needs and the need for other support and intervention, e.g. nursing, medical, therapy, social, etc. However, with the implementation of the Single Assessment Process it is clear that whoever undertakes the contact assessment will be able to make this initial assessment and referral, where needed. There is no doubt also that nursing skills are often significant in the care of older people, and so the need to consider developing these roles is important. The RCN and BSG (2001) identify the key role that gerontological specialist nurses may take, and this is reiterated in the National Service Framework for older people (DoH, 2001i). The specialist nurse can help to support nurses within acute services such as general medicine and surgery, where advice, facilitation or support of staff may help the older person to access the right care or service. It may also be supportive in terms of the older person's autonomy and right to choice and decisions, which are at risk of being neglected or overridden. The nurse is also in a good position to assist in referring older people to other professionals within the acute setting, as well as to assist in assessment for future care e.g. specialist rehabilitation, intermediate care services or nursing and care homes – as discussed in Chapter 3. These nurses will need to have a professional remit to work across the boundaries of agencies and services, so as to promote co-ordinated and seamless care for the individual older person.

With the independent sector becoming the predominant provider of nursing and care homes, access to a multidisciplinary gerontology team could be invaluable, especially access to a specialist nurse. This is not to suggest that nurses in these settings do not have the skills to care for older people, but they often work in isolation, and may find themselves in an untenable situation, while having access to an experienced practitioner provides them with the opportunity to talk through options or concerns, and if necessary have a second voice to support their views. Gerontological specialist nurses can also help in supporting the need to refer to other professions. If the role is undertaken in a facilitative way then it can go a long way in giving confidence to practitioners in these settings and in providing collegiate support. Likewise, specialist multidisciplinary teams and nurses would be able to provide similar support and advice to staff in intermediate care services, again assisting and supporting decision-making and problem-solving, and facilitating referral to other colleagues in the team as well as the gerontologist.

Staff in these roles could have a pivotal role in providing or supporting local needs-responsive teaching and practice development. They could also be involved directly with staff in these settings, working with them and facilitating research activity. Such practitioners would be expected to be an experienced and skilled clinical practitioner in the specialist field of gerontology. They would also be expected to have a first degree in line with UKKC guidelines for the specialist nurse, and be able to demonstrate achievement in the areas of clinical practice, leadership, practice development and programme management. The RCN/BGS statement paper (2001) makes recommendations of the attributes that specialist nurses should demonstrate, as outlined in Table 8.2.

Table 8.2 Attributes and preparation requirements for the older person's specialist nurse

- Sufficient sound clinical experience of working with older people
- Post-registration development in the distinct and 'special' aspects of older people's health and social circumstances and needs (pre-registration education is generally acknowledged to be inadequate in these areas)
- Post-registration development in understanding specific issues of later life, e.g. social and gerontological literature on older people's experiences of later life, the range of living circumstances and personal networks
- Attributes and competencies that enable the nurse to respond expertly to the needs of the older person and professional colleagues

Working practices and challenges of the specialist gerontological nurse

It will be important that there is clarity about the role of the post holder and what is expected of them. In order to maintain clinical credibility, the specialist nurse will need to be able to work in practice and therefore will need clarity as to how this is fulfilled. It will also be important to ensure that they have a sound identified team to which they belong and with whom they can share and discuss ideas and concerns, with explicit lines of responsibility and professional accountability. Because of the autonomous and supervisory role that these post holders are likely to have, they will need to have clinical supervision or a similar mechanism incorporated within their work. There is considerable risk of work overload, and for the boundaries of the role to overlap. There is also a need for effective interdisciplinary and collaborative working. The post holder of the specialist nurse role is at risk of taking over a 'case' where this is not the purpose of the role, unless the role has been developed in a specific way whereby the post holder carries a caseload or holds clinics such as falls or stroke, etc. Thus it is important to ensure there is clarity over who has direct responsibility for the co-ordination of the care of an individual older person, and in most cases this should probably be the main service or care provider.

The way forward

Because of the history of this speciality the provision of planned development and education opportunities for nurses have been quite limited, and as suggested in Part III, the uptake has tended to be poor compared with other specialities. Thus the ability to recruit staff with adequate qualifications and experience may prove to be challenging. Should this be the case, it is imperative that a lead is taken in establishing and developing an appropriate educational and developmental strategy with an appropriate competency framework to prepare staff to take on these roles. The ENB outlined a curriculum framework (ENB, 2001a) before it was disbanded. This could be used as a basis from which to develop and work. The best mechanism to achieve this currently seems unclear, but it would seem sensible if this could be undertaken at a national level which, while not prescriptive, could be consistent and reasonably transferable (see below).

The profusion of titles for senior nurses, such as specialist nurses or nurse practitioner, etc. has meant that roles have often been poorly defined, with practitioners having the same title but performing quite different roles. Prior to its demise, the UKCC worked on standards for 'higher level of practice' and came up with seven standards which it regarded nurses would need to meet if they were to be considered as higher-level practitioners, as shown in Table 8.3 (Gulland, 2002). This begins to develop a framework within which to set the specialist nurse role.

The RCN is also currently working with forums to establish a list of competencies that nurses would need to meet for each grade, and is currently working with the Faculty of Emergency Nursing to develop five

Table 8.3 UKCC standards for higher level practice

- Providing effective health care
- Improving quality and health outcomes
- Evaluation and research
- Leading and developing practice
- Innovation and changing practice
- Developing self and others
- Working across professional and organizational boundaries

levels of competencies for nurses at all levels (Endacott, 1999). These levels go from V to Z, and span from when the nurse first qualifies to the highest level of their speciality – nurse consultant (Table 8.4). The framework has the potential to be adopted by other specialities, and both gerontology and intermediate care would be in a good position to consider the adoption of it since there has been limited or ad hoc work in these fields to date. Careful consideration, however, would need to be given to ensure that it is needs-responsive in these fields. A similar framework may make sense for other disciplines/professions, helping to bring consistency across professions. At present where competency frameworks have been developed, they often centre around the the grading spine and hence pay scale for nurses and for health care assistants. However, the National Service Framework for Older People's Workforce Programme Group is developing core competencies for general and specialist practitioners who work with older people, from all disciplines/professions. These could then be built upon to meet specific disciplines' needs and, indeed, be adapted within the V–Z framework.

Since the role of a specialist gerontological nurse is not well established, and for a long time there has been a lack of clarity around the role of the specialist nurse (Gulland, 2002), it would seem sensible and timely to ensure that any new specialist role that is established should be well planned and evaluated so that learning can be gained and roles refined as necessary.

Table 8.4 The RCN levels of nursing competence

V –	A newly qualified nurse
W –	A nurse who has moved up the ladder and chosen a specialism
X –	An expert in their area who is fairly independent but needs indirect supervision
Y –	A well-rounded autonomous practitioner working at a senior level in their department
Z –	A nurse consultant

Consultant nurse/therapist

The concept

The potential for the role of consultant nurse or therapist within services for older people and intermediate care has much to offer in raising the profile of older people and enhancing services for older people. A key reason for developing this role derived from concerns over the limited clinical career structure for nurses and therapists. For nurses, who were the first occupational group to incorporate this role, it was evident that there was a need to retain experienced nurses in practice and in particular to strengthen leadership (nursing, midwifery and health visiting strategy, HSC 1999/217, NHSE, 1999). This, it was also hoped, would provide a boost to recruitment and retention. In addition, the consultant role is identified as being implicit to the success of the modernization agenda and particularly in the promotion of clinical governance as outlined in *Making a Difference* (DoH, 1999a).

Perspectives on the role

The key functional areas for this role are outlined in Table 8.5. The guidance, however, allows for flexibility, so the way in which these functional areas are interpreted and the format of roles that have been created are wide-ranging and very varied, according to the particular need and speciality. A number seem to be very focused, touching more on the nurse practitioner role, where the nurse adopts elements of the traditionally held doctor's role. At the other end of the spectrum the role seems to have a remit for a wide range of services under the umbrella of a specific client group. It is probably this model that holds the greatest potential for the consultant nurse/therapist within the field of gerontology and intermediate care.

Table 8.5 Key functional areas of the consultant nurse/therapist

- Expert practitioner
- Professional leadership
- Practice and service development
- Education, training and consultancy
- Research and evaluation.

The role needs to be significant strategically and it needs authority.

In all the consultant roles there evidently needs to be something that makes this role special and of value to the organization, and within these specialities it is probably the strategic and cross-boundary/agency working and collaboration that is imperative. The post holder needs to have the ability to take an overview of services across agencies and Trusts, and identify a way forward, working with a whole system approach. The consultant nurse/therapist therefore needs to develop the ability and skill to lead across professional and agency groups, and therefore requires strong leadership skills. Lancaster (2001), in his evaluation of the nurse consultant role, discusses a range of features that emerge where effective partnership working is evident, as outlined in Table 8.6. Thus it would seem that the post-holder needs to have the skills to contribute actively to, or facilitate, the achievement of these if they are to be successful in their role.

Table 8.6 Features needed to achieve effective partnerships and alliances

- Complexity – solve complex problems, working across matrices and other organizational forms
- Connecting – share, spread and learn across a wide range of professions
- Creativity – exchange ideas, innovating
- Continuously developing – learning from one another and self-evaluating
- Collaboration – contribution, interdependency; focusing on the things each member does well
- Emotional intelligence

Lancaster also describes another feature associated with effective partnership working, which he describes as 'emotional intelligence'. This, he suggests, involves individuals behaving in ways that help to build relationships that will strengthen the ability of the alliance in achieving its goals, and in so doing they need to work beyond hierarchies. He suggests that this requires the skills of transformational leadership, while Manley (1997) suggests that there is also the need to display the qualities of a strategist and catalyst. Manley suggests that being a strategist is about behaviour that actively seeks to raise awareness of potential issues and activities that need to be addressed if patient care is to be promoted, while being a catalyst is seen as encapsulating activities which are required for getting things done. This requires commitment and also the ability to give a consistent message. Personal experience suggests that this calls for sensitivity and political astuteness to work with complexity, where knowing when to 'drive' and knowing when to 'hold back' is imperative. The skill of sensitive inaction is sometimes more productive than action, and this requires considerable insight, sensitivity and intuitiveness.

In order to gain insight into this, nurses need to have worked closely in practice in the relevant areas to gain hands-on appreciation of the experience for patients, staff and of the whole system – and hence the importance of direct patient–client contact. They also need to be in a position within the organization where they are able to advise their colleagues at a senior level (Executive and Trust Board) of the recommended actions required to improve services, etc. This is where the nurse consultant role is perhaps at its greatest advantage, because access and involvement at board level are fundamental to the role. Moreover, the link between the board and operational level cements organizational commitment to change. It is also essential that the nurse consultant has the authority and infrastructure to enable them actually to lead the action and developments they have identified and to make changes. This requires a team of practitioners who will be able to work collaboratively within a clear strategy for developing staff and standards of practice such as practice development staff, specialist nurses and the whole spectrum of the multidisciplinary team, etc. Failure of the organization either to hear advice or enable the post holder to implement action puts into question the value of the role for that particular organization.

Organizational fit

It is possible that initially the nurse/therapy consultant posts may not fit easily into existing organizational structures. For example, with the evolution of Primary Care Trusts the importance of collaborative commissioning and service development is implicit. Consultant nurse/therapy roles, among other new roles, have after all been introduced as part of the modernization agenda and are highly recommended within the National Service Framework for Older People (DoH, 2001h). It is likely, therefore, that the longer-term sustainability of nurse consultant posts will be better assured through joint working, across traditional boundaries and into the larger strategic picture – certainly this would seem to be the case for intermediate care and the care of older people.

Nurse consultants/therapists will have to balance their organizational fit carefully, alongside the scope of their role. While the framework clearly provides an outline, in the case of relatively cosmopolitan areas of work (such as intermediate care and emergency assessments) the impetus may be to deliver a huge educational agenda first, to improve understanding before any new service development can be embarked upon (see Figure 8.1). This said, to effectively achieve both, may prove to be a bit of a balancing act!

Support and development

The role of the consultant nurse/therapist is new, and post holders will often find themselves with at least two masters. Initially they may also find themselves in quite an isolated role, as their remit may require them to work across a wide range of teams and agencies, giving them limited opportunity to identify a sense of belonging with any one team. It is thus essential that thought is given as to how this person will function within their role and how they will be supported. Consideration also needs to be given to the challenges that may arise when people identified as giving support find themselves with conflicting agendas to that of the consultant nurse/ therapist.

The way forward

To date, limited attention has been given to addressing the personal development needs of newly appointed nurse consultants. This is going to

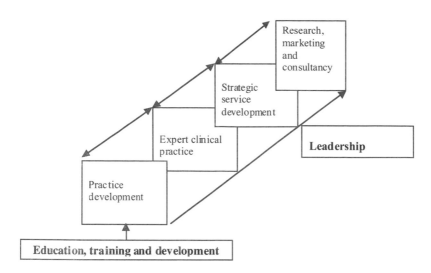

Figure 8.1 Scope of consultant nurse role: framework fit.

become increasingly important as more posts are created among different professionals and the role is seen as part of career progression and planning, for staff 'in the making'. Use of the UKCC Standards of Higher Level Practice could provide a reference point for future appointments from any profession, together with learning from evaluating current posts.

While the Health Service Circular (Nursing, Midwifery and Health Visiting Strategy HSC 1999/217, NHSE, 1999) specifically advises that there is no recognized qualification or experience that the nurse consultant should have for this role, attention needs to be given to this area. One Trust has created competencies and in so doing developed greater understanding and insight of the role when setting up their posts (Reid and Metcalfe, 2001). These competencies are adopted by the post holders in the nurse consultant role and used at Individual Performance Reviews. In the future there is the potential to develop such competencies nationally within the suggested framework by the RCN, as outlined in Table 8.4, and this framework could work for all professions. It is understood that a number of universities have been in discussion or are planning the provision of appropriate preparation for consultant nurses/therapists and those aspiring to be one. This may be through Masters level courses or through taught or research PhDs. Identified competencies and expertise perceived as appropriate to the role could be incorporated within these courses.

With the new modernization agenda and the introduction of CHI, there is a requirement to evaluate all new roles and so the nurse/therapy consultant role comes under this remit. Because the role is new and expectations may be high, it will be important to find a simple and focused way to do this.

Conclusion

There are many opportunities to develop roles within the field of gerontology and intermediate care. Only a few have been addressed here. It will, however, be important to ensure that these roles do contribute in a positive and constructive way so as to enhance the services and experiences of older people. It will also be important to ensure that they complement and support the roles of other staff working in these fields and do not take over, recognizing and valuing the huge contribution that these staff make and the importance of their roles. Some of the ways in which these roles could play a significant and implicit part are in the implementation of some of the recent initiatives that have been introduced or recommended centrally by the government, and which are seen to complement the developments of intermediate care. Care pathways and single assessment along with evaluation include some of these and are addressed in the next few chapters. The staff in these roles will also play a significant role in staff developments, which is the focus of Part IV of this book.

KEY POINTS

- The development of intermediate care and services for older people across the health and social care economy provide promise for improved services for older people.
- To facilitate these developments there is the potential to establish a range of roles which, if implemented with care, will not only be attractive to staff, but will provide a career structure and positive image of these services, so helping to proactively enhance the quality of care for older people.
- Three roles have been described in this chapter, but there is potential for others.
- Establishing new roles is not without its problems, both for the delivery of care or for the post holder. Key features are fundamental to their success:
  - services and care provided for older people must be co-ordinated, cohesive and appear seamless and transparent from the perspective of the older person and their family/relatives/carers;
  - sound staff development and education is a priority with the opportunity to establish a new education and development framework for the care of older people.

CHAPTER 9

Care pathways and intermediate care

LIZ LEES

Introduction

This chapter explores the complexity of care pathways at a macro and micro level, as well as some of the tensions experienced by practitioners while attempting to establish and implement care pathways for intermediate care services (Middleton and Roberts, 2000). It offers a pragmatic perspective and a conceptual model, which may be useful once the tensions have been explored and resolved. Evidence from practice areas suggests the whole process of constructing care pathways is underpinned by healthy professional cynicism, perpetuated by tensions, a lack of resources and in some cases a champion to implement them, all unearthed through the changes pathways pose. Yet, at the heart of those who do believe in developing care pathways is a simple belief – that they are capable of taking the apparently 'subjective or vague' patient journey and transforming this into an 'objective' pathway with a measurable outcome, as discussed by Enderby (1998).

Background

Despite the impetus to deliver a plethora of new intermediate care services (HSC/LAC, DoH 2001e) there appears to be a relative paucity surrounding the development of care pathways to support these. In part, this could be attributed to the magnitude of the job. For example, the scope and complexity of such care pathways is potentially enormous and is exacerbated by the need for them to extend across different organizations and professional roles, all of which have different incentives for their use. Add to this the different focus of intermediate care services/models, such as admission prevention, discharge support or reduction in length of stay, and those responsible for their development seem to succumb to the detail! Recently with the evolution of Primary Care Groups to Trusts, Health Authorities to Strategic Health Authorities and the evolution of Care Trusts, there has been a continual constant shifting ground. The consequence of this has often been confusion, chaos and relative inertia for developments related to intermediate care, let alone developments of care pathways (HSMC, 2001).

What are the potential difficulties in developing pathways for intermediate care?

The concepts of intermediate care and care pathways are not well understood by those who need to access such services frequently (staff) and as a result they are not well marketed to those who stand to benefit the most (patients), whereas the concept of secondary care is a known entity, and is moreover portrayed as a safe environment by professionals, patients and carers alike, providing an abundance of equipment, skills and expertise (Ridley, 1998). The converse could be said of intermediate care, which has often been portrayed and perceived as the poor relation (BGS, 1998).

Different terminology can easily be confused; most commonly 'integrated' and 'intermediate' appear to be used interchangeably. Integrated implies incorporating, in this case other elements of care into the pathway as indicated by condition grouping. However, by virtue of the nature of intermediate care, namely the vast expanse of services it potentially encompasses, intermediate becomes integrated by design.

Having differentiated between 'integrated' and 'intermediate' there is then a need to consider the difference between clinical and intermediate care pathways. For some patients, assessment at the point of entry into a 'clinical' care pathway represents no more than a tick-box exercise to be completed, and to that end is a relatively predictable and minimalist process (Short, 1997; Middleton and Roberts, 2000). The converse may be true of 'intermediate' care pathways, where the emphasis upon criteria to gain access, followed by assessment and reassessment, is pivotal to the success of an intermediate care pathway in practice (Colucciello, 1997). With this in mind it is perhaps best to define care pathways.

A definition

A care pathway determines locally agreed multidisciplinary practice and is based on local guidelines and evidence where available, for a specific patient or client group. It forms all or part of the clinical record, documents care given (to include variances) and facilitates the evaluation of outcomes for continuous quality improvement. (National Care Pathways Association, cited in Middleton and Roberts, 2000)

Hence a pathway can be regarded as a logical framework with which to incorporate evidence-based practice into routine clinical activities. 'There is no place in the modern NHS for the piecemeal adoption of unproven therapies or for hanging onto outdated, ineffective treatments' (DoH, 1998a).

So why develop care pathways?

It is easy to forget that central to the purpose of care pathways are 'patients'. With this in mind, care pathways should be utilized to improve care for patients requiring intermediate care services. At a further level of detail, care pathways can support patients and professionals alike in determining the goals or milestones expected, assessment and reassessments required, which investigations are indicated (at what point), overall care management and the possible variances that might be expected (Middleton and Roberts, 2000). This will also highlight where there are gaps in services and skills. Thus pathways, irrespective of organizational, political and sometimes personal agendas, should be aimed at improving the outcome for patients and carers (HSMC, 2001). What is more, intermediate care pathways should be used to forge positive links and disseminate good practice across all other services/agencies, hopefully reinforcing the place of intermediate care in the whole system of health care delivery (Ridley, 1998).

The impetus to develop care pathways for intermediate care has undoubtedly culminated as a result of the recent rapid growth of intermediate care facilities (HSC/LAC, DoH, 2001e). Crucially, however, at a most basic level, care pathways are required to act as a framework (albeit a baseline) to support audit processes and to prove the clinical effectiveness of intermediate care based upon reliable evidence (*First Class Service*, DoH, 1998a). More recently, this has been reinforced through the quest for national intermediate care evaluation programmes, in particular those focusing upon costs and outcomes. Finally, if intermediate care services are to be sustainable, they must prove their capability by accommodating different pathways, ensuring malleability while governing risk. If not, Middleton and Roberts (2000) argue that relatively typical selected patient groups seen in intermediate care settings will become problematic to manage if they are bereft of supporting frameworks in the form of care pathways.

Is there a difference between care pathways for older people and intermediate care?

Presently, for older people, intermediate care pathways provide the mechanism that legitimizes 'access' and assists navigation into the most appropriate service/setting or scheme. The thrust of intermediate care services tends to be focused round the *complex co-ordination* of services, often heavily reliant upon nurses taking on the greater part of such work (Colucciello, 1997). Although there are similarities, those care pathways that have been developed for older people have tended to focus upon *clinical conditions*; where the pathway provides 'a proactive tool' to determine an appropriate point of transfer out of care or into a plethora of other clinical condition-based pathways (Forkner, 1996). The pathway taken will be dependent upon the diagnosis and variation of multiple patient pathologies experienced (Middleton and Roberts, 2000). For those patients without a reliable diagnosis it may be possible to develop a generic pathway based upon robust assessment and reassessments (Middleton and Roberts. 2000), but nothing more refined.

Implicit in developing combined intermediate care and older people's pathways is the need to consider common groupings used, such as; goals, diagnoses, treatments, stages in care and settings (Middleton and Roberts, 2000). The bulk of the developmental work underpinning the clinical part of the pathways may be focused around locally developed protocols/clinical conditions and charting of the variations through exceptions (Forkner, 1996; Short, 1997). More often than not, a prerequisite of this type of pathway will be a merger of *all* groupings, albeit at an appropriate point in time! Often it is at this level of detail that working groups can effectively dry up through the challenges posed by the sheer level of detail; however, exploring these challenges may assist development.

The key to developing robust pathways for older people in intermediate care settings depends upon the feasibility of developing pathways for commonly presenting co-morbidity and robust patient assessments (NSF Older People, Standard, 2, DoH, 2001j). Hence, while care pathways for intermediate care can perhaps be distinguished from care pathways for older people, there will often remain inextricable links.

Where to begin: mapping

The breadth of these care pathways is likely to be such that they may be multidisciplinary, multi-organizational and have a timespan of about six weeks as originally guided (HSC/LAC, DoH, 2001e), hence it is suggested that it is best initially to consider an intermediate care pathway at the least level of detail (high-level) and in distinct chunks. This process is often referred to as mapping (Middleton and Roberts, 2000). The mapping process will need to be based upon the services available within the remit/scope of the pathway being developed. Following this mapping, the scope, i.e. the start-point, end-point and boundaries with other services, should evolve. The intermediate care pathway should represent a 'continuum of care'; irrespective of where patients are based (primary, secondary or intermediate care) it should be accessible from any source.

Work at a high level

At a high level a model by Godchaux et al. (1997) proves useful in assessing the whole system and the entire scope that an intermediate care pathway may encompass. Five key phases throughout a continuum of care, appertaining to different professional/patient perspectives, defining the key objectives are listed below, with a brief explanation relating them to an intermediate care context, namely:

1. Pre-entry phase (links patient with resources/services prior to admission).
2. Entry phase (agreement made with patients to meet needs/goals).
3. In-patient phase (continuous assessment, treatment and reassessments within the service/scheme).
4. Pre-exit phase (assessment for the need and provision of ongoing care).
5. Exit phase (transfer of care to patients care setting).

Arguably this model simply provides clarity regarding the different phases of care; nevertheless throughout an intermediate care pathway, this model should ensure that the phases of care *do* take place (Godchaux et al., 1997). For example, if the phases are not instigated, or instigated too late, they can delay discharge. Moreover, a further phase, namely Post-Exit, could be added potentially capturing likely readmissions and linking pre-entry with post-exit so as to form a baseline measure to assess the effectiveness of care instigated. Figure 9.1 provides an illustration of this process using the concept of an egg timer. Here time is measured over a defined period, for example six weeks as originally suggested by the government for the maximum length of stay in Intensive Care, with the bulk of the activity focused around the continual flow of patients, assessment, discharge and follow-up.

Adding detail beyond the high level

Several key features of intermediate care services have been identified and are referred to as the six As, which could be further related to each of the six phases of the continuum of care (Godchaux et al., 1997), namely:

1. *Access* (securing a place of care – not always a bed!)
2. *Assess* (linked to diagnosis and Single Assessment Process; clinical, social, economic, etc.)

3. *Appropriateness* (not only patient, but relatives and carers)
4. *Agreements* (reflecting the professionals, patients and carers involved)
5. *Actions* (treatment/goals/variations during the in-patient phase)
6. *Audit* (What was the outcome? Were there deviations in pathway? Has it worked? Can it be improved?)

While these have been discussed separately, it is clear from Figure 9.1 that each of the stages overlaps; moreover, they do not necessarily occur in a linear manner, with older patients perhaps being accommodated flexibly within the intermediate care pathway. For example, the period of recovery/rehabilitation required may take longer than the anticipated six weeks originally recommended (HSC/LAC, DoH, 2001e) according to the number of variances experienced (Middleton and Roberts, 2000).

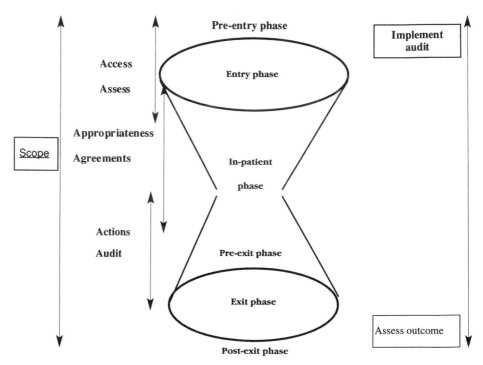

Figure 9.1 The 'Egg timer'. Source: The six phases of care from 'A continuum of care model', Godchaux et al. (1997).

Access

Often, despite service criteria, it is not always clear who can refer or when it is appropriate to refer patients to intermediate care. Consequently, the process of patient assessment for suitability for access into intermediate care services consumes a disproportionate amount of time, with multiple reassessments throughout the decision-making process being commonplace. In part, if intermediate care had been developed in the same era as all services across the continuum of care, instead of being relatively underdeveloped and an apparent 'add-on', the philosophy of identifying or 'pulling out' suitable patients rather than 'pushing out' would assist access considerably.

This said, it is important that the patient is directed towards the correct pathway of care so as to ensure that they are able to maximize their potential and, where possible, prevent admission to long-term care (BGS, 1998, Vaughan and Lathlean, 1999). For example, if a patient who has experienced a CVA is directly admitted to an intermediate care ward instead of an acute stroke unit or a ward/unit with the appropriate expertise and skills in rehabilitation, the chances of preventing admission to long-term care may be significantly reduced (HSC/LAC, 2000; Audit Commission, 1992). The caveat being that these patients are heavily dependent upon the rehabilitation expertise available, irrespective of setting.

Assessment

Several other often invisible factors come to the fore while addressing assessment, namely, where and at what point in their continuum of care (Godchaux et al., 1997) patients are assessed as suitable for intermediate care. All too often, patients are assessed in a busy accident and emergency department or ward, where there would appear to be little correlation between the setting and environment and their potential capability in home surroundings. If the aim of the assessment is to assess rehabilitation potential, for a rehabilitation service appropriately qualified professionals in appropriate surroundings should conduct the functional assessment. In addition, the most basic of factors essential to 'normal' functioning such as footwear, glasses, hearing aid and usual mobility equipment should be in place before an assessment is performed, as alluded to in Chapter 4. Perhaps another invisible element of greater consequence to a longer-term vision of rehabilitation is the ongoing philosophy of enablement, i.e. care of a rehabilitative nature extends beyond the intermediate pathway, in the home surroundings. This should be related to all aspects of ongoing care when handing over to agencies at a pre-exit phase. Attention to this can have profound effects on the well-being and self-esteem of the patient, improving their quality of life, even if not increasing functional ability (Pound et al., 1994).

Agreements and trust

In order for this to happen there is a need to reach agreement and trust between professionals, colleagues in agencies and organizations, for them to accept each other's assessments. This, it would seem, is at the crux of developing intermediate care pathways. For example, on an individual patient level, trust is implicit if they are to agree to transfer into or out of the intermediate care setting initially! At a professional level, trust may serve to legitimize patient assessments and thereby prevent unnecessary reassessments. Agreement and trust, together with the Single Assessment Process (NSF for Older People, Standard, 2, DoH, 2001h; k) should form a powerful tool which has the potential to trigger the need for more specialist or comprehensive assessment. Moreover, this should then be activated more accurately, and equity of access is more likely to be ensured.

Developing care pathways

Creating effective care pathways will require the setting up of a working group/s with multi-professional and multi-agency involvement and representation or links with the various services/schemes that may be involved, along with user representation. There are a number of considerations and stages that will probably need to be addressed in order to achieve a constructive outcome, and these are listed briefly in Table 9.1.

Table 9.1 A checklist of considerations to aid the overall development of the pathway

1. What is the scope (this could be geographical, PCT-based, organizational)
   • Are there any established links with other services?
2. Define the entry requirements (medical stability, etc.)
   • Is there more than one potential entry point on to the pathway?
3. Determine who can refer to the pathway?
   • Define the scope of the professionals' roles (assessment, treatment, evaluation, discharge, follow-up)
4. Define the philosophy (function) of the model (rehabilitation, timescale etc.)
   • What are the service criteria?
   • Will new services developed imply that changes to the pathway are required?
5. Determine the patient's goals (motivation)
   • Define the outcomes desired (measures)

Conclusion

As the pressure on secondary care continues, with escalating emergency admissions, greater demand upon developing intermediate care services and pathways of care should be invoked (HSC/LAC, 2000). Intermediate care service criteria must be clear but pragmatic, in order to make the referral process into services/schemes clearer, and therefore pathways more accessible for patients. Many care pathways remain at a high level of detail representing no more than a detailed process map, virtually skirting the details of what happens to patient and carers alike once they are in the pathway. There is, however, no blueprint for developing a successful intermediate care pathway; the ideas and suggestions made here result from examples of new services trying to establish pathways and from personal experience of managing some of these. At the very least, pathways must provide a level of detail and clarity commensurate with the care that is proposed.

Education regarding the terminology being used is also vital to eradicate ignorance surrounding the development of care pathways. An awareness of the stages involved in setting up pathways should assist in ensuring that they are inclusive, that is, accommodating sufficient breadth to span the continuum required outside of a purely clinical pathway, while integrating social and financial perspectives.

Finally, all individual organizations/agencies need to be developing their own care pathways at the same pace if the 'whole system approach' is to work. This is irrespective of whether they are based in primary, secondary or intermediate care, as only this will facilitate movement of patients seamlessly into and out of a continuum of services as and when required.

KEY POINTS

- Pathways are perceived as having potential benefits in directing patients along the most appropriate pathway of care in order to achieve agreed goals.
- The development of care pathways, while advocated, has in many cases been slow to take off, especially with regard to older people and intermediate care.
- Initially it is probably best to develop a care pathway at a high level – through a mapping process.
- Creating effective care pathways requires multi-professional, multi-agency and user involvement with representation or links with various services/schemes involved.
- It is probably best to work through a series of considerations and stages when trying to create care pathways.

CHAPTER 10

The Single Assessment Process

SIÂN WADE

Introduction

Standard 2 of the National Service Framework for Older People addresses the concept of person-centred care (National Service Framework, DoH 2001h). The stated aim of this standard is:

> To ensure that older people are treated as individuals and they receive appropriate and timely packages of care which meet their needs as individuals, regardless of health and social services boundaries. (DoH, 2001h: 23)

Key interventions are provided for this standard, as for all the other standards in the National Service Framework for older people (DoH, 2001h). As a priority, there is a requirement that specific service improvements are achieved. One of these is the implementation of a Single Assessment Process (SAP), a concept first referred to in the National Health Service Plan (NHS Plan, DoH 2000c). Older people often have a range of both health and social care needs and the Single Assessment Process is regarded as central to appropriate and timely assessment to assist in meeting these. Worth (2001) has described assessment as 'the means by which practitioners ascertain the needs of individuals in order to determine the most appropriate location for care and match services to need' (p. 257).

Highlighting the Single Assessment Process within the National Service Framework for older people provides a clear statement about the importance of effective assessment of need for many older people.

This chapter provides some background to the concept of the Single Assessment Process and describes some of the processes that have been adopted, or need to be adopted, in order to achieve its implementation. It looks at strategies that might be adopted to 'make' the process work but also

154

acknowledges a range of challenges that need to be addressed or overcome if it is to be effective or of benefit to older people.

Background

At the time of the publication of the National Service Framework, the stated date for implementation of the Single Assessment Process was April 2002 (1st milestone). While some initial guidance was provided within the National Service Framework document, this was really only an outline indicating some core principles, and was to be followed by further guidance in the summer of 2001. Initially it was understood that a national Single Assessment Process would be provided from the centre, i.e. by the Department of Health. However when the draft guidance was released in August 2001, this view had changed. There was a statement indicating that the guidance would not recommend any specific process, rather it would provide a rigorous framework that would lead to the convergence of assessment methods and results over time, irrespective of the tools chosen at a local level. This guidance document was eventually issued in January 2002 (HSC, 2002/001: LAC (2002)1, DoH, 2002b). Due to the delay in its release and the changes proposed, the implementation programme and milestones were revised. There remains a fairly robust timetable whereby the progress with its development and implementation are to be monitored, and it is important that this is adhered to and reported on centrally – now to the Strategic Health Authority. The guidance provides details about the process and how it is to be implemented, with individual guidance provided for key staff groups who may be involved in the process (DoH Guidance, Jan. 2002b).

The Single Assessment Process is 'held up' as a means of 'leading to a more efficient assessment process and more effective care services for older people' (HSC, 2002/001: LAC (2002); DoH, 2002b). Three key attributes are identified as central within the Single Assessment Process. These include the establishment of:

* *A person-centred approach*, whereby the older person seeking help experiences a Single Assessment Process that avoids duplication, where a number of professionals may be involved, where the individual's views remain central to the assessment, and where an appropriate level of assessment is undertaken to provide a rounded picture of their needs and circumstances.
* *A standardized approach*, which is supported by an agreed evidence base, builds upon and supports existing good practice, provides information that is useful and is shared between professionals, produces

sets of standardized assessment information with a summary record, and generates information for strategic planning.

- *An outcome-centred approach*, evaluates assessment information, translating it into appropriate and effective care plans, and promotes health, independence and quality of life for older people – helping to fulfil their potential for rehabilitation. (DoH Guidance, Jan. 2002 Annex A – DoH, 2002b).

Central to the guidance, 12 Steps to Implementation of the Single Assessment Process were provided, as outlined in Table 10.1. Each county/locality has needed to benchmark their progress against these steps, evaluate their approach to service provision and commissioning in relation to the provision of future service design and delivery, and then plan how to work effectively towards meeting these.

Two White Papers: *The New NHS: Modern, Dependable* (DoH, 1997) and *Modernising Social Services* (DoH, 1998c) specified the need for closer working between local agencies. Assessment is a key element within the practice of health and social care practitioners (Housten and Cowley, 2002; Milner and O'Brien, 2002) and is perceived as the cornerstone of high-quality care (Parry-Jones and Soulsby, 2001), especially for older people. As such, the Single Assessment Process should provide an effective means for achieving this and potentially be invaluable for older people and intermediate care services. It should help to ensure that patients are appropriately assessed, and then access appropriate services, but should also help to ensure that communication is relayed and shared effectively to enhance the delivery of care and support.

Table 10.1 The 12 Steps to Implementation of the Single Assessment Process – as recommended by the Department of Health

1. Agree purpose and outcome of single assessment process
2. Agree shared values
3. Agree terminology
4. Map care process
5. Estimate types and numbers of older people needing assessment
6. Agree the stages of assessment and care management
7. Agree the link between medical diagnosis and assessment
8. Agree the domain and sub-domains of the assessment
9. Agree assessment and approaches, tools and scales
10. Agree joint working arrangements
11. Agree single assessment summary
12. Implement a joint staff development strategy

The Single Assessment Process is seen as a means of ensuring that a more standardized assessment process is in place and that the same assessment process is used across all agencies. It recognizes that older people often have both health and social care needs (Knopp, 2000) and that agencies need to work together. This requires effective communication and co-operation between health and social care professionals in order for the needs of older people to be appropriately met. It should mean that organizational boundaries become less important, something that has been severely challenged for some decades due to a range of barriers that have impeded effective inter-agency collaboration (Hudson et al., 1997). Lewis (2001) in her review of health and social care provision over the past 50 years, highlighted how the sharp divide between health and social care has particularly affected older people with less acute care needs. She suggests that their care needs have been rationed, ignored or treated inappropriately by both sides of the 'boundary', with care often being passed between different services. This, Lewis (2001) argues, has been perpetuated by different funding streams, administration divides and professional rivalries, as identified by Hudson et al. (1997).

The expectation of the Single Assessment Process is that it will raise the standards of assessment practice so that older people receive a rounded and holistic assessment as identified. Another key aim of the process is to promote inter-agency/professional working, such that no one person will undertake the assessment: rather it will involve all those professionals concerned so as to assist them to share information. This should not only avoid replication and duplication, but also provide a much sounder basis upon which to plan interventions and services, such that the outcome should be an assessment that feels 'single' from the perspective of the older person. Wild (2002) also suggests that it should enable greater equality in access to multi-agency services.

Thus an essential component of the process of developing the Single Assessment Process is the need for all agencies to work together closely to reach mutual agreement on the process, on their values, and on how to make it work. Throughout the guidance the importance of involving older people and their views is emphasized, while acknowledging carers and their needs, and this is crucial if the process is to meet the perceived needs of older people effectively. The Single Assessment Process should cover all areas of assessment for older people, including the Care Programme Approach in mental health services and assessment for admission to a nursing or care home care.

The guidance for the Single Assessment Process indicates that the scale and depth of assessment should be kept in proportion to the needs of the older person, and outlines four levels of assessment that should be available within the process, under four headings:

Contact assessment: including basic information such as name, phone number,
                        address, etc. together with some more detailed information.
Overview: Wider needs assessment – specified domains are detailed.
Specialist: In depth assessment – usually by different professionals/
                        agencies according to need. This is probably where more
                        detailed biographical and life-review information would be
                        collected, if appropriate.
Comprehensive: As full a picture of all the person's needs as is possible. This is
                        likely to involve one or more specialist assessments and will
                        require a team approach. A summary of the person's needs can
                        then be derived from a range of detailed assessments, e.g. a
                        comprehensive gerontological assessment. Comprehensive
                        assessment will need an identified person to co-ordinate the
                        assessment and recommended care – possibly the profession
                        that is most dominant within the care being delivered.

As suggested, the framework around which the process is built should promote the identification of properly targeted assessment so as to ensure that the care and services that the older person receives meet their needs responsively, and promote and maximize their independence (DoH, 2001h). This will be helped if the assessment tools are strongly rooted in evidence and include built-in 'signposts', as this should help professionals make decisions about the domains that need exploring, triggering as suggested where necessary the need for more in-depth or specialist assessment or service need. Through the use of such a process it should be possible to help prevent deterioration in health or social care and manage crises more effectively (DoH, 2001h).

The actual level of assessment undertaken will depend upon the needs of the older individual. The original guidance clearly stated that contact assessment would take place only when there was 'contact between an older person and health and social services and where significant needs are first described or suspected' (DoH, 2002b: 13). Thus, in a way, contact assessment would be the next stage after an initial contact had been made, and when a decision is made that progression to the Single Assessment Process appears appropriate. More recently, guidance has suggested that the information required within the contact assessment is primarily basic personal information. This, it is suggested, would be the normal information sought when initial contacts are made with either health or social service. It is therefore suggested that in most instances this assessment detail should be gathered, and updated on future contacts. It is expected that the need for further assessment within the Single Assessment Process will emerge at contact assessment, although in some cases the complexity of need will be apparent and the need for more extensive assessment will be self-evident, e.g. Specialist or Comprehensive assessment, etc. It is not intended that each level of the assessment is progressed through from level 1–4, but that the appropriate level of assessment is homed in on at the outset. Where there is evidence of presenting problems, or there appears to be the potential presence of wider health and social care needs, the guidance provides a set of suggested key questions/areas that need to be explored at this Contact assessment point if it is suspected further assessment may be needed. These are outlined in Table 10.2 (HSC, 2002/001: LAC (2002)1, DoH 2002b – Appendix E), and help to guide the assessor to the next most appropriate level of assessment, if necessary.

Table 10.2 Seven key issues that may need exploring on contact assessment

1. The nature of the presenting need.
2. The significance of the need for the older person.
3. The length of time the need has been experienced.
4. Potential solutions identified by the older person.
5. Other needs experienced by the older person.
6. Recent life events or changes relevant to the problem(s).
7. The perceptions of family members and carers.

Progression on to further assessment will depend upon a judgment being made by the individual making the assessment at this point. This could mean that the way a person enters the Single Assessment Process may be in question, as it often takes skill or time to realize or appreciate that there is more at stake than the initial presenting problem. There is also the need for skill in assessing if the older person actually wants further help or intervention.

While basic personal information can be collected by a trained but not qualified staff member, the exploration of the presenting and other needs should, the guidance states, be undertaken by a trained and competent single professional, qualified or not, in any one of the settings to which guidance applies. Those people most likely to be involved, and for whom guidance is provided, are geriatricians and old age psychiatrists, GPs, nurses, social workers, therapists and older people themselves.

The Single Assessment Process guidance (HSC, 2002/001:LAC (2002)1, DoH, 2002b) provides a number of domains and sub-domains that should be included within the framework to guide an overview assessment, as in Table 10.3 (Annex F). The guidance suggests that 'in considering whether to explore all the domains or just some of them, professionals will be guided by their judgment, taking in to account service users' wishes and any indications of wider needs that are triggered by the contact assessment'. Again, those assessment tools that are strongly rooted in evidence should help professionals make decisions about the domains that need to be explored.

Table 10.3 The domains and sub-domains of the Single Assessment Process (Annex F)

User's perspective
- Needs and issues in the users' own words*
- Users' expectations, strengths, abilities and motivations*

Clinical background
- History of medical conditions and diagnoses*
- History of falls
- Medication use and ability to self-medicate*

Disease prevention
- History of blood pressure monitoring
- Nutrition, diet and fluids*
- Vaccination history
- Drinking and smoking history
- Exercise pattern
- History of cervical and breast screening

Personal care and physical well-being
- Personal hygiene, including washing, bathing, toileting and grooming
- Dressing
- Pain
- Oral health
- Foot-care
- Tissue viability
- Mobility
- Continence and other aspects of elimination*
- Sleeping patterns

Senses
- Sight
- Hearing
- Communication

Mental health
- Cognition and dementia, including orientation and memory*
- Mental health including depression, reactions to loss, and emotional difficulties*

Relationships
- Social contacts, relationships, and involvement in leisure, hobbies, work, and learning*
- Carer support and strength of caring arrangements, including the carer's perspective*

Safety
- Abuse and neglect
- Other aspects of personal safety
- Public safety

Immediate environment and resources
- Care of home and managing daily tasks such as food preparation, cleaning and shopping*
- Housing – location, access, amenities and heating*
- Level and management of finances*
- Access to local facilities.

Note: the wording of items with a * has been clarified for this guidance.
Source: HSC, 2002/001:LAC (2002) 1 Guidance on the Single Assessment Process, DoH, 2002b.

The National Service Framework (DoH, 2001h) did not recommend any particular assessment process/package/tools to be used, and stated that 'home grown' tools could be used as long as they followed the guidance that was issued in January 2002 (HSC, 2002/001; LAC (2002)1, DoH, 2002b). In September 2002 a further document was released which detailed seven 'off the shelf' assessment processes/packages/tools that were available for national use (DoH, 2002g). None of these, however, had been accredited, as all required further modifications and developments to ensure that they met the requirements of the Single Assessment Process. If these 'off the shelf' processes/packages are used they can be added to, but elements cannot be removed. Alternatively, localities were advised that they could still create their own packages/tools so long as the guidance was followed, and they achieved the required outcomes.

The guidance allows individual agencies and localities to decide which areas or domains should be specified for specialist assessment. A typical range might include those outlined in Table 10.4, and these assessments will be standardized. Where clinical or diagnostic assessments are undertaken the older person will be referred, and the assessor will use their own specialized assessment format. Where comprehensive assessment is required the Department of Health requires that assessment of all the domains are completed. Where the individual older person needs a range of specialist assessments or a comprehensive assessment, there will almost certainly need to be a co-ordinator or key worker identified to co-ordinate the care or intervention provided and to evaluate it holistically.

Where there is a perceived need for nursing or care home placement, additional information should be collected. The information required is

Table 10.4 Possible range of specialist assessment domains specified within the Single Assessment Process.

- Falls
- Continence
- Tissue viability
- Access to other services
- Social care
- Pain
- Cognitive ability
- Depression
- Therapy assessment/rehabilitation potential
- Diabetes
- Palliative care
- Respiratory
- Specialist clinical/diagnostic assessments

outlined in Appendix H of the Guidance, and the assessment should involve input from a range of professionals. Where the placement is in a nursing home a registered nurse employed by the NHS must be involved. Where determination of the registered nurse contribution to care is required, this must be undertaken by a nurse employed by the NHS and will involve the additional RNCC framework for assessment.

Single assessment summary

Once assessment has been undertaken, there is a requirement to provide a selective summary of the assessment with a clear outcome plan using a standardized format that has been agreed by all agencies. Three sets of information must be covered:

- basic personal information;
- needs and health; and
- a summary of the care plan.

The summary care plan should comprise the overall care aims and the needs they are meant to address. There is also a requirement that a list of services is included, with coding to show if the service is currently provided or not (these are provided in the guidance on p.37), together with the name of the co-ordinator or key worker. Further guidance with a suggested pro forma for providing the required summary, evaluation of needs and summary of care plan was provided by the Department of Health in September 2002 (DoH, 2002g).This is the information that will be available to the older person and to other professionals involved in their care. Each person undertaking the assessment will keep his or her own more detailed records.

The Single Assessment Process in itself should act as a care pathway for the individual older person – triggering the need for further assessment if needed, and also triggering the need for services, etc. If utilized appropriately, it should therefore provide the catalyst for entry on to an appropriate intermediate care pathway, where relevant. The synergy of the two should ensure not only comprehensiveness but equity to a range of services and reduce ambiguity of what may be offered to patients. In this way it should also act as a tool to help identify unmet need, highlighting gaps in current provision in terms of service need and skills needs. As such, it should build upon established care pathways in use, and help to build up the health economy in a needs-responsive way, or at least inform commissioning and the LDPs (Local Development Plans) of PCTs, in terms of prioritizing service needs and developments and therefore helping to prioritize bids and funding allocation. Whether this will work in practice will remain to be seen.

Evaluation

The Department of Health guidance (DoH, 2001j) provides criteria against which localities have been required to check and evaluate their progress. This is provided on page 5 and there is a recommendation that other local stakeholders and older people themselves are asked to evaluate the proposed approach and progress. The advice is that the answers to the questions outlined should be 'yes' or 'with very few exceptions', and that all the criteria should have been achieved by 2004. Progress milestones are provided with different target dates to help facilitate this progress. Where consensus has not been reached by June 2004 there is the possibility that the Department of Health will prescribe one of the recommended Tools/processes that were made available in September 2002 (DoH, 2002g).

Implementing the Single Assessment Process

Implementing the Single Assessment Process is a huge undertaking and the process of involving staff and users from across the whole health and social care economy cannot be overestimated. It will change the way we work together, how we record our findings and how patients/clients access services. It is evident that for the Single Assessment Process to work, all those involved in its use need to work together to establish a common understanding and clarity of its purpose, its values and the expected outcomes of the process. For this reason, early work has involved stakeholder forums in various forms, involving health, social care, voluntary agencies, older people and carers. The initial purpose of such forums has been to begin to establish inter-agency working where this was not previously occurring, and to further develop joint working where such collaborative working has already been established. Localities have been required to address and report their progress on three overarching activities:

- to look at the process involved;
- to decide and agree on an information technology tool;
- to decide on how staff are going to be trained and supported with this process.

Since the level of partnership working has varied across the country, progress with the implementation of the Single Assessment Process has also varied. This may well account for the reluctance of the Department of Health to impose a standard assessment tool nationally. This is something that many feel would have been more appropriate, bearing in mind some of the obstacles faced by the introduction of a whole range of different processes nationally. This, however, will not be the only reason for not choosing one specific nationally recognized tool, and there is probably a range of other reasons for not taking this route. One of these may be that by imposing a specified tool the Department could be criticized for supporting a monopoly for the company licensing that particular tool/process. Another reason, and probably a much more important reason, is that by requiring each area to develop their own tool/process, stakeholders have been forced to engage in the process in a proactive way. This will have provided the opportunity to explore and debate the pros and cons of the Single Assessment Process, and work through the challenges encountered, so helping to avoid the whole concept just becoming a paper exercise, which would not work.

By requiring stakeholders to engage in the process it is much more likely that a common understanding of its purpose and value is reached and that the adopted process, when implemented eventually, will be owned and signed up to by all those who need to be involved. This has inevitably been a slow process.

It is probable that across the country various steering groups have been working to find effective ways of implementing the process. As work has progressed, organizing workshops has provided a means of enabling stakeholders to engage in the process so as to gain an understanding and some clarity about it, and to gain insight into the progress that is being made. Such a forum provides the opportunity for participants to explore the potential outcomes that might be achieved through using the Single Assessment Process, to examine how patients can best be engaged in the process, and to discuss why agencies should 'buy in'. This kind of forum also provides the opportunity to address issues related to implementation and to agree on the principles of assessment, as shown in Table 10.5.

Table 10.5 Principles of assessment

- Values
- Outcomes
- Access to services
- Processes
- Mapping
- Who undertakes

Table 10.6 outlines a wide range of potential outcomes that could be achieved by introducing the Single Assessment Process, with a suggestion of who might best benefit from each of these, although ultimately all these outcomes should improve things for the older person.

Trying to introduce anything new is time-consuming and likely to meet resistance, especially if it involves such a fundamental cultural change as

Table 10.6 Potential outcomes of single assessment

Potential outcomes	User	Staff	Organization
Speed up assessment and planning process	✓	✓	
Unnecessary duplication	✓	✓	✓
Reduce waiting time for assessment	✓		
Allows effective use of resources	✓	✓	✓
Appropriate referrals ▼ Inappropriate ▲	✓	✓	✓
Avoid scatter-gun effect	✓	✓	✓
Universal language	✓	✓	✓
Trigger for service need			✓
Streamlined service delivery with cohesion between services	✓	✓	✓
Clarity of pathway – progressive, productive		✓	✓
Clarity to user	✓		
Reflects performance targets			✓
Assessment delivered and patient guides patient to right place, at right time with right skills	✓	✓	✓
Client satisfaction with pathway of care	✓		
Minimize starting points for assessment		✓	✓
Robust enough to work at times of pressure as well as other times	✓	✓	
Assessments should improve solution/care plan	✓	✓	
Supports decision-making – informed process		✓	✓
Improve trust between assessors		✓	
Real time updated		✓	
Triggers relate to eligibility for services and need	✓	✓	✓
Describes need in realistic terms	✓	✓	
Informs more accurately about unmet needs		✓	✓
Flags up resource and service development needs and could guide SAFF Bids and negotiations			✓
Engages staff in informing commissioning and the SAFF Rounds	✓	✓	
Drives development of better tailored services	✓	✓	✓
Gives transparency	✓	✓	✓

that involved with the Single Assessment Process. It has therefore been essential to try to identify benefits that can be shared with stakeholders so as to 'sell' the concept. These 'selling benefits' might include those listed in Table 10.7.

Table 10.7 Selling benefits of Single Assessment Process

- Enhances person-centred and focused care
- Allows practitioners to influence and shape the process
- Accessible shared information and provides an overview of all records
- Effective use of time – enabling practitioners to provide direct care
- Improved care planning
- Reduces paperwork
- Smarter not harder
- Joint and partnership working and valuing of each other
- Financially cost-effective
- Performance information
- Provides opportunity to allocate resources appropriately
- Provides performance information

Making the Single Assessment Process work

Having a Single Assessment Process will mean that a range of practitioners, or indeed older people themselves, may be involved in undertaking assessments or self-assessments that they may not have previously been involved in. While these may not be in-depth assessments they should be at a sufficient level to act as triggers to identify if there is a need for another service or for a referral to a more specialist practitioner where the need emerges, as already described – see Table 10.2. This should help to avoid individuals being referred inappropriately, as often occurs at present – with the individual sometimes attending a range of appointments before they reach the right person or service. If this is to be achieved, however, the questions involved in the assessment will need to be reliable enough to identify the need. There will also be a need for practitioners to establish trust with each other and with older people in undertaking this assessment, if referrals are to be accepted from any member of the multidisciplinary team. Considering the present culture, relying on a colleague from another profession to undertake this level of assessment is likely to lead to some concerns, at least initially.

While engaging key stakeholders in the planning and process of implementing the Single Assessment Process is one step, engaging all those who may be involved in understanding it, participating in it and undertaking it, is even greater. This will involve an agreed strategy for education, which will not be easy to achieve when practitioners are so busy, and will require protected learning time. While inter-agency/inter-professional workshops may be the most appropriate and beneficial approach, there will be times when the education will have to be taken to the individuals in their own workplace if it is to reach those who need to be involved. This has huge resource implications for those delivering the training and in providing protected time out for those who will be undertaking it, for which funding is inevitably needed.

Using the Single Assessment Process should, as suggested, help to identify gaps in service provision. In order to do this there is a need to know what services are already available. As services have developed, for example in intermediate care as identified in earlier sections of this book, it has been difficult for staff to keep abreast of them. This may also relate to other services that staff may not currently utilize or refer to. With the wider remit to undertake initial assessments and refer on, it will be important to have some means of informing staff effectively of the availability of a whole range of services. As with access to intermediate care services/schemes it would seem that some form of single point of information or resource centre may be necessary. Where gaps are identified it is likely that there will be conflicting demands for development, and so it will be necessary to identify ways in which agreement on priorities can be reached so as to inform PCT commissioning.

Progress to date and challenges faced

As indicated, progress with the implementation of the Single Assessment Process varies greatly across the country. While some areas are already actively engaged in piloting or using, others are still at the stage of engaging stakeholders and reaching agreement about the value of the process and the expected outcomes and benefits. Wherever people are in the process of implementation there are a range of challenges involved in implementing the Single Assessment Process, in addition to those already addressed, which are important to consider. Some of these are considered here.

The Single Assessment Process has been singled out for use with older people, yet if we are to ensure we have a non-ageist approach to care, using chronological age is inappropriate. If this is the case, there will be a need to establish how adults of all ages will be eligible to benefit from the use of the Single Assessment Process if it is deemed appropriate. It could be argued that, as with so many attributes required in relation to the care of older people, the use of, and skills involved in, the Single Assessment Process should be transferable and therefore used for any individual as and when needed, to the level it is needed. This would help to ensure that anyone with more in-depth, specialist or complex needs would receive an appropriate level of assessment.

One of the key challenges faced in developing the Single Assessment Process is reaching an agreement about the documentation format and 'tools' used to assess the different domains used. This is why establishing inter-agency workshops and forums is so important. It is likely to require the use of pilot sites to test out tools and various assessment formats, even if these are recognized tools/processes. Along with this challenge is a concern about how the information will be shared among practitioners. While the older person will be able to hold their own personal records, if these are still available only in paper format, they may not always be easily accessible to them, especially in an emergency or if they are away from home, when requiring help. This is likely to be the very time when to have access would be most timely and helpful.

There is quite a strong view that single assessment will really work effectively only once the Single Assessment Process records can be kept electronically and accessed by all. While most GP practices use electronic records, this is only just gradually being implemented within most social services and Hospital Trusts, and while there is a requirement for all to implement Electronic Patient Records (EPR) eventually, this may be some years away (DoH, 2002f). Even where these records are in use, it is almost certain that Health Care Trusts and social care services will not utilize an integrated information technology system. However, there is the potential for the different systems to be programmed so that they can 'talk' to each other. Another major concern is the lack of IT skills among many practitioners, suggesting that considerable work is required in order to train staff adequately if they are to engage effectively. It is evident that there is much work to be progressed before there is a system that will lend itself to the Single Assessment Process, and in many Trusts considerable investment is required to provide technical support to these systems if they are to be relied upon.

There is an added concern about confidentiality related to both paper and Electronic Patient Records (EPR). Paper records are likely to cause more concern as anyone can read what is written within them, if they gain access to them. Although there is also concern related to access to information held in Electronic Patient Records, it is probable that this can be managed more effectively, as individuals will be required to have access to a PIN number for access, and further controls will be in place to limit access to specific sections of information. Older people themselves will also be able to access their Electronic Patient Records, at least their summary and care plans, and will have a PIN number of their own.

By engaging in the implementation of local Single Assessment Processes, problems are envisaged where patients require care across geographical service boundaries within other localities, either because they live near geographical boundaries or because they are away from home. Since each locality may well be using different Single Assessment Processes, the out-of-locality care settings or services will not be able to access the records from another area. It seems that there is little that can be done about this, although it may be that some solutions are found. What needs to be acknowledged is that at present there is no such system to share information and avoid duplication or replication locally. Requests for notes have to be made, and delivery of these may take some days, depending where they need to come from, so any new process will be better even if there are limitations.

Where there is access to a Single Assessment Process for an individual, there will always be a need to check that the details and assessments that have already been undertaken are still viable and valid, if the patient is encountering a new episode of care. It will be necessary to check that information is still correct and that things have not changed, but at least a foundation will be there, and if it is held electronically it will be quite easy to update, by adding new information. What is evident is that with current electronic systems in use, another practitioner coming afterwards cannot delete information that has been collected and recorded previously. Their new or updated information can only be added, so that in effect an historical record builds up about the individual.

Conclusion

The value of the Single Assessment Process for intermediate care has become increasingly evident as it develops. In the past, most care pathways have involved the transfer of patients either into hospital or home from hospital, with perhaps one additional service involved. With the introduction of the concept of intermediate care and the wider range of services being developed, which may be accessed at different stages of a pathway of care and via a range of routes, pathways could well become more complex. This has therefore added complexity to assessment and complexity to the range of services that might be accessed. The Single Assessment Process should help significantly in making appropriate assessment and in directing individual older people to the service most appropriate to their needs, and in helping to ensure effective communication.

KEY POINTS

- The Single Assessment Process is seen as a process that will enhance person-centred care, using a standardized approach by all involved in assessment of an individual.
- The Single Assessment Process should ensure that assessment leads on to effective care planning with planned intervention.
- The Single Assessment Process involves a series of levels of assessment which will be undertaken according to the presenting needs of an individual older person.

- The Department of Health outlined a specific process that localities have had to demonstrate they have followed when implementing the Single Assessment Process – with explicit deadlines and progress milestones.
- The Single Assessment Process will require skilled and knowledgeable practitioners to ensure it is used appropriately.
- Implementing the Single Assessment Process involves a range of challenges which need to be addressed or overcome for it to successfully help and benefit older people.

CHAPTER 11

Evaluating intermediate care services and schemes

SIÂN WADE

Introduction

Evaluation of any new service is essential if its planned purpose is to be realized and its value recognized. During the 1980s, as increased attention was focused on the services provided for older people, concern about evaluative research of new developments became increasingly important (Challis and Darton, 1990; Lazenbath, 2002). This concern has continued, and within the HSC/LAC Guidance (DoH, 2001e) and National Service Framework (DoH, 2001h) there is a requirement for all intermediate care schemes and services to be evaluated. It is therefore appropriate to include a chapter in this subject within this book. This is incorporated for example in the statement 'service design should include evaluation and audit to help inform future investment decisions for 2002/3, Standard 3 of the National Service Framework for Older People' (DoH, 2001h: 47).

Why evaluation?

Goldberg and Connelly (1982) identify five reasons to support the importance of evaluation. These are:

- public accountability;
- deployment of resources;
- effectiveness;
- cost-effectiveness;
- safeguarding against over-enthusiasm for the new.

What is evaluation?

The term 'evaluation' implies the use of criteria in order to make a judgment of the efficacy of a service or mode of care. This seems a highly appropriate requirement if new services are to be developed, especially as so many new and different schemes and services can be expected with the 'emergence' of intermediate care. It is particularly important, but ironic, for the Department of Health to make this recommendation, since within Standard 3 of the National Service Framework (DoH, 2001h: 41–50), it is acknowledged that evidence to support many of the early models of care was rather limited, even if there appeared to be good support for the service.

Evaluation in intermediate care services/schemes

Most early evaluations of intermediate care schemes involved the use of randomized controlled studies such as that by Shepperd et al. (1998). This scheme involved patients who had undergone either a hip or knee replacement or a hysterectomy, and who received either routine care in hospital or an intensive 'hospital at home' service. Shepperd et al. (1998) showed that there was little difference in health outcomes, that most patients preferred the treatment at home, and that while the cost shifted from hospital to the community, it also increased. Another scheme run in Bristol was also evaluated using a randomized controlled trial approach (Richards et al., 1998). Here patients with a similar mix of clinical problems as those in the Shepperd et al.'s study, were involved in a similar kind of 'hospital at home' scheme. In this study again no overall health differences were found and there was no difference in patient satisfaction. However, length of stay was shorter than for standard hospital care although costs were slightly higher. Thus, in both these schemes costs increased. In an early discharge/domiciliary rehabilitation scheme for stroke patients in London, outcomes were similar, but hospital bed use was reduced by 15 per cent (Rudd et al., 1997).

It is important to consider the views of informal carers and the level of stress they experience when evaluating intermediate care schemes. This is a highly important consideration when setting up these schemes, as their success often depends upon the availability of carers, as evidenced in Chapter 12, since it is these informal carers who tend to provide the main 'load' of the care. With lifestyle changes, informal carers may not be available and with an ageing population these carers may well be quite old or disabled themselves. This may mean that if the service is to be extended to larger populations of patients it may be more problematic, and early findings may not be so transferable. The concern about carers' stress and acceptability was addressed in both the Richards et al's (1998) and Rudd et al's (1997) studies, where on both occasions the views of carers were mixed. It must be remembered, however, that patients were able to enter the scheme only if they met certain criteria, which included having someone to help in their care.

Some of the criticism centring around these early studies is that the evaluations focused on schemes that addressed a single problem or pathology and, as suggested, certain criteria had to be met before patients could be accepted into the service or scheme. This may limit the perceived benefits that these services/schemes can achieve if, when extended to more complex care needs or populations, the criteria cannot be met (Shepperd and Illiffe, 1998b). A study by Steiner et al. (2001) of a nurse-led unit led to much less conclusive findings than those cited in the studies above. Also, randomized controlled studies are limited in the variables they can account for and this may lead to difficulties when a range of uncontrollable factors may be impacting on the success or otherwise of an evaluation. Other randomized controlled evaluations of nurse-led units have failed to show effectiveness in either organizational or patient outcomes (Griffith and Wilson-Barnett, 2000; Alfano and Hall, 1969). While Steiner et al. (2000) see a place for randomized controlled evaluative studies with regard to intermediate care schemes, Vaughan (1998) is much more sceptical as she believes there are too many variable factors influencing the outcomes and that these risk being overlooked.

Martin (2001) warns that despite the optimism that seems to be centred on the success and value of intermediate care, doubt remains about the evidence of the clinical effectiveness and financial saving of the more general schemes as suggested by Shepperd and Illiffe (1998b). He also warns that there are considerable methodological problems in doing a cost/benefit analysis of such intermediate care schemes/services as found by Hensher et al. (1999). What Martin (2001) does suggest is that there is better evidence of success where teams have focused on rehabilitation of specific conditions such as hip fractures or strokes. He suggests that there is a need for more evidence of the effectiveness of schemes involving a clinical mix of patients, especially those set up set up to avoid acute hospital admission. He also warns of the need to consider the effect these schemes might have on the local health economy.

One of the challenges when trying to evaluate some of the more recent schemes, especially those designed to avoid acute hospital admissions and where funding was through the use of Winter Pressures monies, was that they were often set up in great haste. As a result, it was difficult to establish an effective method for evaluation, as funding was often so short term that the service had hardly been established when it was being withdrawn. This meant full and effective evaluation was almost impossible. This is not a reason to dismiss the value of many of these schemes and services, if set up appropriately. It is a reason, however, to ensure that effective evaluation processes are in place when establishing them, and to ensure that the service can be sustained long enough for evaluation to be effective. This certainly justifies the importance given to evaluating future developments as recommended by the DoH (2001h).

Strategies for evaluation

It is evident from the discussion so far that it is important to find effective ways of evaluating these new services/schemes. Suchman (1967) describes evaluation as 'A method for determining the degree to which a planned programme achieves its objective', and while this might be regarded as an outdated piece of work, in principle it still holds true. There is, however, a need for clarity and specificity about goals or objectives, inputs and outputs, and as Challis et al. (1988) state, this needs to include consideration of the resources available and therefore a cost/benefit analysis.

A range of strategies may be utilized to evaluate services and these can be accessed from a variety of sources and literature. It is intended here to provide some limited suggestions and initial guidance of how evaluation might be approached. This, however, is by no means comprehensive and does not carry critical rigour.

The Department of Health NHS Executive (1999) provide six key areas for assessing a service or scheme:

- health improvement;
- fair access;
- effective delivery of appropriate health care;
- efficiency;
- patient/carer experience;
- health outcomes of NHS care.

Martin (2001) suggests that there are a number of questions that need to be asked and answered when evaluating schemes. These he outlines as:

- Do the right people get to use the services, according to need? i.e. the right people in the right place with the right skills;
- Are they (the schemes) effective at what they were set up to do?
- Do the services operate efficiently (use of resources)?
- Are they popular with patients and carers, including comparisons with alternatives?
- Do they deliver health gain, however defined?
- Does the overall local health economy provide better outcomes with these services as a part?

- Does the overall local health economy operate more or less equally efficiently with these services as a part? (This question includes the consideration of whether new services are a substitution for or additional to existing provision.)

The Clinical Governance Support Unit (Oxford Radcliffe Hospital NHS Trust, 2002) has provided a toolkit to assist practitioners with the evaluation of a health service. While not directed towards intermediate care services, there are some core principles that may well be worth considering.

Why are you evaluating and who is it for?

Having first established why you are evaluating a service it is then important to consider who the evaluation is for. While the Department of Health has requested that these intermediate care schemes are evaluated, and will no doubt monitor these closely, decisions about the future of the service will be made at a more local level, and therefore the evaluation needs to tailored to what the reader is wanting and is interested in. In the case of intermediate care this is likely to be a PCT, who will be judging if the service/scheme should continue and, if so, if any changes/developments are needed. It is therefore useful to have established before the evaluation those aspects of the service that they see as most important, and will look for in a final report.

Project planning and who will be involved

Undertaking an evaluation can be very time-consuming, so it is important to identify people and resources that can assist and decide who will be involved in the process of planning the evaluation, collecting and analysing the data, and producing the final report. Planning is best established before the service/scheme is set up so that the situation before and after can be demonstrated. This will require project planning, which will involve a number of possible stages such as:

- background information;
- aims and objectives;
- study design;
- proposed data collection, recording and processing;
- how data will be analysed;
- how confidentiality will be maintained;
- timetable;
- statement of who is responsible for each aspect;
- estimate of resources required.

Drawing up such a plan helps to clarify the ideas of the evaluation process, and should highlight weak areas as well as give an idea of the work and time involved. It also serves to assist in explaining the evaluation process to others.

Identify other comparable services/schemes if provided

If you have not already done so it will be important to find out if similar services/schemes are provided elsewhere, and if so to see if they have been evaluated and if this model may be of help to you. Comparison with other service providers is a good method of displaying the quality of a new service/scheme, as is a comparison with what was provided before the new service/scheme was introduced.

What to evaluate

When considering what aspects to evaluate it is useful to utilize the Structure, Process and Outcome format that was proposed by Donabedian (1980). This process might involve:

1. Identification of aims and objectives

When starting out it is important to identify clearly the aims and objectives of the proposed service/scheme, and fairly clear criteria for judging expected outcomes. Where there have been previous evaluation reports, reference to these will probably make this easier.

2. Demonstrating achievement of objectives

Actually finding ways of demonstrating that objectives have been achieved may not be easy. Where this is quantifiable then the data can be quite easily collected and an appropriate method of presenting the data chosen. Where services aim to improve the health status or well-being of the patients, criteria to measure these may not be so easy, and several methods may need to be considered and used. The kind of approaches that may be utilized include:

- audits against guidelines or protocols;
- patient, carer/relative, staff views sought through questionnaires, interviews, focus groups or meetings;
- analysis of complaints;
- any other source of data collection that may be available, e.g. patient stories, observation studies, etc.

Structure and resource data

When considering the resources being used or needed, information about equipment and costs, staffing levels and grades, and hours/shifts worked will be important. There will also need to be data collection about the number of patients using the service, their age, referral source, details and diagnosis/ needs. Details of the assessments and investigations, etc. performed for each patient and the care they received will be important, while data about the length of time patients waited to access the service/scheme and length of time in it, will be necessary. Planning this kind of audit information into any documents where information is collected anyway will ease the work required to effectively collect these data. Noting reasons for delays or improvements in accessing, using or transferring out of a service will provide important qualitative data to support the way a service/scheme is being used.

Reporting and displaying your findings

When the information and data collected have been analysed, they need to be reported in an easily accessible way using appropriate bar charts, pie charts, etc. where amenable. As already suggested, the way the findings are reported will depend upon the person requesting them, but when considering an intermediate care service or scheme this is likely to require both quantifiable and qualitative elements. In order to demonstrate benefits it is best to focus on any substantial changes first, with less important information possibly going into the appendices. It is also beneficial to focus on consistency as this gives a good indication of reliability, while showing that everyone involved in the data collection consistently used the same criteria when recording data. Response rates and other quantifiable measures used should be transparent. Where bias or potential bias may have been present in data collected, this should again be made explicit as should any other factors that may have affected data collection, such as human error.

Where comparisons are being drawn with previous or other services it is useful to demonstrate these, identifying if these are (statistically) significant or simply due to variation of a relatively small sample size.

The main purpose of the evaluation report will be to demonstrate the present quality of a service/scheme and also to demonstrate a comparison with others or with the situation before it was introduced. It should be an honest account and if problems have emerged these need to be acknowledged with some discussion about how they may be addressed; they should not, however, become the focus of the report. Demonstrating that thought had been given to how these problems will be tackled, however, will give credibility to the study and add to the overall quality of the service/scheme once addressed. Table 11.1 provides a framework that was

Table 11.1 A framework for monitoring and evaluation

Pathway	Objectives	Measures	Data collected
Referral to intermediate care (GP/RRT/A and E/ Community geriatrician, etc.	• Prevent admission	• Correct use of protocols • Immediate (speedy) • Response/assessment/triage • Application of criteria correctly	• Person carrying out immediate assessment • Date of assessment/referred to intermediate care – (Y/N).
Assessment for rehabilitation/CA(R)T	• To be able to provide a timely assessment for all referrals • Produce an individual rehabilitation programme with a short period of time for every patient • Ensure involvement of user and carer in development • Provision of good-quality programme assessment	• % of relevant target population referred • Time between referral and assessment • % appropriate referrals • % with individual rehabilitation programme • Appropriate professional undertaking assessment • Audit of assessment/ team-based	• Intermediate care assessment date • Length of assessment progress • Professional/team member undertaking review • Outcome of assessment, i.e rehabilitation programme • Number progressed/refused. If refused, reason and destination

Table 11.1 (contd)

Pathway	Objectives	Measures	Data collected
Service provided e.g. CART/beds/equipment only	• Deliver effective rehabilitation programme with measurable improvements for patients • Increase in independence • Reduction in admissions to care homes	• Time between assessment and commencement of rehabilitation programme • % receiving service agreed in the programme • % with no package • Use of resources available • Improvement in patient ability/ independence (Barthel score)	• Service admitted to • Admission date to service • Length of stay • Review of programme undertaken – date • Barthel at end of programme • Equipment
Overall pathway issues	• Effective user/carer involvement • Effective delivery of pathway, i.e. delays minimized	• Satisfaction survey • Time between pathway stages	• Name • GP • Date of birth • Sex • Address and postcode • Tel no. • Ethnic group • Religion • Patient/carer questionnaire • (Signatures on programme)

drawn up by Birmingham Health Authority as a pilot to guide practitioners on how to monitor and evaluate intermediate care services and schemes, as they developed (Main and Lees, 2000). It demonstrates the objectives that could be set for each service/scheme, the measures used to collect data, and identifies by whom and how these data might be collected.

Conclusion

A brief overview of the importance of evaluation in relation to intermediate care services or schemes has been provided here, with some ideas of how to undertake an effective evaluation suggested. This section is intended only to alert readers to the key place of evaluation. Further examination of approaches and methods should be undertaken before commencing such a study. Most practitioners will now have access to clinical governance and clinical effectiveness teams within their organizations, and their skills and advice should automatically be sought at the outset of any plans to set up or evaluate a service/scheme.

Seeking the views of older people and carers remains implicit within developments with intermediate care, as identified. In the next chapter the findings of a study exploring the views of carers involved in providing support within intermediate care services and schemes within the home are described.

KEY POINTS

- Evaluation of early intermediate care services/schemes was often patchy and poor.
- The Department of Health has stipulated that evaluation of intermediate care services/schemes is mandatory.
- Evaluation of intermediate care services/schemes is not easy due to a range of uncontrollable variables or factors that may impact upon the service.
- It is important to be clear about what you are evaluating and, wherever possible, to plan this in with the planning and development of new services/schemes.
- There are various frameworks and approaches that may be adopted to evaluate new services/schemes; however, with the emergence of clinical governance support units, etc. their advice, support and expertise should be sought before commencing.

CHAPTER 12

Home: a refuge from the chaos

SHEILA BEGLEY

Introduction

When planning and introducing new intermediate care services or schemes that are provided within the home, the role of carers, particularly lay carers, is usually implicit and can often be pivotal to the success or otherwise of the service. This chapter explores the findings of a study undertaken to explore the experience of both lay caregivers and staff caregivers involved in providing support and care within intermediate care schemes following hospital admission. The study reveals the benefits and value that lay caregivers and staff caregivers place on providing care at home. While at times the demands on lay caregivers can be quite great within the home, this in no way compared with the stress and sense of loss of control when care recipients were in hospital. The findings of this study provide an interesting discourse for those involved in providing care in both hospital and community settings.

Background

As pressure increases to use hospital in-patient resources efficiently and effectively, continuing treatment and rehabilitation in the home is an increasingly important feature of National Health Service Planning (DoH, 2000b, 2000c, 2001h). The use of the home as a site for continuation or completion of treatment has been described as an 'intermediate zone' (Stacey, 1993: 209) for the provision of 'intermediate care' (DoH, 2001e; Vaughan, 1998). In shifting recovery and treatment aspects of care into the home from the hospital, there is unexpected and unexplored potential to disadvantage home lay caregivers unjustly (Stacey, 1993).

This concern over the potential to disadvantage home lay caregivers prompted an exploratory study of caregivers' perceptions of their roles in intermediate care. The study revealed that unexpected serious illness interfered with established life patterns and expectations, which disrupted long- and short-term plans for both the care recipient and their carers (Begley, 2002). The caregiving relationship often existed as part of closely entwined biographies within family relationships of spouse, daughter or son. Disruption in the biography of one within these relationships had an inevitable effect on other associated parties. The occasion of unexpected illness caused a shift in family relationships, which was accompanied by varying degrees of lifestyle change, depending upon the severity of the illness (Begley, 2002; Conger and Marshall, 1998; Corbin and Strauss, 1988). An important factor in regaining control over the disruption in lifestyle was found to be the domain in which caregiving was conducted. It is this aspect of intermediate caregiving which is discussed in this chapter.

Study background

The findings discussed here formed part of the findings of a larger study. The study involved open-ended interviews with 13 lay and 29 staff carers from the full range of disciplines involved in intermediate home care provision across eight care schemes. While the main study involved the perceptions of lay and staff caregivers, this chapter limits the discussion mainly to the perceptions of lay caregivers in intermediate home care. In this chapter quotations are used to enhance the discussion where appropriate, C indicates the quotations taken from lay caregiver interviews and S from those of staff intermediate caregivers. Any names used in this chapter have been changed to protect the identities.

A Grounded theory method was used to guide data collection and analysis. Data were categorized into three 'timelines' which described the variations in intermediate caregiving experiences in which lay caregivers particularly expressed how the usual patterns of their lives were suspended during unexpected severe illness. The concept of caregivers' lives being conducted in relation to metaphorical timelines related to the normal, often rhythmic, patterning of aspects of the daily life, which was often disrupted by the onset of severe unexpected illness. Disruption in normal lifestyle patterning was exacerbated by the need for patients to be transferred from home into the hospital (Begley, 2002). Disruption in this context was described in terms of 'Timeline Destabilization', which focused upon three main areas where destabilization occurred in caregivers' lives:

• *Bureaucratic or organizational destabilization* – whereby caregivers' existing life patterns were reconstructed to fit into an established bureaucratic or organizational structure. An example of this was scheduled visiting hours, which required caregivers to change the patterns of their everyday lives to fit in with hospital-imposed schedules. Caregivers complained that activity in the hospital responded to a bureaucratic control over time rather than responding to the needs of the patients and their families.

- *Personal destabilization* – whereby caregivers described losing their sense of place in the world through changes in work role, reduced personal contacts, and loss of companionship from the patient now in hospital. All these resulted in feelings of caregiver isolation and loss.
- *Social destabilization* – which occurred through changes brought about in relationships and interactions with others. These changes were marked primarily by changes in the usual pattern of dependency between lay caregiver, patient and other staff caregivers.

Caregivers' need for stability and security

The concept that intermediate caregiving can be described in terms of the three timelines was built from interview data which showed that caregivers strove to re-establish a sense of control and stability in their lives which had been disrupted by illness. This drive for stability in personal biography is not a new concept and is not related only to the caregiving situation. Allatt (1992), for example, in an examination of unemployment identifies people's innate need for stability in their lives. This is identified in parents' desires for their unemployed children to be 'settled', 'secure' and 'settled down'. These sentiments reflect parents' desires for stability and ordered progression in their children's lives, with events occurring at the right time and in the right way.

Intermediate care in the study followed an episode of illness and subsequent hospitalization of the care recipients. It was the period of hospitalization that was identified as the most destabilizing issue in all three timelines. It was during this period that lay caregivers' perceptions of control over their lives were at their lowest, leaving them feeling excluded from caring, lonely without their normal course of companionship, and isolated from their normal everyday life. Most of the lay caregivers experienced the hospital period as highly stressful and described the period as one in which their perception of personal control, and control over what was happening to the care recipient, was at its lowest.

Stability through control

Control can be seen to be highly significant in lay caregivers' perceptions of their role in intermediate caregiving. All of the lay caregivers referenced back to the hospital period and their relational perceptions of control in the home and the hospital domains.

Control, traditionally, is discussed in nursing and non-nursing literature in relation to power, authority, patriarchy and hegemony (Connell, 1987; J. O'Connor, 1996; Rafael, 1996). In psychology, control is defined through individuals' perceptions of their potential to undertake some action to alter the outcome of an adverse stimulus (Miller and Combes, 1989). Perceptions of control relate in psychology literature to emotional well-being and increased success in coping with stressful situations, making behaviour changes and improving personal performance (Cook, 1993; Helgeson, 1992; Seligman, 1975; Thompson et al., 1993). Thompson et al. (1993) suggest that powerful situations in everyday life can threaten the sense of control. The onset of illness in a loved one, for example, forced alterations to established work or lifestyle patterns, and resulted in high stress and low control being experienced by lay caregivers in this study.

Lay caregivers employed a range of strategies to control events and limit their impact. Intermediate home care served as a compensatory strategy through which the event of illness in a loved one could be more controlled. Generally, illness was a situation over which caregivers had little control. However, there were aspects of illness, which could be stabilized through various caregiver strategies, which were facilitated by intermediate home care.

The relationship between domain and controllability of the caregiving experience

Intermediate home care provided caregivers with the potential to conduct care in a domain that related to the normal patterns of their daily lives. Draper (1997) provides powerful arguments of the importance of the caregiving domain in influencing perceptions of control and stability. Control and stability in people's lives are closely related to the identification and location of identity through places and things. Draper (1997) suggests that the location of identity in places occurs through three basic areas:

1. The static physical setting
2. The activities that are associated with the place
3. The meanings that the place holds (adapted from Draper, 1997: 101).

Hospitalization and control

The importance of these aspects of domain featured strongly in lay caregiver data. The hospitalization aspect of lay caregivers' experiences indicated high levels of instability and thus low perceptions of control. These feelings of instability and lack of control were attributed to caregivers' separation from their normal daily rhythms; this was particularly evident in the hospitalized phase of the care recipients' illness. Threat was perceived to be more severe in the hospital environment than in the home because of the hospital's association with acquired infection and staff shortages, which were related to concerns over the quality of caregiving, as illustrated in the following quotations:

> C: The sputum jar in the room was never cleaned, the room was never cleaned properly, there were no paper towels and there was no mouth care. He was supposed to be turned every two hours but he was lucky to have been turned every 6-8 hours because there was just not enough staff. They're [the ward] so busy and they had lots of incontinent patients and patients that called out so mournfully ... when he came home with the IHSS he got better quicker.
> C: The nurses in the hospital were obviously very stretched, there wasn't enough staff to cope with what they had. There was a lady in the hospital with my husband she wouldn't have food. Some of the nurses tried ... but they really didn't have the time to feed her properly, she died and I thought at the time if there were more nursing staff she could have had more attention.

Lay caregivers were concerned that the care recipient was stripped of personal control while in hospital and that staff were unable to take the time to get to know the care recipient as a real person. Patients were often referred to as 'the gall bladder' or 'the diabetic in bed 3'.

This depersonalization in hospital care is most notably discussed in Goffman's (1961) old but still valid conceptualization of the total institution. Goffman (1961) describes the hospital as governed by rigidity of routine, block administration of treatments, depersonalization and social distance between staff and clients. More recently, hospital care is interpreted in an industrialized context whereby treatments are conducted in terms of time economy by herding together those with similar needs (Gibson, 1994; Farrell et al., 2001). While providing care over the 24-hour period, staff have contact with the patient for only 'a minute at a time' (Gibson, 1994: 115). Begley (2002) describes these aspects of hospital care were described through the concept of the bureaucratic timeline, which was perceived by intermediate caregivers as having broad effects on how care was delivered. Lay caregivers expressed their perceptions of threat in their concerns that care recipients' identities were being subsumed to the needs of the institution. They often felt that this accounted in part for their poor relationships with the hospital staff, which were perceived as affecting the quality of care the recipient received.

According to Helgeson (1992), the severity of the threat directly correlates with how important it is to the individual to control it. However, control strategies have to be determined in relation to how controllable the situation is perceived to be. So, it is not surprising to find that, while hospitalization was perceived by lay caregivers to present a considerable threat, caregivers also saw this period as one over which they had low levels of control. Low personal timeline control resulted in caregivers' feeling that they were helpless in influencing hospital caregiving activity.

> C: The worst thing was feeling that they could refuse to treat him or they could make us wait all night if they wanted to.
> C: We noticed that Dad had a temperature and told the nurses, of course she didn't believe me until she took his temperature. She phoned the doctor and it took about four hours for him to come, I saw him standing at the desk reading the notes and I thought, fine he'll be in soon. I waited another hour then asked the nurse, she said he was in to see your father an hour ago. He had gone into the wrong patient, even took blood from him there was nothing wrong with that man, then it took him another four hours to come back.

These feelings of helplessness were often exhibited in feelings of anger and dissatisfaction against hospital staff. Hospital staff were perceived as enforcing bureaucratic control. Frankenberg (1992) suggests that hospitalization itself is a major mechanism of control, not only of time but of the activities undertaken there. Frankenberg concludes by arguing that the hospital, in 'claiming to act in the interests of the subject, does not detract from its exercise of power' (Frankenberg, 1992: 27).

Home care and control

Intermediate care, in contrast, was conducted in a domain facilitating the perception of high levels of control in both groups of caregivers.

> C: Every day at the hospital there was a problem, but having him here I have peace of mind and nothing and no one can harm him. When you're a carer you do more than just administer, you have to make sure the food is done, their medications are given on time. You owe it to them to make sure that they're not sitting in faeces and wet. Where in the hospital do you get that sort of care?

Stability in lay caregivers' personal timelines occurred through what Rowles (1983) describes as *insideness* which stemmed from people's attachment to their home. Insideness linked lay caregiving to places, possessions and relationships which drew upon the past, present and future of both the care recipients and lay caregivers in assisting with regaining a sense of stability in their lives.

> C: It's much better being a relative of somebody at home, you are so used to your own surroundings.
> C: You have much more control over your life at home, you can eat when you like sleep when you like.
> C: Sarah came on so much better at home. They got the care in straight away and all the care was here for her. When you get one-to-one care at home it is much

more effective because you know they are in the house just for you, you don't
have to share them.
S: If you are on a limited time you just go in and do things as quickly as you can. I
don't put time restrictions on the staff by supporting the patients; their confidence
increases and that's what it's all about.

Caregivers, while arguably unable to control the illness to any greater extent
in the home, perceived that they had more control over caregiving, which
made the situation less stressful.

The identification of the home as a place of perceived stability and control
is examined in the literature (Draper, 1997; Rutman and Freedman, 1988). A
notably insightful account of the significance of personal control over space
is provided by Porteous (1976) who supplies detailed support for the notion
that personal control can be located through attachment to the home
domain. Porteous (1976) sees control as secured through two major means,
personalization of space and the defence of space. Personalization acts to
promote identity so that one is not only known by oneself but also by others,
which in turn enhances self-determination.

The appearance of the home is constructed and reconstructed to reflect
the self-perceived identity of the owner, decorative style, ornaments, pictures,
etc. In the home, caregivers identified links with their past through material
objects which held memories and meanings of significance, which helped to
reconnect with, and give a sense of order to, their personal timelines (Twigg,
1999; Jeon and Madjar, 1998; Kellett and Mannion, 1999). Often lay
caregivers would take out old photographs of themselves and the care
recipient, their wedding, the birth of their first child, him in the army, all
important clues to the person with a significant timeline.

S: You are working in an environment where there is Mrs Smith's furniture, Mrs
Smith's photographs, Mrs Smith's garden as opposed to Mrs Smith's hospital bed.
C: It was a different atmosphere at home, as a relative of someone at home, you are
so used to your own surroundings. If you get back home again it's a booster.

These material objects helped staff caregivers to connect with aspects of care
recipients' personal timelines, identifying them as individuals with different
needs and interests from other care recipients. Both staff and lay caregivers
felt that these differences were unnoticeable in the hospital setting but
would have had a significant impact upon care provision.

C: The IC team consists of some very caring ladies. They would ask my Dad if he
wanted a shave, they would ask if things were good, they would communicate
with my Dad, they had time for him. They would ask if he wanted the football on
now and they would talk to him like he was a human being.

> S: I went to see a 92-year-old, who had a mild stroke. He was able to do the stairs, get around and I couldn't understand why he had been referred. He hadn't received physio in the hospital because he was mobile. Then he said, when we were having a cup of tea, that before the stroke he used to play golf three times a week and I said 'Hang on a minute, he's not ready for discharge'. So we went into the street, did kerbs and up hills. If he had been referred to the hospital for physio it would have taken weeks to get it and he may never have got to play golf again.

In conducting care in the home, therapies and treatments could be undertaken to adapt to the physical environmental differences from one home to another. A general view of intermediate care staff was that the home was a much more appropriate environment than the hospital to conduct rehabilitation or set up long-term therapy.

> S: Let's face it, if you're trying to rehab someone in hospital to do the stairs they get these three little stairs to go up and down and nobody's got stairs like that at home, they've got huge long Victorian stairs. It's more realistic rehabbing someone in his or her own home, getting out of his or her own bath rather than doing it in hospital. In hospital they may be able to walk around because they have nice shiny floors with no clutter, you've got to teach them to do it at home.

In the home, strategies could be put in place to support normal family activity. One couple, for example, usually prepared dinner in the kitchen together. Prior to his stroke, Ben would prepare the vegetables while Sue prepared the remainder of the meal. It was a time in the day where they talked, laughed and shared a task together. Once home from hospital it became obvious that all Ben needed was a perching stool in the kitchen for them to continue to undertake this daily activity, to return their lives to as near to normal as possible. Simple things like this were often not identified in the hospital because the environment simply did not relate to individual lifestyles.

Twigg (1999), in exploring the spatial ordering of care, also identifies the importance of dignity and privacy in the home and the capacity of caregivers to construct stability in their lives by controlling who enters and when. This idea was confirmed by lay and staff intermediate caregivers.

> S: When they are in hospital, I wouldn't say it's power but it's the nurses' domain and they have to adhere to the way that things are done in the hospital. Whereas in the home it's their (care recipients) domain and you are more relaxed about what they are doing. You are a guest in their home and the roles are reversed, you have to respect their privacy and it's a better way of working.

In the home, control over domain is inverted from the pattern of the hospital. The staff caregivers entered the home as an invited guest, bound by the confines of social convention, with lay caregivers controlling access to private spaces.

These observations highlighted the importance of lay caregivers' need for control in caregiving and identified the home as a significant factor in their search for stability, security and identity, not only for themselves, but for the care recipient. These revelations were seen by staff and lay caregivers as increasing shared control over caregiving. Intermediate care is found to enable a more meaningful understanding to be developed of both the home caregiving situation and relevant aspects of the care recipients' and lay caregivers' personal timelines.

Lay caregiver involvement in care provision in relation to domain

Intermediate care acts as a vehicle for empowering care recipients and lay caregivers to have more control over the context and content of care provision. In intermediate caregiving, choice was an important factor in influencing caregivers' perceptions of control. Rodwell (1996), in an analysis of the concept of empowerment in health care, suggests that the present economic climate, which emphasizes self-reliance and self-care, increases control by lay caregivers. However, control in this context can be achieved only when caregivers are able to make choices and influence their own future. In intermediate care, choice is not available to all people and may be constrained by many factors. While it is argued here that intermediate care invoked empowerment through the ability to choose the domain for care provision, this applied only to those judged able to meet scheme criteria. So, although intermediate care could be seen as promoting lay caregiver empowerment and thus control and stability, it was achieved through the implementation of staff control, through the application of scheme criteria. Scheme criteria acted as a system of bureaucratic control over resources and aimed to be selective over those admitted to the schemes.

To some extent scheme criteria also linked to a bureaucratic division of labour, with one group endowed with the power to admit or deny admission to the scheme based upon professional status. Casey (1995) observes that the bureaucratic socialization of nurses requires that they perceive themselves as experts in controlling the care situation, with lay caregivers acting as passive recipients of advice. This was certainly true in terms of admission criteria and assessment. However, once admitted to the scheme, intermediate care staff were often found to be willing to relinquish control over direct care encounters, although they still perceived themselves as professionally responsible and accountable for care provision.

> S: Me coming in offering professional advice with all the risks that it involves for me. Giving you advice that goes wrong means that I have to do it and be responsible to accept the liability of giving that advice.

In the intermediate home care context some aspects of bureaucratic control appeared to be welcomed by lay caregivers. Lay caregivers felt more involved with care planning and often referred to themselves as part of the intermediate care team.

> C: I could say she needs so and so and they would write it up, you felt part of the team you were involved.
> C: The nurse puts the ones [dressings] in the morning and I sort out the night time ones. The nurse comes in and says 'Can you continue?' It's very reassuring. They are very good.

Lay caregivers were often happy to work within the team and gained physical and emotional support from the interaction. Being associated with the team, lay caregivers felt that they were supported in caring and at times were also relieved of some of the responsibility for home caregiving.

Casey (1995) argues that nurses feel threatened by knowledgeable and experienced caregivers and act to limit their involvement in formal care settings. This notion was replicated in many lay caregiver stories when referring to the hospitalized aspect of care. Lay caregivers often felt that their expertise in caring was often dismissed in the hospital setting, to the detriment of care standards.

> C: In the hospital his [husband's] blood glucose was going high and we didn't know why. It turned out that they were giving him ice cream. They didn't know that he was a diabetic. It was a bit careless they should have put a sign above his bed or something. At least now I have him at home I can monitor what he eats.

However, intermediate care staff were conscious that the service was time limited and that any treatment that was intended to be long term should, where possible, be managed by the care recipient or the lay caregiver in order for them to maintain as much control over their lives as possible.

> S: There really isn't a need for a nurse to carry out this type of treatment [peritoneal dialysis]. I don't think it's an underhand method of reducing the workload of the nurse, it's simply that it's a treatment where the patient [or lay caregiver) can be independent and take responsibility for their own care.
> S: You have to get back to people taking responsibility for their own health.

Once home, with intermediate care, patterns of care and dependency could be re-established. Mary had looked after Tom all of her married life and was used to caring for him 'in sickness and in health'. When he was taken into hospital she felt disconnected from her normal caring role and was lost and isolated until he returned home. Other lay caregivers perceived that their timelines were more stable and predictable at home and their sense of control over their own, and the life of the care recipient, was increased.

C: I feel important looking after him. Everybody else that comes in has their own job to do but I am most important because I am here all the time. I look after all aspects of his care. I am here all the time.

C: If she had gone into hospital I would have been at a loss, I wouldn't have been able to do for her in the same way. I wouldn't have liked her being in hospital.

Lay home caregivers felt more able to direct aspects of care. This was directly related to the shift in domain and the consequent increase in lay caregivers' sense of control. Intermediate care had the potential to change assumptions about the power dynamics of care provision. In intermediate care the caregiving domain, being another person's home, was clearly more controlled by lay caregivers' than scheme staff and as such shifted the power dynamics in the interactions. Intermediate care, while still redolent of aspects of Goffman's (1961) total institution, in the requirement for assessment of appropriateness to scheme criteria, staff shift patterns and staff time schedules, also endorsed caregiving partnerships and facilitated direct lay caregiver control of decision-making and management of care.

In summary

Many lay caregivers experienced low control with high levels of stress during the hospital period of care provision. In the hospital, lay caregivers conducted their relationships with the patient in small snapshots of allocated time during visiting hours. Other activities in the home were disrupted in order to allow hospital visiting, with lay caregivers often having to negotiate unfamiliar travel arrangements, etc., all increasing the sense of loss of control over their lives. During this period lay caregivers felt separated from their normal routines and activities, such as work, domestic activities and interests. They were also often separated from their usual networks of community support through these changes in routine.

In the hospital, lay caregivers felt that their competency in providing care and support was often dismissed or questioned. This was associated with a bureaucratic division of staff and lay caregiving roles. Many lay caregivers also experienced distress related to the levels and standards of care they observed in the hospital, and associated with this was a sense of trivialization of their concerns by hospital staff.

Once care was transferred into the home, lay caregivers felt that their lives were more stable. Intermediate home care acted to promote increased caregiver control through shifting care into a domain which held connotations of security, privacy and personal identity. The home domain provided lay caregivers with a sense of familiarity and security. They were often able to resume many of the activities associated with their everyday lives and re-establish normal relationships with the care recipient and the community they lived in. Through caregiving in the home, lay caregivers were able to project to scheme staff a sense of themselves and the care recipient as individuals with a past, present and future through the display of mementos of significance, thus promoting a sense of personhood. Often other family members became involved with care, shifting the balance of caregiving relationships from the hospital into the home.

In short, intermediate care in the home was more real and relevant to the lives and aspirations of not only the care recipient but the lay caregiver and their wider social context, and provided the means to gain a sense of stability in their personal and social timelines. Intermediate care was found to be a significant development in placing the care recipients and lay caregivers at the centre of care planning and care provision and is a step forward in the provision of person-centred care. Furthermore, the application of the concept of theoretical timelines to the planning and provision of intermediate care services can be used to enhance the development of person-centred care. Timelines focus on each individual as having a past, present and future related not only to the person as an individual, but also in relation to the society within which he or she lives and functions.

KEY POINTS

- When illness occurs in a family or relationship it can disrupt the established patterns of daily lives, especially those of lay caregivers.
- Providing care in the home was much less stressful and disruptive for lay caregivers compared with care in hospital.
- While care recipients were in hospital, lay caregivers experienced a sense of low control and high levels of stress – much of which related to standards of care, and they felt that their competence in providing care was often dismissed or questioned.
- At home, lay caregivers felt that their lives were more stable and that they had much more control over events, while also retaining a sense of normality and personhood.

PART IV

Delivering Intermediate Care: Preparing Staff for Delivery

CHAPTER 13

Developing staff

SIÂN WADE

Introduction

So far this book has provided a background understanding and insight to intermediate care and some of the various services that it may constitute, along with other issues that concern older people receiving care. The first three chapters in Part I provided an examination of the concept and context of intermediate care and its evolution and development, along with an exploration of how services for older people may develop and evolve. Part II (Chapters 4 and 5) provided an introduction to the ageing process and how it may affect older people - a key client group within intermediate care - along with an examination of perspectives of older people within society, and especially within health care. The focus then moved on to examine the planning and development of intermediate care services and initiatives associated with these services/schemes that may help to promote their effective delivery.

In this part, the focus shifts to centre attention more on the delivery of services for older people. While focused on intermediate care, much of this has equal relevance to staff in other settings and services. The emphasis here is on the importance of the preparation, development and education of staff working within intermediate services/schemes and with older people. This chapter provides an initial overview of some of the preparation and development needs of staff. Some of those elements that have not already been covered so far are then enlarged upon in ensuing chapters.

Background

As is evident, the planning and creation of a new intermediate care service/scheme are complex, especially where a new building is involved. It is a considerable undertaking and requires immense time and energy. This, however, is really only the beginning, for the process of getting a service off the ground operationally is another very significant stage, and needs to be thought through and planned very carefully if success is to be achieved. It is unfortunately this stage of a new development that often falls down and sadly it is this stage, in particular, that may account for the difficulties of some of the early intermediate care service developments. This may also be the case where new intermediate care services have been developed within existing services, such as care homes or district nursing services that are required to extend their current practice to incorporate the concept of intermediate care. While careful planning of the what and how of the service may have been undertaken, it may be that, once commenced, the staff in a home or service have then been expected to deliver the service without adequate, if any, preparation. This comes down to expecting staff to change the culture and approach to the way they work, without knowing or exploring how. Steiner (2001) discusses this issue in her article exploring intermediate care. She also discussed it in the evaluation of the service she was involved in setting up (Steiner, 2000), recognizing that the way staff worked may have been influential in the way the service was provided and in the subsequent outcomes and effectiveness of the service. Thus this stage is equally as important and crucial, if not more so, than any other stage in the success of a service. It is emphasized throughout much of this book and this signifies its importance.

Team-building of staff working within intermediate care services

As identified, however well planned a new service is premeditated, it is essential that the staff who are going to operationalize it are prepared. In relation to the staff working within the service/scheme, team-building is really a prerequisite so as to promote clinical effectiveness and high-quality care. Those involved in the planning and creation stages, are not usually those who actively provide the service, although some of those who have been involved may hold senior positions in relation to the new service, and practitioners may also have had some involvement.

It is almost an inevitable part of the evolutionary process of service development to appoint staff at a later stage, i.e. after it has been planned and is being established, with a clearer idea of its purpose. This can have its problems, because when it comes to operationalizing the newly created service with the intended outcomes, planned care, pathways of care, and protocols that have been produced, there are bound to be challenges and the need for review. New staff, or staff transferred from other services, need to have the opportunity to develop an understanding about what their new service is all about, through exploration and debate, as at this stage it may be that some rethinking and revision are required. This is crucial when a new service is being developed, and will need to be supported with ongoing integrated team-building, as suggested by McCormack (2001b) (see Table 13.1).

Table 13.1 Some strategies to promote effective teamworking

Clinical supervision

Mentorship/preceptorship

Regular multi-disciplinary staff team meetings

MDT case/patient reviews

Individual personal development plans

Reflective dialogue

Conflict management

Patient/user forums

Follow-up team-building sessions to allow review, ongoing clarification of team values and consolidation

It is also important for any new member of staff coming into a new post to have a substantial induction with ongoing development, and within this there needs to be the opportunity to discuss in depth the aims of the service and expected outcomes together with working practices. Preparation for all staff appointed to an intermediate care service should involve visiting and gaining insight into the services and situations from which patients may be referred to their service. This enables them to appreciate the situation or setting from which referred patients may come. It also provides the opportunity to meet those staff they may work with at a distance, so that they can start to develop working relationships with these staff and begin to network. Knowledge of staff in other services seems to greatly enhance the care that patients experience – mainly because interpersonal communication and know-how is usually improved.

Initial team-building provides the opportunity to plan team objectives, systems and processes, and to begin to establish relationships. An initial approach is to provide a forum to create a team philosophy for staff and for patients. The key purpose of this is not to create a glossy, framed statement written in jargon, but to reach an agreement together about what the service aims to provide, and the approach to care. This should then be reflected in the whole working culture of the service. Within contemporary service provision, this needs to take a person-centred approach so staff will need to explore what they mean by this – see Chapter 14. There will need to be an agreement about how the multi-professional team members will work and this will need to be explored so that there is common understanding of what this means and how it will affect working relationships and working patterns within traditional roles, as discussed in Chapter 16. If new roles have been introduced, such as generic workers or rehabilitation assistants, these roles will need to be discussed and examined, as indeed will traditional roles, with all team members. Adopting a culture of rehabilitation is no easy task and again this will need exploration – see Chapter 16, along with developing skills of looking after and understanding the care of older people (see Chapter 4). There will be a need for general and specific skills acquisition and extended roles to be assessed and addressed for individuals, along with individual personal development plans, although this has not been addressed here. There are also key areas such as discharge planning, decision-making and problem-solving, that are of particular significance to staff working in these areas; hence these are addressed in more detail in Chapters 17 and 18.

An initial introductory programme and development plan is suggested in Table 13.2 for staff who are starting with the implementation of a new intermediate care service. The importance of the logistics of delivering this cannot be over-estimated, because however well planned recruitment is, it is almost certainly going to be staged, i.e. all the new staff will not start on the same day. Similarly, pressure to commence and operationalize a new service will probably be an imperative. Somehow this all needs to be juggled to ensure that staff have been adequately prepared to commence the service, which is then built upon through ongoing staff development. Some of these areas have already been addressed in earlier chapters and can be used to provide the foundation for some of these sessions, while others identified are addressed in later chapters.

Induction provides a basis from which to work and continue staff development, and this ongoing development may incorporate the following areas:

- more in-depth exploration of areas covered in induction;
- visits to identified services involved in patient care pathways;
- specific care needs and required extended roles;
- individual personal professional development plans.

Preparing supporting staff

While very careful attention must be given to the staff working within a new intermediate care service/setting, attention also needs to be given to those

Table 13.2 Staff induction and development programme – suggested areas

Setting intermediate care in context – the political scene and policy issues

Creating a draft philosophy for staff and patients

Exploring what is meant by person-centred care/life review – how do we do it?

Exploring roles and multi/interdisciplinary teamworking

Rehabilitation – what is it? what is our role within it? How can we promote it?

The experience of transition for patients experiencing lifetime changes

Introduction to ageing (to be addressed in more depth through ongoing staff development)

The Single Assessment Process – to include comprehensive geriatric assessment

Care pathways

Discharge and transfer process

Risk-taking throughout the patient's care pathway

Decision-making and problem-solving

Revisiting original philosophy

Emerging issues

---

staff who will be involved in the referral of patients. A key challenge faced by those involved in setting up new services has been related to under-utilization or inappropriate referral. This may be due to a range of reasons. It may be that the referral criteria are not clear, or can be too loosely or too strictly interpreted, although it has to be kept in mind that the care needs of older people in particular can change quite rapidly. Equally, it may be that staff who are required to refer to the services do not have these services at the front of their mind. This may be because they do not know about them, because they are very busy (which is no doubt the case), because they cannot remember what all the new and newly developing services are for, or indeed what the criteria for referral are. In hospitals this difficulty can be assisted by developing a single point of referral with designated staff such as discharge liaison sisters, who can be contacted and who can then advise on the appropriate referral destination. Similarly, a specialist nurse or integrated multidisciplinary teams of staff in A&E and MAU (Medical Assessment Unit), and perhaps across wards and clinical units for older and vulnerable people, can assist staff in their decision-making and also in providing appropriate care – see Chapter 18. The mandatory introduction of the Single Assessment Process should also help to direct patients to the right service, as discussed in Chapter 10.

Finding effective ways of informing staff about the services available needs to be identified and addressed, e.g. providing flow charts in A&E cubicles and ward offices, while short road-shows or presentations can help. However, the reality is that even with these prompts, the presence of specific staff and regular visits by others, as suggested, is probably essential if referral is to be maintained and staff are to find out about and remember the services. Within contemporary health and social care there are just so many staff coming and going within care settings and services that it is perhaps unreasonable to expect them to remember or keep informed about all these services. What they do need is to be alert to the fact that there is probably a much greater range of service options now available and that they need to be considering these for their patients and seeking advice about the most appropriate referral destination.

Another unfortunate reason for the underuse of new services seems to have arisen when GPs, nurses or other staff have made referrals, and their referral has been rejected. This needs to happen only once, or at most twice, for confidence in the service to be lost, leading to a reluctance to try to refer again. Rectifying this situation certainly presents as a challenge, for reassurance that the next referral will be accepted is unreasonable if not appropriate. Spending time with a referrer, or working through case examples, may be the best way of helping them to understand, but this is a hugely time-consuming activity for all those involved. What is clear is that the preparation of staff who are potentially going to refer to these services needs very careful thought and consideration, and the time involved must not be underestimated.

Conclusion

This chapter has provided an overview of some of the developmental needs of staff who work with older people and who work within intermediate care. As identified, some of these areas will be explored in more depth in the remaining chapters of this book.

Key points

- The preparation and development needs of staff involved in intermediate care is as important as the planning and creation of the service – all too often this is given low priority in the guise of 'getting the service into operation'.
- Practitioners providing an intermediate care service need a carefully planned orientation and induction together with ongoing development – this should form the basis of the development needs of any new staff in the future.
- Practitioners utilizing intermediate care services, i.e. those who may wish to refer patients or who receive patients from the service also need to be carefully prepared so that they understand the expected purpose and outcomes of the service, and the criteria for referring.

CHAPTER 14

The crux of person-centred care

SIÂN WADE

Introduction

Providing person-centred care is fundamental to effective recovery and rehabilitation for the older person, and for their continued well-being and peace of mind, when receiving help and support from any health and social care service. As discussed in Chapter 4, helping the older person make transitions at a time in life when personal control may be most challenged and compromised is also imperative, and this can best be achieved by taking a person-centred approach. This chapter provides some background to the concept of person-centred care and this is then built upon in later chapters, and in particular when looking at rehabilitation and helping the older person through transitions.

Background

While person-centred care and concepts such as respect, dignity, independence and autonomy should be inherent within health and social care provision, evidence clearly suggests this is often not the case, with ageist practice still existing (Social Services Inspectorate, 1997; HAS, 1998; Barber, 2001; DoH, 2001h; Help the Aged, 2000). As Hughes (1995) discusses, the values seem 'simple in their expression but highly complex in their translation into behaviour and practice'. Within intermediate care and those services involved in providing care for older people, person-centred care is imperative, for it is not possible to work towards rehabilitation goals unless these are agreed and known by all involved – particularly the patient. This emphasizes the importance of the team working collaboratively within intermediate care if effective high-quality care is to be experienced by patients.

This chapter explores central features of person-centred care and discusses ways in which staff may be assisted to gain insight into effective ways of delivering person-centred care. There is also some discussion around the attributes that staff need to enable and help them to promote person-centred care.

Hughes (1995) identifies three key values that may help to challenge an ageist perspective:

- The belief in personhood of all. The value of personhood ascribes to people of all ages the authenticity of being alive and having lived.
- Citizenship concerning the relationship between individuals and society, and how that relationship is defined. Here the concept of citizenship emphasizes the rights of individuals and the reciprocal responsibilities for both the individual and society, whereby the older person is validated not only as a person, but as an equally valued member of society.
- Celebration of later life and the richness of a long life, where life expectancy has increased significantly in just 50 years (Coleman and Bond, 1999).

The key principles of anti-ageist practice embrace the concepts of empowerment, participation, choice, integration and normalization – as outlined within the *National Service Framework for Older People* – NSF (DoH, 2001h). This in effect requires the practitioner to enter into partnership working and is perceived as central to providing high-quality of care. While these are all good principles, and rightly so, they are in practice very hard to fulfil for many reasons, and publishing a framework such as the *National Service Framework for Older People* is not a simple answer, although it may help to drive changes and raise awareness.

Partnership working is something that has not come easily to practitioners or indeed to some older people (Biley, 1992a; Wade, 1995b). It requires 'changed thinking', as reflected very aptly in the quote by the Department of Health (1998a):

> The drive to place quality at the heart of the NHS is not about ticking checklists – it is about changing thinking.

Developing a person-centred approach to care involves shifting the power base from the health care professional to the older person, and as such listening to the voices and aspirations of older people and their carers.

Quality of life

A key challenge for those working with older people is to establish how older people measure quality of life and successful ageing. The effective use of assessment and comprehensive assessment is seen as key to being able to appreciate what is important to an older person, and therefore to guide their goals and aspirations with appropriate intervention. As indicated, what the professional perceives as important may not be the case for the older person. While an emphasis on promoting independence and getting older people home may be a measure of quality of life for the professional, the older person may have different priorities. As Nolan et al. (2001) point out, the preoccupation with objective measures of success and the importance accorded to the functional abilities of the older adult, as with activities of daily living, has tended to dominate perceptions about their quality of life. They argue that there are 'striking discrepancies' between the views of professionals and those of disabled people, such that, as Peters (1995) suggests, 'professionals and users often have significantly different understanding of the phenomena that initially brought them together' p. 8. For older people, the use of life review or biography is key to gaining insight into what indicators constitute 'quality of life'. This provides the opportunity to gain a sense of the past, present and future for the individual, so shifting the emphasis away from a problem-orientated model of care to focus on a much more holistic approach, taking account of psychological, social and emotional needs such as hopes and aspirations. Thus the emphasis on biography, continuity and meaning seems to become central to quality of life indicators in later life.

There are a number of ways that practitioners may be assisted in enhancing the way they work with older people. Older people should have been involved in the original planning of new services – a requirement within the *HSC/LAC Intermediate Care Circular and Implementing the NHS Plan* (DoH, 2001e, 2002f), and supported by the Better Government for Older People initiative. This involvement should continue once the service has been set up and is operational, and may be in the form of patient forums as discussed in Chapter 7 – perhaps supported by the work of PALS (DoH, 2002f).

Life course review or biography offers a personalized account of an individual's life course. This focuses on the individual's interpretation of their own experiences and events throughout life, from their own world view and lifetime perspective. The concept of life review and biography helps to provide an understanding of the ways in which different structural or social factors interact with the experiences of an individual – influenced by their own personality and interpersonal experiences throughout life. This helps to create insight into the individual and offers the opportunity to appreciate the unique response to, and patterns within, old age for different individuals. Personal biography does not negate the common experiences of older people within their cohort experience, but allows for the expression of the individual and their experiences within this and throughout life. This provides an approach to exploring how different older people interpret, negotiate and respond to old age. Thus, as Johnson (1988) contends:

> just as societies are currently analysing current events in terms of their own history, so individuals are in a state of lifelong self-reflection and reassessment of who they are and where they are going. (1988: 139)

Life review has become recognized and valued for its role in the practice of health care. Apart from often providing an effective form of therapy through reminiscence, it also provides an approach that can be adapted and adopted to enhance assessment and the negotiation of unique care, acknowledging the individual's own beliefs and values, as identified by Leininger (1985). How it is utilized is up to the practitioners concerned, but the Burford Holistic Model of nursing (Johns, 1991), Appendix 14.1, and the first question, 'Who is this person?', provides a template from which to work and can be utilized by all practitioners, not just nurses.

As Denzin (1989) suggests, life review provides an opportunity for a wider recognition of the uniqueness of people's lives and personal experience. This can give insight into how an individual has managed during their life, and therefore how they may manage or cope with their life now and in later life, especially if faced with life changes and transitions. It can help explain how and why people may behave as they do as older adults and perhaps while in care. Life review can also provide insight into how wider social, political and environmental events can powerfully impinge upon and influence the course of peoples' lives. While not addressed here, life review has also provided an approach to research methodology that can be used by practitioners in a very productive way, and which has relevance to their day-to-day work (Leininger, 1985; Stanley, 1993). In exploring the experience of those with dementia, Lynott (1983) found that biographical work by friends or relatives of those with dementia was very effective. It revealed the persuasively social character of the disease, the diverse nature of their related experience, and how much biographical work can bring people together when attempting to make sense of their experience.

In order to use life review with patients, it is important for practitioners to have utilized the concept to some extent experientially themselves. This gives them an appreciation of the very personal and sensitive nature of using life review and helps to highlight how it may arouse memories and emotions for patients. Thus it is an approach which, while it may be very useful and beneficial for the patient, should not be entered into lightly. It is not intended here to cover the use of life review, more than to suggest a way in which it may be used with staff experientially. Undertaking any activity in relation to

Kivnick and Murray (1997) believe that such relationships are dependent upon 'interpersonal mutuality'. Williams and Grant (1998) support this, believing that there is a need to have 'knowledge of people as individuals', and to 'explore and recognize their ideas, beliefs and lay knowledge'.

Brändstädter and Greve (1994) identify three processes that people may adopt to sustain psychological well-being, which is helpful when considering quality of life, especially with those whose abilities and control on life are being compromised. These processes are described as:

- *Assimilation* – where the individual makes efforts to sustain current activities/interests by, for example, maintaining levels of fitness or using aids and adaptations.
- *Accommodation* – where the individual endeavours to replace current activities/interests with equally valued new ones, or to maintain current interest but in a more achievable way.
- *Immunization* – where the individual either ignores certain evidence that threatens strongly held beliefs or places more importance on the past rather than present achievements. This provides support for the sensitive use of reminiscence in a therapeutic way – especially for older people where their accounts of past activities and achievements help to confirm their present personhood.

An example of how this model might be demonstrated is when considering someone who has a real interest in cars and driving. It may be that for some reason their muscle strength is compromised – perhaps due to a degenerative illness. This challenge may be overcome initially by purchasing an automatic car so that they can continue to drive (assimilation). Eventually it may be that this is no longer sustainable, but the individual may be able to become involved with some activity that involves cars, such as selling cars, or managing a transport or driving company, thus maintaining their interest (accommodation). Eventually the individual may no longer be able to undertake this role, so may now enjoy watching car programmes, attending car events and, when in company, talking about cars and particularly about their knowledge and what they did and achieved when involved themselves (immunization).

Interpersonal competence

It is evident that if truly person-centred care is to be provided for older people within intermediate care services, staff need to have enhanced interpersonal skills, so as to gain both personal knowledge and to give confidence to patients. This takes as much precedence as the competence in technical skills and knowledge about health care needs, as well as therapeutic care. Hinshaw and Atwood (1982) demonstrated that of 14 predictor variables used to assess patient satisfaction, 10 related to affective variables and four to technical variables. Both Fossbinder (1994) and Tarlow (1996) identified attributes needed by staff to demonstrate interpersonal competence. In Fossbinder's (1994) ethnographic study, she demonstrated that when patients were asked 'what happened when the nurse was taking care of them' they described overwhelmingly the interactive style of the nurse. Thus interpersonal competence was the primary focus of their comments, not the task the nurse was doing. From her study, Fossbinder (1994) identified four emerging processes to provide a framework for interpersonal competence, as shown in Figure 14.1. Other key interpersonal attributes that seem significant include taking a genuine interest in the patient, their concerns and their carers, and demonstrating an understanding and appreciation of 'how it is for them'. These later skills are very much reflected in the therapeutic style attributed to a Rogerian person-centred approach to care, as described by Thorne (1984).

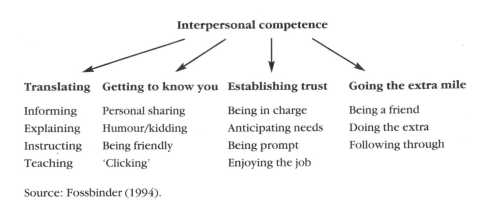

Source: Fossbinder (1994).

Figure 14.1 Emerging theory of interpersonal competence.

Conclusion

Taking a person-centred individualized approach to care, where patients are involved in choices and decisions and shown respect at all times, provides a mechanism to avoid ageism. Practitioners need to be able to understand and know each of their patients as an individual by really getting to know them, as discussed. They need to know how much to involve an individual patient and when and how. They also need to understand how to involve relatives and carers sensitively so that they feel valued and acknowledged. Taking a person-centred approach will also help the practitioner to find ways to assist the older person address transitions that they may be facing, as discussed in the next chapter, and to be able to better manage the demands associated with the work of rehabilitation – see Chapter 16.

KEY POINTS

- Within any service, the importance of keeping the person at the centre of our thinking and care is imperative.
- Working in partnership and respecting the individual seems an obvious aspiration for practitioners but in reality it is challenging to achieve. It requires 'changed thinking' and 'a shift in power' for both the practitioner and the patient/user.
- What constitutes quality of life for the user/patient may conflict with the perceptions of the professional, and this needs to be recognized and acknowledged.
- Appreciating an individual's life course/review will go some way towards seeing them as a unique individual person.
- Drawing on a range of theories and frameworks may assist us to gain insight into the wishes and views of those we care for. This can help us to explore what is important to each individual so that care and interventions can be modelled around these values and aspirations.

Appendix 14.1 Life review and transitions

Consider your life-course please. Think of times or situations when your life course has changed. You may consider such events as going to secondary school, becoming a student, becoming a qualified nurse, leaving home, moving house or job, marriage, starting a family, etc.

Having identified these events/situations, please give thought to the following:

- How did you feel when faced with undertaking this activity?
- Did you have difficulty remembering key events?
- Were you able to influence the event or situation, e.g. did you choose them, initiate them, organize them or did they happen by chance, or were they forced upon you?
- Can you identify any form of process or stages that you experienced as a result of this change?
- Can you remember/describe any of the feelings that you experienced at the time of this change in your life course?
- Now consider the kind of changes that older people may experience in their life course in later life.

- Can you identify any differences or similarities between the changes you identified and those that older people may experience?
- What skills and strategies might you adopt/develop to assist an older person to make these changes?

Appendix 14.2 Burford Nursing Development Unit Holistic Model of Practice

Core question

What information do I need to able to care for and nurse this patient?

Cue questions

- Who is this person?
- What health event brings this person into my care?
- How is this person feeling?
- How has this event affected their usual life-pattern and roles?
- How does this person make me feel?
- How can I help this person?
- What is important for this person to make their stay comfortable?
- What support does this person have in life?
- How do they view the future for themselves and others?

CHAPTER 15

A world of transitions

SIÂN WADE

Introduction

When considering person-centred care, quality of life and life review, the concept of 'transition' plays a significant part, as already identified. As individuals, we experience transitions throughout our lives, such that they are an inevitable part of our life course. Consideration of the experience of transitions when working with older people and those who have experienced a life-changing illness is of particular importance and relevance within the context of health and social care in promoting quality of life. In this chapter the concept of transitions will be explored, looking at how older people may cope with transitions, the kind of transitions they might experience and how health care practitioners can help facilitate such transitions. Individuals may need to come to terms with some significant changes in their lifestyle, where plans for the future are completely shattered. Skill in recognizing and understanding the effect of such transitions for patients, and in helping patients through these transitions, therefore has a significant place for staff working within intermediate care settings/schemes, and they need to be equipped to sensitively undertake this.

Understanding transitions

A transition has been said to be 'a passage from one life phase, condition or status to another' and as 'a process that forms a bridge from one reality that has been disrupted to a newly constructed or surfacing reality'. The task of the individual experiencing a transition is to incorporate the disruptive event and its consequence so that personal integrity and a sense of self and wholeness are maintained or regained. Thus a transition extends the concept to some kind of movement, involving a process of entry, passage and exit, which takes place as a three-part psychological process where the individual moves from one state to another, as portrayed in Figure 15.1.

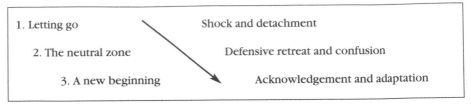

Figure 15.1 Stages of transition.

A key feature of a transition is that there is no going back, therefore there is a need for the individual to accept the change and find a way of incorporating it into their life course without its compromising their self-esteem and personal integrity. This may be a very significant challenge causing considerable stress, for it may be that the individual experiences some life-changing event, such as compromised mobility, or some disability which means they have to rethink the way they work or live. Holmes and Rahe (1967) found that, compared with younger people, older people assigned greater magnitude on a Social Readjustment Rating Scale to life events, and therefore concluded that change is perceived as more difficult for older people. This could be because the older person feels they have less control over such changes, and this demonstrates the importance of practitioners having the skill and insight to help older people adapt.

The effects of stress on the individual have been well investigated and researched, and it is well recognized that it can lead to both physical disorders (Eysenck, 1990) and psychological distress such as anxiety, depression and anger, as well as negative social behaviours (Sarafino, 1998). The level of stress experienced may be relieved or eased if the individual can be assisted to adapt to stressful events or activities; thus adaptation is an important feature in dealing with transition. Adaptation may be defined as:

> an anatomical, physiological or psychological response to changes in an individual that occur as a reaction to stress

or

> defences with which the individual attempts to counter a stress by limiting its site, lessening its impact or neutralizing its effect so that the body (and mind) can continue to function. (Saxton and Hyland, 1979)

Coping

The way in which an individual deals with such an event may vary, but it is likely that some coping mechanism or strategy is required, and this may be adaptive or destructive. Lazarus and Folkman (1984, cited in Atkinson et al., 1985) suggest that coping is aimed at reducing or managing stress, while Sarafino (1998) suggests that the word 'manage' is significant as it indicates that effort is required to cope and that this can be quite varied and not necessarily lead to a solution of the problem. Sarafino (1998) also sees the coping process as not just one single event but a concept that involves a number of ongoing transactions with the environment. Lazarus and Folkman (1984) concluded that coping served two main functions:

- *Problem-focused coping* – the individual focuses on the problem, evaluates the situation and does something to avoid change, such as being proactive. This is aimed at reducing the demands of the stress situation, extending the resources to deal with it or finding alternative interventions/activities. Examples may include leaving a stressful job, seeking private medical advice, choosing a different career, etc.
- *Emotion-focused coping* – the individual focuses on the emotional response to the problem, where the aim is to control the emotional response such as trying to reduce anxiety without dealing direct with the anxiety-producing situation. Thus the individual may try to distract their attention from the problem by watching TV or going out with friends. It is believed that people tend to use emotion-focused approaches to coping when they believe they can do nothing to change the stressful situation (Lazarus and Folkman, 1984), e.g. the exam is tomorrow and I haven't done any revision – it is too late now!

As practitioners, being aware of the impact lifestyle changes may have on an individual is fundamental to having the insight and ability to help the individual recognize what is happening and to help them find ways of 'dealing with it'. Being aware of how an individual has coped in the past may help us to appreciate a patient's behaviour and how this may reflect their way of coping, and inform us on how we might be able to help them. If, for example, it has been a characteristic for an individual to avoid challenges when faced with them, it is possible this is how they will deal with challenges presented when in care. Thus if an older person/patient is worried that a home visit will fail, they may introduce a range of mechanisms to prevent it happening, maybe trying to delay it. The home visit inevitably needs to be faced, so the practitioner needs to find ways that will best help the patient through this challenging event, showing empathy but being realistic at the same time and giving support. This could be described as 'problem-focused' coping. Alternatively a patient may realize that they will need some help if they are going to be able to go home. Because this is something they find undesirable, they may try to suggest alternatives that are unrealistic, or avoid talking about it in the hope that maybe the reality will go away or they can perhaps stay in hospital. This may seem a more desirable alternative at the time, perhaps because of the security felt while there, and the familiarity of the staff. Here again the practitioner will need to draw the patient round sensitively to face up to and discuss the reality of managing at home, and will need to try to find ways of reaching a mutually agreeable solution that enables the patient to go home and manage without feeling compromised.

Freud, and later his daughter Anna Freud, proposed a series of mechanisms described as defence mechanisms, which may be adopted by an individual when reacting to change or stress, some of which are outlined in Table 15.1.

Table 15.1 Examples of use of defence mechanisms within our practice

Rationalization - Don't worry, my neighbour will help, she always has. However, the neighbour has told nursing staff the demands upon her are becoming too great and she is unable to continue with her help.

Projection - Relatives complain about care due to own guilt of being unable to offer care themselves.

Denial - Patient with severe arthritis is unable to get out of bed without a hoist, and insists at a case conference that she will be able to get up herself when she gets home as she desperately wishes to go home and genuinely believes that she will be able to manage there.

Displacement - Patient is angry with nurses because they are unable to do something themselves. This may lead to a complaint such as the dust collected on the radiator or blaming the practitioner for some action they have or have not taken.

Controlling - Patients who are very dependent, e.g. MS/arthritis, become very particular about the way things are placed around them, as they are unable to have any control themselves.

The patient/carer may be totally unconscious of what is happening when they adopt and display defensive behaviours and tactics. They may feel they are in a desperate situation and are subconsciously dealing with it in the only way they can relate to. For the practitioner, it is important to be able to recognize what is going on, for it can help them understand and appreciate the behaviour of the patient/carer and take account of this. It can also be useful in helping them recognize that they should not take personal offence and enables them to handle it in a calm and reasoned way. It is useful to quote complaints and critical incidents in staff training, as analysis of some of these will display evidence of defensive behaviour and can be used to help prepare staff in how to prevent and deal with such behaviour and how to cope with their own feelings.

Patients receiving care in an intermediate care service or setting may have experienced any one or more of a range of transitions, as outlined in Table 15.2. In later life there is a tendency to relate transitions to deteriorating health and the subsequent effects of this on other aspects of life, such as relocation. The practitioner needs to be able to acknowledge this where it is the case; however, it is not inevitable and the transitions experienced by older people may be very positive life course events. Patients within an intermediate care setting may also have been unwell and away from their home for some length of time. It may well be that they are able to return home, but this may be together with changed circumstances, such as a deterioration in health or a disability, or with services visiting at unexpected times. Even if the individual has regained their health in general, the whole experience of returning home after a long period away may be quite distressing, and staff need to be aware of the need to provide support and understanding of the anxiety and concerns that patients may have in order to help them. Services such as the Red Cross and WRVS often provide valuable support to patients as they go home, and help them make this transition.

Table 15.2 Transitions that patients in intermediate care may face

Change in health status/illness – abilities/independence

Change in individual/role developments – mid-life to later life

Change in relationships/family developments – mother/grandmother/ daughter/carer

Death of a loved one and bereavement

Organizational transitions – policy changes that affect lives, e.g. Community Care Act/eligibility criteria

Changes in expectations/aspirations of achievements

Situational transitions – day care/widowhood/relocation to a nursing home/relocation or needing care

When considering how an individual is coping, there are a range of features that may influence and affect this coping. This is where an understanding of the individual from a life course perspective can be of help and value to the practitioner and may help them to predict reactions and understand them – see Table 15.3. Similarly, drawing upon the principles of giving person-centred care, as discussed, will have significance.

Table 15.3 Features that may influence ability to cope with transitions

---

Past experience of how the individual has dealt with significant life changes or transitions

The characteristics of the particular transition and recognition of the significance of the
transition to the individual's change in lifestyle and functioning

The pre-morbid character of the individual and ability to deal with the transition

The support mechanism that may be available to individuals to help them through the
transition and in their future life course

Previous coping mechanisms

The who and why of the person and their selfhood

The characteristics of the pre- and post-transition environments

---

Transitions and chronic illness

Anton Antonovsky (1984) has examined in great depth the way that people
cope and adapt to transitions related to chronic illness. Within his work he
describes the concept of a '*sense of coherence*' (SOC), which he uses to help
explain how people come to terms with their illness and some of the factors
that may influence their ability to respond and cope. He defines the concept
as involving three elements, and this offers a useful framework to consider
when working with patients and older people:

- *Comprehensiveness* – making sense of chronic illness by asking questions
  such as 'why me?', 'why now?' and then understanding how the emergent
  illness is unfolding. Reviewing one's health history and its cause and effect
  can start to give sense to a situation, while an eventual clear diagnosis can
  give validity and reassurance that there really is something wrong. Then,
  however, there is the uncertainty of progress of the illness, as chronic
  illness can often have an uncertain trajectory, and this can cause anxiety
  and problems. Furthermore, there may be a powerlessness to control
  symptoms. Here a narrative reconstruction may help, by helping to
  ensure that the challenge is understood, so demonstrating appreciation
  and empathy by the practitioner.
- *Meaningfulness* – the meaning of both the illness and transition may
  change as a result of its changing course. Establishing what the chronic
  illness means to people in terms of its effects on their body, their minds
  and their social situation is important if they are to be able to manage and
  adapt to these changes. Meanings are culturally significant, but most are a
  threat to the individual's competence with the significance of becoming
  an invalid and therefore IN-VALID, accompanied by the threat of social
  stigma. Where there is uncertainty and ambiguity, the individual may feel

vulnerable, and if the condition is denied little progress may be made, e.g. with rehabilitation or physiotherapy, etc. Giving hope and the motivation to wish to try will be an important role for the practitioner.

- *Manageability* – the ability to manage one's own life may be difficult, especially due to the uncertain prognosis and trajectory. A perplexing state of being neither sick nor well may account for some of the variation in adaptation. There is often uncertainty of the relative effectiveness of recommended medical regimens, and health promotion behaviours carry no guarantee. The problem with chronic illness is that it involves not just pain and psychological distress but also for many, as Charmaz (1983) describes, 'a crumbling away of their former self-images without simultaneous developments of equally valued new ones'.

A process of reconstruction may occur within the context of uncertainty and unpredictably of the course of illness. This may involve remissions when hopes and expectations rise, only to be later dashed when the individual regresses again. Charmaz (1983) identified four ways in which the self is under assault due to chronic illness or disability, shown in Table 15.4.

Table 15.4 Ways in which the self is under assault due to chronic illness

Having to lead a restricted life

Being discredited

Social isolation

Being a burden to others.

For the practitioner, it is useful to consider the stages that an individual may go through during a transition such as outlined in Table 15.5. This may help them recognize the different stages so as to provide appropriate support and understanding of the older person and their experience.

Table 15.5 Stages an individual may go through during transition

A need to face up to the change, to recognize and accept the symptoms/problems as they are in order to be able to manage them, i.e. perception of the event.

A need for time to reflect and think it through, to redesign lifestyle in order to mitigate these changes. This may require pacing oneself or balancing activity due to the often-unknown trajectory. It may also affect issues of compliance with treatment.

A need for support.

The ability to become aware of oneself and the environment, and to incorporate new experiences into past identity, such that it may be a time for personal growth when the individual is able to make sense of, and derive meaning from, the experience.

Transition and relocation

There will inevitably be times when the patient or individual who is receiving care within an Intermediate care setting or scheme, needs admission to a care home. Relocation to a care home can be a very traumatic transition for an individual, and the ability to deal and cope with this may be influenced by the individual's perception of the move, their coping mechanisms and their situational support (Holmes and Rahe, 1967; Young, 1990; Morgan et al., 1997). This may also be influenced by other losses or transitions occurring concurrently and as such these may need to be dealt with at the same time, e.g. the effects of a debilitating illness and/or the possible loss or death of a loved one, etc. Chenitze (1983) examined the experience of relocation and described three basic conditions that affect the response of the individual to relocation, as outlined in Table 15.6. Placing this transition within a framework related to the process of relocation, as in Table 15.7, may be useful to the practitioner in helping to facilitate the older person with this.

Table 15.6 Three basic conditions affecting response to relocation

Centrality – refers to the significance of the move

Desirability – a measure of the willingness

Legitimization – reflects the perception that the relocation is warranted, e.g. for financial, physical or social reasons

Table 15.7 Framework of process experienced when relocating

Ending of previous lifestyle/environment/friends, etc.

A neutral zone – is a time of limbo, characterized by a disconnectedness from both past and future. This requires time to reorientate to the new situation, and work through emotional upheaval.

A new beginning – realigns expectations with reality and engages with new activities (may be influenced by other transitions which may have led to the need to relocate – so could have implications).

The role of the practitioner in relation to transitions is very much a facilitative one to support the individual and help to give them confidence and assurance. This can help to enhance a sense of well-being and can be assisted by preparing the individual for the continuity of care, helping them to understand what is happening, and showing understanding and insight into the transitional experience.

Thus, when relocating, the older individual may be helped by:

- having knowledge of the precipitating event;
- having the opportunity to ask questions about the home and being enabled to visit it and meet staff and if possible other residents, so that they can participate in deciding where they would like to go and also so that they are informed of where they are going and feel they know some people prior to their move;
- being assisted to maintain contact with their previous lifestyle as much as possible, such as engaging in previous interests and activities, seeing friends, telephone calls, etc.
- being able to bring some personal possessions;
- giving help, time and counselling if needed to facilitate reflection and evaluation of life – just having someone who cares and is willing to listen or spend time may be of value;
- having activities or developing new interests once settled.

It is important that the practitioner is aware of the support and care needed by relatives/carers at this time, as they may experience 'a range of emotional reactions' as suggested by Dellasega and Nolan (1997: 445). There may be a range of reasons that lead them to feel a sense of guilt when the decision is made for a relative to go into a home, and this may mean they will feel a sense of having to 'live with the consequences' as described by Nolan et al. (1996) cited in Dellasega and Nolan, 1997: 445). The admission to care does not mean the end of caregiving for relatives/carers, but may be the start of a different form of caregiving that they may need to adapt to and engage with so that they still feel involved. Thus they will need time to begin to adjust to the changing circumstances, and it may be most appropriate to try to begin this process prior to the move, by beginning to broach the subject, as suggested by Dellasega and Nolan (1997).

Practitioner skills and attributes in facilitating transitions

Thus practitioners need to be aware and be concerned with the process and the experience of human beings undergoing transitions where the promotion of health and perceived well-being is the outcome. This requires skill and attributes, as outlined in Table 15.8, and knowledge of the process of transitions (see Table 15.9).

Table 15.8 Skills and attributes required of practitioners

Listening and having empathy, with good communication and counselling skills – anticipatory counselling may be important

Offer understanding and help when individual trying to make sense of a situation

Support to problem-solve, clarify understanding, thoughts, and gain increased insight into own experience

Offer knowledge about available resources and information

Skills of organization of work and time

Table 15.9 Knowledge required by practitioners to undertake this facilitative role

The processes and experiences of human beings who are in transition

The nature of emerging life patterns and new identities

The processes and conditions that promote healthy outcomes

Environments that constrain, support or promote healthy transitions

Structure and components of nursing therapeutics that deal with transitions

Knowledge related to transitions into new roles and new skills

Conclusion

Older people entering intermediate care service/schemes will very often be experiencing transition, which may have a very significant life-changing impact for them and their carers, and can be traumatic. Helping an individual psychologically and practically to deal with such events is crucial, for failure to do so can impede their progress and well-being. Developing and fine-tuning the expertise to help patients address the challenges presented are an important element of the work of staff in intermediate care, and it is therefore important to include this in staff preparation and to identify ways of continuing to develop their skills.

KEY POINTS

• Older people entering intermediate care may be faced with significant life-course transitions which may cause distress and trauma.

• In particular, these transitions may relate to the need to face up to, or come to terms with, a chronic or debilitating illness or to accept the need to relocate to a new home environment.

- Practitioners providing care in intermediate care services/schemes therefore need to have an understanding and appreciation of what this may mean to those in their care and how this may be manifested in their behaviour.
- Practitioners can help and facilitate those in their care by helping them to understand what is happening and by showing understanding and insight into what is happening.

CHAPTER 16

Rehabilitation and team-working for effective outcomes

SIÂN WADE

Introduction

As outlined, the promotion of independence is a key objective within the health and social care policy agenda, leading to an increased interest in rehabilitation and thus the interest in intermediate care (DoH, 1998a; DoH, 1998c; HSC/LAC, DoH, 2001e; DoH, 2001h). Because of this underlying and fundamental link between intermediate care and rehabilitation, it is appropriate to devote a chapter to rehabilitation and multidisciplinary/ inter-disciplinary teamwork, in more detail. The intention here is to examine the concept of rehabilitation and how this relates in particular to older people within intermediate care. Teamwork goes hand in hand with rehabilitation and is crucial if both rehabilitation and intermediate care are to succeed.

Background

Grimley Evans and Tallis (2001) lament the demise of interest in rehabilitation over the past two decades, prior to contemporary policy. They describe how specialist geriatric rehabilitation was gradually eroded within acute hospital care, with its place as an element of the comprehensive care of older people marginalized. This shift, as discussed, seemed to be associated with the preoccupation with bed-management and capacity, and the drive to reduce patient lengths of stay. They also warn of the danger of confusing convalescence (spontaneous recovery) with comprehensive, complex and specialist rehabilitation that is required to 'make non-spontaneous' rehabilitation happen. Rehabilitation, they argue, is of course costly and can take time. They believe that such specialist care and rehabilitation cannot be transferred to intermediate care. What needs to be addressed, therefore, is clarity about those older patients who require specialist rehabilitation and those who will benefit more effectively from general rehabilitation in intermediate care.

Defining rehabilitation

A wide range of definitions for rehabilitation have been proposed, such that the ability to reach a uniform understanding is problematic (see Table 16.1). The reason for this can probably be attributed to the fact that effective rehabilitation seems to mean different things to different people. Although there are certainly similarities, the perceived disparity of views has contributed to confusion over the actual purpose and process of rehabilitation. Becker (1994) argues that rehabilitation remains centred on the ethic of medicine and the doctrine of cure. The focus on quantifiable and measurable outcomes such as survival, functional ability and discharge destination, which dominated the ethos behind early definitions, may in no small way account for this – particularly when referring to older people. For older people, such a focus may not be their greatest priority, and indeed may not be a realistic goal. Robinson and Barstone (1996) argue that the extent to which an older person will benefit from rehabilitation will depend very much upon the way that rehabilitation and its aims and purpose are conceptualized. The concept of frailty often associated with older people is a further complexity. Young et al. (1999: 184) describe frailty as being related to 'true' or biological ageing (as opposed to age-related disease), which leads to compromised physiological/functional reserve, as discussed in Chapter 4. The

Table 16.1 Definitions of rehabilitation

'An active process by which those disabled by disease or injury achieve full recovery, or if a full recovery is not possible, realize their optimal physical, mental and social potential and are integrated into their most appropriate environment'. (WHO)

Rehabilitation is... 'the whole process of enabling and facilitating the restoration of a disabled person to regain optimum functioning (physically, socially and psychologically) to the level they are able or motivated to achieve' (Waters, 1994).

'An educational, problem-solving process aimed at reducing disability and handicap' (D. Wade, 1996)

'A process of aiming to restore personal autonomy in those aspects of daily living considered most relevant by patients or service users and their families' (Sinclair and Dickinson. 1998).

'Rehabilitation focuses on re-enablement, facilitating and trying to recapture motivation so as to help people to adapt to changes in their life and circumstances. It must be of therapeutic value to the older person with the ultimate aim of maximizing social well-being' (RCN, 2000).

effect of this is that minor stress events result in 'disproportional functional consequences' which lead to 'unstable disability' and resulting fluctuations in functional ability – evident when working with frail older people.

The need to take into account the holistic needs and wishes of the older person and what they perceive as important for their quality of life cannot be over-estimated. This is where the goals of the professional and those of the patient may well show some disparity. The emphasis on addressing disability, where there is a restriction or lack of ability, rather than focusing on the perceived handicap, or the level of inconvenience and interference with personal fulfilment of the patient, can be a major flaw in the aspirations of the purpose of rehabilitation. This can lead to some of the dissonance that arises, and unless well addressed can lead to incompatible goal aspirations. Redfern and Norman (1999) discuss the importance of creating a therapeutic environment and culture when promoting rehabilitation with older people that is responsive to their needs. Thus, the importance of creating therapeutic relationships and recognizing the emotional needs of older people in planning care and interventions is crucial, as discussed by Nilsson et al. (1998).

A survey of multidisciplinary staffing profiles within specialist rehabilitation services for older people, compared to rehabilitation services for younger people, could well reveal a relatively poor skill mix and staffing level ratio to the number of patients when balanced against the dependency and rehabilitation needs of the number of patients. Where this occurs it could be argued as tantamount to older people receiving a second-class service, where staff have lacked the time and often the skills to give the level of person-centred therapeutic care that the older person deserves. Waters (1994: 242) describes the 'persuasive organizational routines' often found in rehabilitation settings for older people, where each discipline undertakes activities in isolation and there is no goal-directed person-centred care. Although her work is now almost ten years old, the findings of a study undertaken for the ENB (2001b) confirmed this concern. They found that 'even in specialized rehabilitation settings time constraints, work priorities and skills were crucial hindrances to the nurse working in a rehabilitative and individualized way' (ENB, 2001b: 3). Thus, ensuring appropriate staffing and skills acquisition is essential if Intermediate care is not to become a Cinderella service, although with the current recruitment problems this is no easy task. The situation can, however, be improved by paying attention to the preparation, development and education of the staff and their approach to work.

Young (1996) argues that the main aim of rehabilitation for an older person should be to realize their full potential, to resettle in the community and to find role fulfilment. While these may not be the aspirations of all older people, they provide a good framework from which to work and complement the principles of those models described by Brändstädter and Greve (1994), Stevernick et al. (1998), and Nilsson et al. (1998), as discussed in Chapter 14. To achieve this, the importance of appreciating the meaningfulness of any rehabilitative activity and addressing emotional needs becomes paramount, with the importance of instilling hope, as described by Spencer et al. (1997), as a key aim. Understanding rehabilitation in this way allows for a whole range of rehabilitation needs, including those of people who have mental health needs and those with cognitive impairment, as may be the case for older people. Of significance here, the need to give attention to social and recreational interventions is implicit, yet these sadly are often invisible or almost invisible in many settings. In the case of patients with cognitive impairment, using the work of Kitwood (1997) and principles of Dementia Care Mapping may also be very helpful in achieving these interventions.

The wide-ranging needs of the older person signify the importance of effective teamwork within rehabilitation when it comes to discussing and agreeing collaborative goals with the patient. This way, all can work together to help achieve these. Here again, the importance of comprehensive individual assessment is paramount in identifying the needs and the aspirations of the older person. Their life-course experience and their personality will influence this, hence the significance of obtaining a life-course perspective of each individual older patient we care for (McCormack, 2001a). As discussed, this does call for skill and expertise and highlights the need to have skilled practitioners involved in the care of older people. Failure to identify the rehabilitation potential of an older person not only compromises the opportunity to improve the quality of their life, but can actually lead to ineffective care and inefficient use of beds – possibly extending patients' length of stay in hospital inappropriately and in some cases affecting their discharge destination. Such an outcome is an indictment of health and social services and of the use of public money. Young (1996) also criticizes the tendency to time-limit rehabilitation, and the imperative position that professionals find themselves in, in trying to identify an end-point. Grimley Evans and Tallis (2001) confirm this concern. Rehabilitation is an ongoing activity and almost never ends. The preoccupation and focus on time limits is a challenge for any rehabilitation service, since they are constantly under scrutiny with imposed pressures of limiting length of stay, although at some stage an end-point does need to be agreed. It is no less of a challenge for intermediate care services. In some cases very short timescales are imposed (some rapid-response services have a five-day commitment) with the goals of intermediate care tending towards six weeks, although the onus on this may be more relaxed than the original guidance implied (HSC/LAC Guidelines, DoH, 2001e). While such constraints may have a place, they may also be compromising for older people who, due to their frailty, may reveal a recurring history of fluctuating good and poor health, which directly affects the process and progress of their rehabilitation trajectory.

If staff are to support rehabilitation they need to have had the opportunity to discuss and explore what it is, as well as to have training in certain skills and to have practised these. While the priorities of rehabilitation for each individual may differ, there are a range of principles and attributes that are of significance to staff involved in rehabilitation. First, it is important to remember that it is the patient who is the key person in rehabilitation. They can be helped immensely by staff who work with them, but it is the patient who will have to do the work and therefore they need to want to do it. This will require considerable energy as well as patience and perseverance. For this reason, reaching mutually agreeable goals with the patient is essential, and these need to be appreciated, acknowledged and accepted by all staff working with them, as well of course by the patient. Failure to do this may mean that the patient does not know what their own goals are – not an uncommon feature of some rehabilitation services. Similarly, if each staff member has different goals they will be working to different interventions and could compromise the continuity of care. This will lead to confusion on behalf of the patient and indeed may lead to a situation that might be interpreted as non-compliance. It is also important to involve the family and carers, where appropriate and possible, especially if they are to play a part in the ongoing care on discharge from the service. However, the importance of respecting the older person's wishes and views is significant, so at times this may need to be handled with great care, sensitivity and honesty.

Rehabilitation can be described as an active process that is deliberate, planned, skilled and continuous. It may be regarded more as a function of services, not necessarily a service in its own right (Nocon and Baldwin, 1998). It is not so much what we do, but how we do it. Rehabilitation with older people may be multi-faceted and, as identified, may mean different things to different people. It may involve focusing on functional ability, i.e. about lessening disability, maintaining ability and preventing its deterioration. Indeed, it may mean lessening the rate of further deterioration, for it has to be acknowledged that some illnesses are deleterious and the effects of their continued deterioration can only be slowed and not prevented. It may be more about restoring well-being and regaining or maintaining social roles, so as to enhance quality of life. The aim will usually be to maximize potential and abilities, while preserving dignity and personhood. For older people there is often a need to find ways to adapt to and integrate changes brought about by old age at the same time as those brought about by illness, for sadly the environment is not always amenable. To help the older person achieve this requires practitioners to act as enablers in the process of re-enablement. There are a number of attributes that are imperative in achieving rehabilitation goals. As identified, the need to establish a relationship and take on board the emotional needs are important. The importance of instilling hope and enhancing motivation may also be very influential in the success of ongoing rehabilitation.

Three key foci of rehabilitation may be helpful for staff to keep in mind, as listed in Table 16.2, while Young (1996a) summarizes a number of key purposes of rehabilitation – see Table 16.3.

Table 16.2 Three key foci of rehabilitation

- Enhancing and maintaining quality of life
- Restoring holistic well-being
- Preventing further illness/disease or deterioration

Table 16.3 The key purposes of rehabilitation

- Realization of potential
- Re-enablement
- Resettlement
- Role fulfilment
- Readjustment

Source: Young (1996a).

As discussed, rehabilitation involves a much wider remit than improvements in functional abilities. It involves addressing a broad spectrum of problems and needs that include physical, social, psychological, spiritual and emotional factors. These therefore need to be identified through effective assessment and will be interlinked in the rehabilitation process (Figure 16.1).

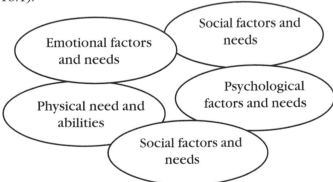

Figure 16.1 Factors involved in rehabilitation

Young (1996) describes rehabilitation interventions as being either 'hard' or 'soft' (Figure 16.2). Hard interventions are those that are more objective and observable, such as 'hands on' intervention. 'Soft' interventions are those that are not always easily recognizable or evident, but involve great skill. They are the therapeutic skills related to interpersonal interaction and involve the development of a relationship and trust. 'Hard' and 'soft' interventions and techniques are closely interrelated and dependent on each other.

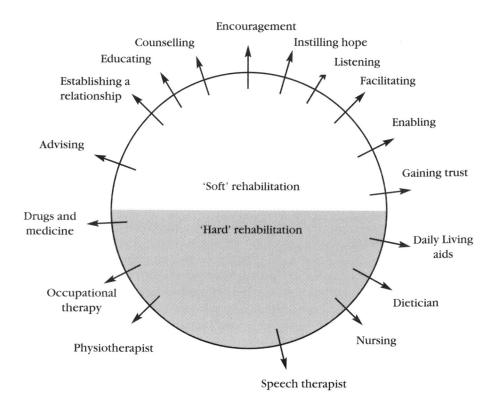

Figure 16.2 Common rehabilitation interventions.
Source: Young (1996).

While the patient is the key player in rehabilitation, there is a misapprehension that the activity occurs only when the therapist is with the patient. This idea completely negates the whole process of rehabilitation. Rehabilitation should be occurring 24 hours a day, and should occur with every activity that the patient undertakes (assuming this has been agreed and they are not too tired). This highlights the significance of the nurse in the whole process of rehabilitation, for nurses are present throughout the 24-hour care cycle. Waters (1994) describes the lack of clarity of the nurses' role within rehabilitation, and yet she argues they have enormous potential to make a significant contribution. She suggests that this state of affairs arises from the lack of preparation and teaching of the principles and techniques of rehabilitation, demonstrating the need to invest in this aspect of the nurses' role, especially within intermediate care.

The RCN (1997) identified a range of key functions of rehabilitation for nurses (Table 16.4), as well as four key activities that they become involved in, as indeed do all team members (Table 16.5).

Table 16.4 Key functions of rehabilitation

- Supportive functions
- Restorative functions
- Educative functions
- Life-enhancing functions/risk assessment
- Teamwork

Source: RCN (1997).

Table 16.5 Activities undertaken by practitioners

- Actual assistance
- Directive assistance
- Supervisory assistance
- Management assistance

This may focus on:
- Improvement – even if slowly
- Maintenance
- Slowing progressive deterioration
- Prevention of secondary problems

In a study undertaken on behalf of the English National Board (ENB, 2001b) before it was disbanded, a comparative analysis of the findings was used to help to articulate the role and contribution of the nurse within rehabilitation. Six key activities were identified (ENB, 2001b: 3):

- *The role of assessment* – especially initial assessment. This is often performed by the nurse, and used to devise the care plan from which first referrals to other members of the multi-professional team are made.

Through their ongoing assessment they provide up-to-date information for other team members and can prevent potential problems.

- *The role of co-ordination and communication*: This embraces responsibility for co-ordinating a whole range of activities, including gathering, synthesizing and disseminating information, liaison, negotiation, and in hospital settings running the ward and co-ordinating discharge planning, as identified in Chapter 18. It also involves accessing other services, and requires good relationships with team members and insight into patients' needs. In this study it was evident that the nurse provided feedback to other therapy staff on the progress of patients and how they were responding to treatments, so enabling these therapy staff to adapt their care plans.

- *The role of providing technical and physical care*: This comprises a large part of the nurse's so-called 'routine work' and provides the opportunity to integrate therapeutic intervention with physical care. This, however, is often delegated to auxiliary or support staff, and highlights the importance of preparing these staff well for their role within rehabilitation.

- *The role of integrating therapy and therapy carry-on*: This requires the nurse to adopt the philosophy and practice of rehabilitation, along with additional skills and knowledge. *Therapy carry-on* has limited focus and in essence involves the nurse carrying out 'prescribed' therapy exercises etc. *Therapy integration* is broader and involves two interconnecting aspects:

1. the nurse's attempts to create an environment which itself is therapeutic and facilitates rehabilitation – seeking ways to minimize physical, emotional and social barriers to rehabilitation;
2. the nurse's role in building on the work of the therapist: taking time to correct transferring or positioning techniques, coaching and supervising the client to the table, using the same technique as the occupational therapist when aiding the patient to wash and dress, etc.

This approach helps to provide continuity of patient care together with more effective rehabilitation.

- *The role of the nurse in providing emotional support*: This tends to be an informal activity, and often involves nurses finding out about worries and fears, and providing advice and reassurance. This takes time, and lack of time by nurses was noted in the study.

- *The role of the nurse in involving the family*: This involves part of the activities of providing information, emotional care, communication and co-ordination. Since nurses tend to be the most accessible practitioner, and the one patients are usually most accustomed to, they tend to be the 'first port of call' when relatives seek information or advice.

There are suggestions that therapists should work across the 24-hour care cycle. However, the reality of this, with the current staffing and recruitment crisis and when the basic daytime hours are hard to fill, seems unlikely. Nor indeed is it probably necessary within intermediate care. Therapists will be giving only a specified length of time to each patient and this is probably best achieved when the patient is up and alert during the daytime. During this time, however, the therapist's time must be focused and well planned. They will need to assess and reassess the patient's progress and their needs. They then need to work with the patient to teach them skills, activities and exercises, etc. as well as to explain and give information. Thus the role of the therapist is very much one of assessment, education, evaluation and reassessment. During their time with their patient they may well need to concentrate on certain work and techniques. Older people, in particular, can sustain only short periods of intense therapy interspersed during the day, and while some of this will need to be undertaken by the expert, aspects can be seen through by nurses or support staff, if understood. If the patient is to gain maximum benefit, this intervention and care will need to be shared with the nurses and ward staff, within the collaboratively agreed goals, in an effective way. They will then be able to continue the intervention, or help and support the patient to achieve their rehabilitation throughout their 24-hour day.

This is where a key role of the nurse emerges – that of continuation of, and building upon, the therapist's work in their absence. This is the aspect that is often poorly addressed, for a range of reasons. Lack of time, as identified, is often expressed as implicit, and may well be the case, where staffing levels are compromised. Other factors may well be related to skill mix and preparation of the staff, as already highlighted. It is, however, this element of continuity that is imperative if the patient is to make headway and progress in a timely way, and must be addressed by providing adequate staffing with appropriate preparation, competence and attributes. It will be important, though, for the therapists to be clear about any activities or techniques that should still only be undertaken in their presence with their skilled supervision.

Often rehabilitation can be reflected in very simple interventions or activities, and yet go unrecognized by staff, patients and relatives. This can result in the failure of nurses to encourage or promote these interventions and the inability to identify and articulate them to patients or their relatives – see Table 16.6.

Table 16.6 Features of everyday rehabilitation

Rehabilitation can involve very fundamental activities, such as:

* walking to the toilet instead of having a commode by the bed
* sitting out for breakfast and being positioned and facilitated so as to eat as independently as possible at all times, with appropriate aids as necessary
* encouraging the older person to wash themselves and going to the bathroom to wash as one would at home
* working in every way to maximize the individual's independence as is reasonable and desirable

In particular, rehabilitation involves facilitative and educative skills, such as:

* allowing time
* being supportive but enabling and encouraging, and at times walking away to allow the patient to be self-reliant and use self-initiative
* using effective skills of communication and education and motivation with patients and carers/relatives

Of equal importance is the need to make sure that the rehabilitation needs of the patient at night are assessed and addressed. As stated, this is when therapists are rarely present. It is also when the patient is most likely to be either tired or drowsy, so that abilities are most compromised. Thus the role of the night nurse is paramount in the successful rehabilitation of patients. An effective means of communicating what the problems and needs are is essential, so that the therapist can begin to work with the patient and begin to address them and draw up a plan of intervention that can be followed by staff at night.

It is of interest to note that specific specialist rehabilitation tends to be synonymous with the view that it involves more therapy time, and yet studies have shown that this is not the case, and it may in fact be the reverse (Young et al., 1999). Young et al. (1999) cite studies which show that around 4 per cent of the waking day of a patient is spent with therapists, irrespective of where they are – acute or rehabilitation settings. This same finding has been revealed within the trials of stroke units. It has also been shown that patients are less likely to die if cared for in a designated stroke unit rather than in a medical ward (Dennis and Langhorne, 1994), and that outcomes for these patients are improved. The actual factors that contribute to this are not clear for, as suggested, therapy time is unlikely to be greater than in a general ward. This raises the interesting question as to what it is that does make the difference in a stroke ward and what is it that is of significance in the process of rehabilitation. It suggests that structure plays an inherent and imperative part in 'cementing' rehabilitation (Young et al., 1999). This relates to the highly individualized nature of rehabilitation treatment and intervention required by each patient.

The process is highly complex, usually involving the integration of a unique set of individual but diverse activities and interventions to reach a positive outcome for the patient. It is this individuality that seems to 'make for' successful rehabilitation, and is closely related to the culture and philosophy adopted by the team and the way they work. Dennis and Langhorne (1994) suggest that for stroke units, effective communication between health professionals, patients with stroke and their carers is fundamental in achieving this way of working, and they propose that this is one of the key factors in the success of a dedicated and integrated stroke unit. It would seem that this is just as important and crucial for the success of any rehabilitation service or setting and it emphasizes the role that inter-disciplinary/trans-disciplinary working can have in contributing to this success, as discussed later in this chapter.

There also seems to be a view that not only does rehabilitation occur only with the therapists, but that this needs to be in the gym, OT department or other specialist setting. The ward or home setting are often not perceived in themselves as central to rehabilitation activity. Thus, if patients are to participate as well as they are able to, it is important to be clear with them that rehabilitation does not just occur when the therapist is present and while in therapy departments, but that it is an ongoing activity involving the whole team, and most importantly the patient throughout most activities of the day and night, wherever they are (Seymore, 1988). It is paramount that an understanding of what to expect is gained. Where a patient is transferring from another service to a rehabilitation service it is important for this to be discussed carefully prior to transfer, as it should go some way to avoiding misunderstandings. If patients have been in an acute setting and are then transferred to a rehabilitation setting or service, the level of activity and sense of intensity may seem very much reduced. If the patient does not understand what is involved they may feel let down and feel they are not receiving the level of service that they were before transfer – and certainly not more, as they may well have been expecting. It is not uncommon for patients to complain that they are not getting the same level of intervention as they had expected, as they had been told they were coming for 'rehabilitation' and that this would involve more therapy.

It is also worth considering the views of Pound et al. (1994). They suggest that with patients who have had a stroke, the patient or their relatives may well complain that they have not had enough therapy. This, they suggest, may well be an expression of disappointment with the amount of recovery they have made, and it focuses on therapy as this is the only treatment they

perceive they have received. Pound et al. (1994) also suggest that
dissatisfaction may well arise from the lack of information given to patients
and relatives about the likelihood of recovery, and argue for providing more
information. This, however, needs to be given sensitively and in a timely way
– although there is possibly never a right time. They go on to suggest that the
very process of undertaking exercises and tasks set by therapists gives
patients and relatives something tangible to work on, so giving them some
sense of control and hope. They thus suggest that if this is the case then the
work of therapists could be built upon by encouraging nurses to develop and
learn the skills to fulfil rehabilitation tasks throughout the 24-hour day (as
should happen anyway) with the patient. Therapists can also train patients to
carry out appropriate exercises on their own or when at home, and advise
carers how to continue the role of the therapist. They suggest that a
challenge for the health services is to recognize the possibility that patients
may gain non-specific benefits from treatment that may not be demonstrated
by functional improvement but may be associated with greater well-being
and hope for the future. Taught treatment, exercises and tasks can be carried
on without therapists present if taught to those who are involved in the care,
and this should be part of the culture within any rehabilitation setting, but
also within longer-term settings, or at home once discharged.

As discussed, rehabilitation settings for older people of any kind often
seem to lack recreational activity. Lack of staff and time is often the reason
given for this. In some settings this is undertaken by occupational therapists,
but due to other more pressing demands upon their time they may need to
concentrate their efforts and time on activities such as assessment of
activities of daily living and home visits, etc. Nurses are also likely to identify
lack of time to undertake such activity. While this may be more to do with
differing priorities about how they work, there is no doubt that nurses are
busy and find it difficult to provide even essential care. Another reason to
account for this is that developing and providing recreational activities that
benefit the process of rehabilitation is really very skilled and certainly
requires a creative leaning. Playing bingo or quizzes may meet the needs of
some patients and may ensure that they are actively engaged for a short time,
but these are not directed towards individual patients' own interests and self-
esteem nor towards assisting in their rehabilitation. In Canada there is a
recognized discipline of recreational therapists who are trained to degree
level as a minimum. Visiting one of the resource centres in Canada, such as
the Baycrest Centre in Toronto is living proof of what this profession can
achieve (Wade, 1995a). Activities will be found that are not only of personal
interest to the patient, but which will provide therapy and use, for example,
of a weak arm or hemiopia following a stroke. Generic workers could be
involved in this kind of activity, and even voluntary helpers, but good

leadership and supervision is needed as well as designated time, preparation and development.

Barriers to rehabilitation

There are a range of challenges or barriers that may be experienced when trying to provide rehabilitation. These includes medical instability or unidentified medical problems which can slow rehabilitation quite significantly, and as already identified, is an issue with older people who may have co-morbidity or compromised functional reserve. Conditions that may not be recognized may include anaemia or heart failure causing the patient to feel fatigued and compromised in their ability to participate as actively in the demanding challenges of rehabilitation. Indeed, rehabilitation activity may be contraindicated if the diagnosis is known. This highlights the importance of a medical overview of patients in intermediate care settings/schemes. There may also be other undiagnosed conditions, such as Parkinson's disease, hypothyroidism or arthritis, etc. Side effects from medications need to be observed, and consideration of these need to be accounted for when working with patients. Some anti-depressants, hypotensives and anxiolytics can cause postural hypotension and dizzyness – especially on standing. It is important to be aware of this and allow the older person to get their balance on standing before expecting them to participate in other actions or activities. Similarly, some medications cause fatigue, as do some treatments, and again consideration needs to be given to this.

It may be that patients are experiencing elements of cognitive impairment or depression which may not have been previously recognized. This may become evident only when the individual is being required to become actively involved and participate. This will inevitably compromise their ability to participate in, and benefit from, rehabilitation. It is important, however, not to exclude them, although the approach and pace of progress may be altered, as may the interventions used.

Failure to achieve rehabilitation may occur where the environment is disabling and may be related to the use of an old or discarded building. This may occur within an institution or in the patient's own home. Alterations to either will not be easy to achieve and will probably take time, if possible at all. Some minor ad hoc alterations and adaptations may be possible; otherwise consideration of these will need to be given in rehabilitation goals and interventions.

As already discussed, rehabilitation is unlikely to be successful where the goals are inappropriate, irrelevant or not mutually agreed or important. Similarly, timing is crucial, as being over- or under-optimistic about the patient's readiness or abilities may be detrimental to their motivation and enthusiasm.

As addressed in Chapter 4, older people may have communication problems which, if not recognized and acknowledged, may compromise their rehabilitation potential. This again asks for skill and effective assessment of each individual. Knowing your patient is important as not all patients may wish to engage in rehabilitation for, as discussed, motivation and self-determination on behalf of the patients is an inherent requirement if they are to benefit fully. Thus earlier knowledge of a patient is important, as it guides the practitioner to appreciate what their strengths and limitations are and to what extent they are going to respond to rehabilitation and therefore help judge how to involve them effectively. There are times when it may become fairly evident that the older person does not want to participate in the activity and process, even when it is explained that they may regress and indeed may be subject to risks, e.g. pressure sores, etc. This calls for a very considered approach when addressing the rehabilitation potential of such a patient, for it is important not to exclude or neglect the patient, although compromise will probably be needed. Skill is required in assessing just what can be achieved and in looking for interventions or ways in which the patient can benefit. Thus a positive attitude has a significant role to play, as does an insight into the patient's life history – see case study (Aunt B).

Case study 16.1 Aunt B

An aunt of mine had a life history of apathy. She had in effect been a 'lady of leisure' and her personality to some extent was one that allowed her to sit back and let things happen to her. She lacked perseverance, and when in her sixties she broke her hip she inevitably developed a dropped foot. Repeated efforts and explanations made by staff to prevent this were to no avail at the time, as were any efforts to promote her independence. In the latter stages of her life her independence became compromised. She persistently refused to use a pressure-relieving cushion, despite a range of different cushions being offered and tried. Knowing her life course and personality helped to explain these reactions, and from a professional perspective made it easier to accept that these decisions were hers and were made with full cognitive appreciation, while interventions that were acceptable were sought. Unfortunately she did not seem very happy and was always complaining so it seems doubtful if she experienced much quality of life – although complaining had been a way of life for her, so it was difficult to judge.

Preventive care

A key feature of rehabilitation for the older person is the implementation of preventive care (Swift, 1988). The severity by which the health of an older person can be compromised due to normal ageing changes or pathology, along with sociological and psychological challenges, can be unpredictable (Herbert, 1986; Herbert, 1992; Dunbar, 1996). This makes older people particularly vulnerable to complications of their health, even when attending to daily needs such as washing skin, taking meals, undertaking activities and resting. Older people are at particular risk of acquired complications, such as infections, constipation, dehydration, fluid overload, electrolyte imbalance immobility, pressure sores and malnutrition, especially when in hospital, i.e. *Clinical Iatrogenisis* as described by Illich (1975). Lack of mobility can lead to many of these complications.

Birchall and Waters (1996) assert that lack of attention to the particular activity needs of older people in acute settings contributes to their increased dependency and subsequent 'delayed discharge'. Yet in these settings the needs of those more acutely ill may take priority over those of older people who no longer need acute intervention. Older people may then become regarded as problematic, and are often referred to as 'bed blockers', once their care needs have altered. This in itself can lead to resentment and tension in staff, and may be picked up by patients, thus inhibiting their recovery. This supports the need for alternative settings such as specialist rehabilitation services or intermediate care services/schemes.

Staff in settings such as intermediate care settings/therapeutic units or care homes also need to be alert to ensuring adequate activity. Seligman (1975) describes the concept of 'learned helplessness' while Baltes and Barton (1979) showed that dependent behaviour of nursing home residents is frequently directly maintained by nursing home staff. Avorn and Langer (1982) reaffirmed this notion in a study to assess residents' ability to learn and maintain an activity, and so warn of the importance of encouraging independence and activity. This may, however, be difficult if the older person is fearful of falling, is in pain, is breathless, stiff, or indeed simply does not wish to partake. It is therefore essential that appropriate treatment and intervention are provided, so that activities can be promoted, requiring great skill on behalf of the nurse and staff.

Complications can be very costly to the quality of life of an older person, let alone to the health service, and at this stage of life may even be life-threatening (Swift, 1988; Robertson, 1990), as outlined in Table 16.7. The skill of identifying and dealing with problems quickly, to prevent deterioration, promote quicker recovery, prevent hospitalization and help reduce the length of hospital stay, is paramount (RCN 1993). In the past, however, UK health education activities and screening programmes have not focused on older people. Similarly, attitudes towards the value of active intervention and treatment for older people has not always been forthcoming, possibly leading to the increased costs of their care and loss of quality of life in the later stages of illness (Legge, 1996). It is for this reason that health promotion is one of the key themes and standards within the *National Service Framework for Older People* (DoH, 2001h).

Table 16.7 Costs to older people and the health service that could be avoided with effective preventive care

- Osteoporosis-related fractures are estimated to cost the NHS in excess of £640 million per annum and are most significant in terms of morbidity, mortality and expenditure (Leyland, 1994).

- Trauma is within the top ten causes of death for those over 65 years of age (Robertson, 1990).

- The incidence of strokes and myocardial infarction both increase in cold weather and are often directly related to hypothermia (Watson, 1995), which could be prevented.

- The incidence of cancer is recognized as increasing with age, occurring in 70% of those over 60 years of age in the UK, and accounting for about 50–60% of all deaths from cancer. It is not usual practice to call older people for mass screening, as is the case for younger people – although changes are impending with regard to breast cancer screening.

Risk-taking

There will inevitably be a need to take risks when involving older people in rehabilitation, if they are to maximize their abilities and regain and retain control over their lives within the limits of their potential. Risk-taking is therefore an important element within rehabilitation and cannot be avoided, although practitioners will need to make decisions related to the level of risk that they feel should be incorporated into a plan of care (Cook, 1996). Cook (1996) acknowledges that for nurses the UKCC Code of professional conduct (1984), now superseded by the NMC (2002), presents a dilemma. The UKCC advised that the nurse should do the patient no harm, but should also act in the patient's best interests (Cook, 1996). These same sentiments are reflected within the NMC code of conduct for nurses (2002), yet taking risks and promoting abilities and functions may lead to injury.

Within current health care, sadly, awareness and escalation of legal action as a result of injury sustained while in care may make practitioners very wary. This may compromise their willingness to be as proactive as they could be in promoting rehabilitation activities and abilities. Equally so, to avoid risks may in the long run mean that the patient may be in danger of hospital-acquired infections/problems as described by Illich (1975). This could not only compromise their immediate quality of life, but could be influential in their future ability to rehabilitate and even in whether they will be able to go home.

Risk-taking will often relate to what may seem like simple activities or interventions, such as whether a patient needs supervision when walking to the toilet, or help to wash and shave. It will apply to almost every activity the individual is involved in, and will inevitably carry the risk of injury or harm. This will be an issue within rehabilitation, whether it occurs in an institutional setting or in the patient's own home, and indeed may be influential in deciding whether or not to admit a patient to a unit at this stage for rehabilitation, or to pursue this at home. Unfortunately there is a general belief that once in hospital the patient is safe! – nothing could be further from the truth, for the ward environment is unknown and may have many unexpected obstacles to the patient, which could impede success with rehabilitation. Thus the practitioner is constantly 'walking a tightrope' when making decisions related to rehabilitation.

Effective management of intervention, anxiety and fear are essential to gain confidence and will need continuous assessment and reassessment. Careful and reasoned discussion with the patient at all stages is necessary, providing information and offering the opportunity to enter into discussion and negotiation. This allows for mutually agreed goals to be set and for activities to be undertaken, but also provides them with the opportunity to recognize, acknowledge and accept the risks involved. Involving relatives as appropriate is also important and may go a long way to avoiding complaints at a later stage should an injury or problem occur. Thus there is a need to be aware of the risks involved and to be proactive in raising awareness in a sensitive but realistic way, entering into discussion and reaching an agreement about those risks being taken, and how these will be managed and addressed. Open and honest discussion among team members is also desirable, although it is almost inevitable that different professions will have different values and different perspectives, which will need working through.

Risk-taking will be high on the agenda when making decisions about patients going home. It will often involve risk-taking, with the possibility that it may not be successful. While again the patient has rights in terms of taking risks for themselves, these cannot be considered in isolation – for their own risks may impose risks to others. For example, setting light to a saucepan and causing a fire may well create danger for others if living in a shared living complex such as sheltered housing. Similarly, where others are providing care or support, their safety must be considered, and again a risk assessment may help. Psychological risks also need to be considered, for example where a relative is required, or is offering, to give extensive help and has little or no support with little or no relief – not uncommon within contemporary health and social care scenarios.

Due to their altered situation, an older person may no longer be able to live independently in the community without the help of others. Help and support need to be discussed and planned with those who will provide it, yet this needs to be undertaken while respecting and involving the older person.

The decisions that practitioners need to take in relation to risk-taking are considerable within rehabilitation and intermediate care services. Risk-taking is 'part and parcel' of successful rehabilitation and needs to be accepted and addressed in a recognized way that forms part of the clinical governance agenda. The decisions related to risk-taking supplement the many other decisions that often need to be made, and should not be under-estimated in this arena of work.

Developing a successful rehabilitation culture is fundamental to the concept of rehabilitation, re-enablement and addressing quality of life issues. Fundamental to this is effective team-working as discussed in the next section.

Team-working

Throughout the text, reference has been made to effective team-working. Effective rehabilitation requires the skills of a range of different disciplines and professionals – some examples of which are indicated in Table 16.8. The composition of the team should depend very much on the needs of the particular patient and the functions of the team members. Both the structure and function of teams can be critical factors in determining patient outcomes. Intermediate care services tend to be associated very much with nurses, with an emphasis on being nurse-led. This perception lies partially with fact that such services are regarded as taking a more socially or therapeutically orientated model of care, where the dominance of medicine and the medical model of care is not so evident. It can also be attributed to the fact that nurses tend to outnumber other disciplines and there is no doubt that it is usually only nurses and assistants who are present over the 24-hour day. There is no reason, however, why a therapist or social worker should not in fact take the lead, although there is a need to clarify how health care needs and staff competence will be met within this more social model of care. The general ethos, however, is one of team-working involving members of all the disciplines, where there is no dominance of anyone – or, if there is, that it derives from patient need as available. Unfortunately, with the current recruitment and retention problems it may well be that recruitment to therapy roles is challenged, as it is with most disciplines.

A team approach involves the team members working together with the united purpose of effecting rehabilitation outcomes for clients. Regardless of the team mix, the critical members are the patient and usually their carer/family members.

Table 16.8 Potential rehabilitation team members

- Occupational therapists
- Physiotherapists
- Social worker/care manager
- Podiatrists
- Nurses
- Speech and language therapists
- Orthotics
- Dietician
- Psychologists
- Community psychiatric nurse
- GP
- Consultant/geriatrician
- Generic/rehabilitation assistants.

McGrath and Davis (1992) argue that rehabilitation can be usefully viewed as a goal-driven problem-solving activity. A vital part of rehabilitation is the mutual moving closer together of clients and professional's goals and, as discussed, this involves partnership working and negotiation to reach agreement. The process of negotiation involves at the very least systematically both ascertaining what the client's desires and expectations are and acknowledging them. McGrath and Davis (1992) suggest that 'goals that are acceptable to both client and therapist must be negotiated. Where this can be done successfully problems of compliance and motivation and secondary behavioural problems which accompany them are largely solved' (1992: 227). The contemporary term for this coming together to reach agreement is known as concordance (RCP, 1998). This requires taking a person-centred, holistic approach to each individual client, as discussed, and will require all team members to work collaboratively to reach an understanding of these mutually agreed goals in order to contribute to their attainment.

Teams may works differently in terms of their philosophy, structure, leadership, goal-setting practices and goal-attainment strategies, and there are perhaps three recognized approaches – multidisciplinary, interdisciplinary and transdisiplinary.

Multidisciplinary teams

Multidisciplinary teams combine the efforts of each member of the team. Their work is characterized by working towards discipline-specific goals, with clear boundaries between disciplines, such that the teams' outcomes are the sum of each discipline's efforts (Figure 16.3 and 16.4) (Hoeman, 1996). To achieve this, effective systems of communication need to be established. There is a risk, however, that such an approach does not allow for the holistic needs of an individual to be met, since the efforts of each team member is addressed individually with each isolating their goals and taking responsibility only for that goal, failing to integrate them. The scenario in hospital of the physiotherapist or porter coming to take the patient to the therapy department and later returning with no communication or discussion is not uncommon. The therapist will write in their notes but how the progress is communicated to the ward staff and team members may not be clear, and may not happen at all. This means that ward staff and other therapists cannot engage in helping, assisting or re-enforcing the activity being implemented in the therapy department. Success may therefore depend very much on the ability of the patient to continue their therapy and/or convey their needs to other staff, which is unsatisfactory and may impede continuity of care and progress.

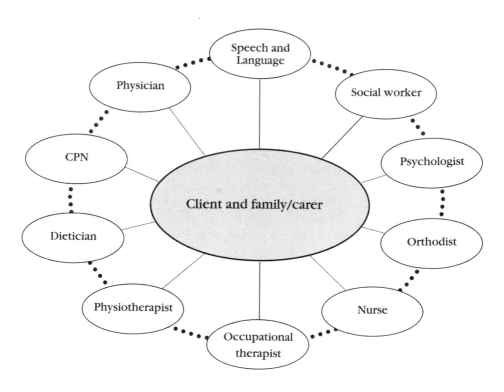

Figure 16.3 Multidisciplinary team-working.

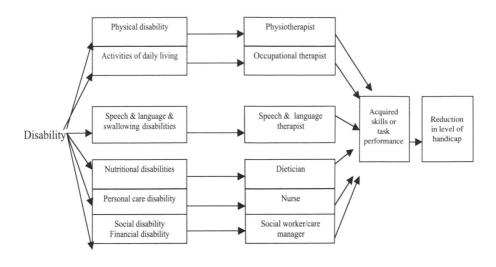

Figure 16.4 Multidisciplinary approach to rehabilitation.

Interdisciplinary teamwork

As identified, a collaborative and co-ordinated approach to this may be more effective. Collaboration is key to successful interdisciplinary team-working. Here the team membership will probably be the same, but the way they work differs. Rather than each team member identifying their own discipline-specific goals, the whole team identifies client goals and therefore strives to avoid duplication or conflict in goals. This involves expanded problem-solving beyond the discipline boundaries and confines. Using these agreed goals, each team member then works to identify how they will contribute to goal attainment within the parameters of their discipline (Figures 16.5 and 16.6).This will lead to greater synergy in the way the team works and interacts, so that more comprehensive outcomes are achieved than would be possible for any one discipline. To promote effective collaboration in this approach to team-working it may be beneficial to have a key worker or named person. This person can be from any discipline and may be the person who has a key role to play in the particular patient's rehabilitation, although it is not unusual for it to be a nurse. Successful interdisciplinary working is not easily achieved or maintained, for it requires a high level of teamwork, where team members work together with shared goals and philosophies. This requires mutual respect and trust, with a clear understanding of the expertise of each discipline and team member. This requires a willingness to share, adapt and communicate effectively (Sellick, 1985: 35) – an approach to working that has not been well reflected within health and social care in general.

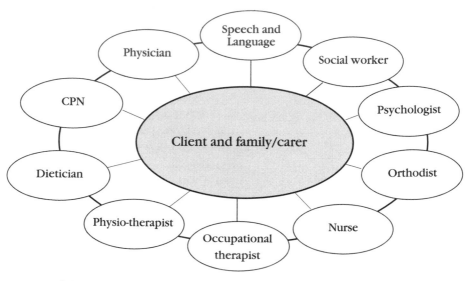

Figure 16.5 Interdisciplinary working.

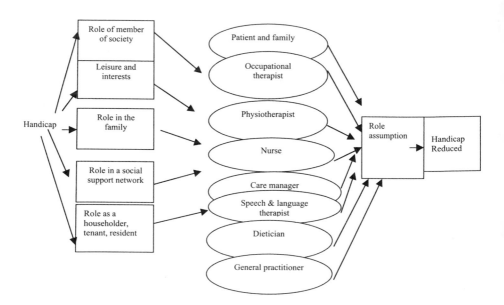

Figure 16.6 The interdisciplinary approach to rehabilitation.

Transdisciplinary teamwork

Transdisciplinary team-working is a development of interdisciplinary working, and is not dissimilar, except in this case the key or named worker adopts a more significant role, and team members communicate information and advice via or through this person, as shown in Figure 16.7 (Hoeman, 1996). This provides a means of planning and implementing care, but reduces joint collaboration where one team member can effectively achieve the task, irrespective of their actual discipline. This approach may be particularly effective where staff resources are limited, and it does involve a blurring of discipline boundaries. This model, or a hybrid of interdisciplinary team-working and transdisciplinary working, may be the best approach in intermediate care services where the extent and human resources of the team concerned may be limited and the logistics of all the team meeting together may be difficult. It will, however, require team members to be flexible and require cross-training. Thus team preparation is essential, and is best incorporated within induction and team-building. It will be very important for the roles of each team member to be clarified and understood, so that members can be clear about when and how they need to draw upon their colleagues' specific skills. It will require team members to be receptive to learning to cope with a wider domain of functioning (Hoeman, 1996) and able to recognize each other's capabilities. This demands a cultural shift, and it can be challenging for professionals to accept that others may perform aspects of their role, for they may fear that their roles will be eroded or diluted. If managed appropriately this will most certainly not be the case, as each team member will learn to respect and value the expertise of their colleagues and recognize when to call upon them to assess and plan care.

This approach will apply to whatever model and approach to team-working is chosen by the service, and addressing an understanding of the team membership, culture, working relationships and patterns of work cannot be over-estimated if a service is to function effectively. Time spent at this stage of the introduction of a service, will 'serve dividends later', with ongoing review arising from an initial fundamental understanding.

The role of the nurse and those supporting this role as care assistants, generic workers, etc. within the rehabilitation team has often been unclear (Waters, 1994). For this reason it would be important to explore the views of the role of the nurse within rehabilitation with team members during the induction and team-building period. This is important because, as identified, nurses are present throughout the 24-hour day, and their role is therefore crucial. They will need to be involved in the identification of patient goals and aspirations – indeed, it may be the nurse who identifies the need to refer to another team member for their expert opinion and involvement. It is often other team members who need to assess and prescribe care and treatment

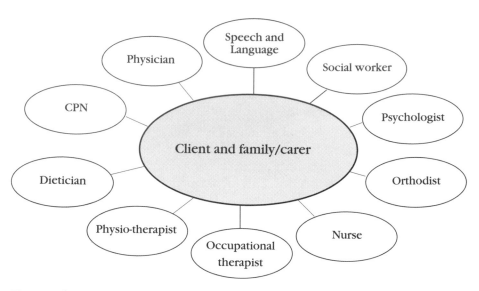

Figure 16.7 Transdisciplinary working.

for certain rehabilitation goals, but the nurse may need to be facilitated to help and support the patient to continue with treatment over the rest of their day. As discussed, rehabilitation occurs over the whole day and night and involves many of the daily activities that the patient may be involved in. The nurse and supporting staff can contribute a great deal to meeting the other holistic needs and goals of patients, and this role is implicit to successful rehabilitation. One of the challenges for the nurse and staff on duty is being able to address all these needs, where they lack either the skills or staffing. They can also be challenged in this if there is a lack of understanding about the culture of rehabilitation. This can be a particular problem in acute settings where the emphasis is on acute care. It can, however, also be an issue in intermediate care if skills attainment, staffing and organization of time are not addressed.

The other key feature of successful interdisciplinary or transdisciplinary team-working is the use of shared or collaborative care plans, where all team members work to the same agreed goals and communicate in the same documentation and in the same area of that documentation. It means that any team member can identify goals and that, once the goal has been agreed, all team members can contribute to the intervention, evaluation and updating as required. It also means that all know where to find the goals and plan of care, and they cannot be criticized for not working towards these. This means that there are no specific or coloured pages allocated for each discipline, as is sometimes found (such that true interdisciplinary communication is compromised) and it also means that each discipline does not keep a separate set of 'their documentation'. Apart from promoting collaborative working, this approach means that all the information about the patient is in the same set of records, and is not dispersed around in different places. This information can be accessed easily and will be stored together for review or even audit. The approach helps to promote open and honest communication with patients, but it will be necessary to discuss with patients where they wish their documentation to be kept to ensure confidentiality. At times this will present as a challenge for professionals, where the handling of sensitive information may be of concern to them, and open discussion will be required.

Explicit goal-setting will be a central task if patient and team members are to be able to ensure a consistent and coherent approach. At the heart of rehabilitation lies an iterative cyclical process based upon identification of goals. Assessment, as always, is central and essential before planning goals triggering selective interventions, and will be followed by evaluation of the outcome and reassessment. The patient must agree these if they are able and feel motivated to participate. Young et al. (1999) identify that this process is effective in improving outcomes for the older person, providing the assessment process is closely linked to appropriate interventions. This is where comprehensive assessment is so important and, while some objective assessment measures such as the Barthel Score, etc. may give some guidance, the most important element is the opportunity to engage in exploratory discussion with the patient, seeking to identify patient-related problems. This requires the combined skills and time of team members.

Young (1996, p 679) suggests that successful goals are recognized as being:

- meaningful – i.e. appropriate to the problems and circumstances of the patient;
- agreed – by all involved through concordance;
- clearly communicated;
- realistic – achievable, but sufficiently challenging.

Achievement of this can be facilitated if goal-setting is explicit and the following principles are met:

- who will do what;
- under what conditions;
- to what degree of success.

This will allow evaluation and progress to be assessed.

Conclusion

Providing and achieving successful rehabilitation involves a great many interrelated factors and features, all of which need to correlate. It is not a straightforward activity but very complex and dependent upon so much. Most of all, it requires skills or attributes of those involved in assisting with the process. This cannot be over-estimated and it is particularly important to address with staff who have often not been well prepared for this approach to work.

KEY POINTS

- With a focus on promoting independence, the role of rehabilitation has taken on a new role within health and social care, and in developing intermediate care.
- Rehabilitation tends to mean different things to different people, but to maximize success the patient and their goals need to be at the centre of decision-making, interventions and activity, with all practitioners working to the same goals.
- For the practitioner, rehabilitation involves a wide range of skills, functions and activities which extend throughout the 24-hour day, involving the patients in all their activities in any environment or setting.
- Rehabilitation will inevitably involve some risk-taking if an individual's potential is to be realized, but this will need to be assessed, considered and agreed by those involved, with attention given to the rational support of those risks taken.
- For effective rehabilitation to be provided, there is a need to identify and acknowledge an approach to teamwork that takes account of person-centred goals and ensures effective collaboration and communication between all involved, utilizing each other's skills – being best achieved through single assessment and shared or collaborative care planning.

CHAPTER 17

Decision-making and problem-solving

SIÂN WADE AND LIZ LEES

Introduction

Problem-solving and decision-making have constantly been referred to throughout this book. This involves skills that are not unique to practitioners in intermediate care, and in choosing to allocate a whole section to this subject within a book related to intermediate care it is important to acknowledge this. No apology, however, is made in choosing to do this here, for as Lipman and Deatrick (1997) confirm, significant changes in health care services and delivery have placed an increased emphasis on the place and effectiveness of decision-making abilities. Henry et al. (1989) concurs with this view, concluding that knowledge, skills and ability to manage rapidly changing situations are consistently necessary for clinical decision-making within contemporary health care. High-quality information, co-operative action and open channels of communication are needed to assist an effective decision-making process. Marquis and Huston (1996) describe this process as 'the cornerstone of professional working practice and the criteria management expertise is judged upon'.

Background

In their work looking at community-nursing practice, Bryans and McIntosh (1996) argue that nurses working in community settings often face different decision-making challenges to those working in hospital settings. Their arguments bear relevance to staff working in the whole range of intermediate care services, who often have to address a wide range of decision-making situations. This all provides justification for designating this chapter to the subject.

The terms 'decision-making' and 'clinical decision-making' are used interchangeably, and refer to those decisions that relate directly or indirectly to patient care and outcomes. Much of the discussion here derives from nursing literature, but the focus will be upon the kind of situations found within intermediate care services/schemes, most of which have as much relevance to members of all the multidisciplinary team as to the nurse. The focus on nursing derives from the fact that nursing has been closely associated with this kind of service; however, depending on the intermediate care service/scheme and the make-up of the teams, many of the decisions undertaken may be by any one of the team members.

What are we talking about?

A range of definitions of what constitutes decision-making have been proposed, some of which are outlined in Table 17.1.

Table 17.1 Definitions of clinical decision-making

'discriminative thinking, used to choose a particular course of action'
(Griffith-Kenny and Christensen, 1986)

'the act of choice following deliberation and judgment'
(Schaefer, 1974)

'situations in which choice is made from among a number of alternatives, often involving a trade-off among values given different outcomes'
(Baumann and Deber, 1989)

'A clinical decision is a decision taken by a nurse (practitioner) to influence patient care. It is based on his or her knowledge of the patient's circumstances and arrived at through a cognitive process, the aim being to influence the patient's well-being'
(Bulmer, 1998)

'Decision-making is the process of selecting one course of action from among alternatives, based on collation of information, and is the essence of leadership'
(Huber, 1996)

The context of decision-making within intermediate care

Within intermediate care the significance of decision-making is important, because although staff may have the opportunity to come together as a team at times, each individual with their own discipline will often find themselves on their own in many situations where problems need to be solved and decisions need to be made, there and then. They may also often find themselves as the only representative of their particular discipline when involved in team-working, and will wish their professional beliefs and values to be considered among those of their colleagues when involved in decision-making or problem-solving. Teams will be made up of a range of staff, and a number of these will be unregistered staff to whom work will be delegated. Thus registered staff will need to have the skills to decide how and to whom to delegate – this is all the more critical when such staff will be working alone in other people's homes or possibly care homes and not directly supervised. Furthermore, throughout this book the importance of involving patients in partnership working, where they are encouraged to engage in decisions about their care, has been promoted. Ensuring patients are enabled to make informed decisions is no easy attribute, and thus warrants exploration.

Decision-making and problem-solving tend to go hand in hand. Lipman and Deatrick (1997) contend that the ability to think critically is a requirement for decision-making, where a process that uses critical thinking and judgment is used to solve emerging problems. When trying to solve a problem it is usually necessary to consider a range of options and how they interrelate in order to reach a decision as to which option to take. Alforo-Lefeveve (1994) regards critical thinking as requiring 'careful, deliberate, goal directed thinking based on principles of science and scientific method' (1994: 4). Thompson et al. (2002) argues that the significance given to the use of research-based knowledge has become increasingly important as the evidence-based culture of health service delivery has evolved during the past 12 years, following a series of NHS policy initiatives. Additionally, Watson and Glaser (1964) believe attitudes, knowledge and skills are encompassed in decision-making, and that this requires the practitioner to question practice in an organized manner, which leads to clinical decision-making. Jones (1988) proposes that segments of information are accumulated over time, and that when faced with a decision, choices are made from the alternatives identified and recombined into a logical chain. Expertise is thus developed from a holistic network of content knowledge, which can be integrated rapidly and significantly to reach an appropriate decision. English (1993) also identified expertise as the ability to view situations holistically from a knowledge base embedded in practice.

On reviewing the literature it becomes very clear that these skills need to develop, and that the experience of the practitioner greatly affects clinical decision-making. Benner (1984) demonstrated that nurses with more experience are more likely to intervene and make decisions without consulting others than less experienced nurses, while Paniagua (1995) suggests that the more experienced the practitioner is, the more extensive, accurate and rapid their reasoning abilities become. The significance of this experience and expertise is often, however, related more to the way the practitioner has developed and their related experience than the actual years of practice experience. Thompson et al. (2002), for example, contend that while experience is a necessary source of information for making decisions, it is not sufficient by itself. Jasper (1994) suggests that this is linked to a knowledge base, where the practitioner possesses extensive practical knowledge as well as theoretical knowledge, and is able to generate new knowledge. This, in turn, may relate very closely to their ongoing education and development, and their ability to question, challenge, analyse and reflect on practice. Thompson et al. (2002) go on to propose that a 'good decision from an evidence-based perspective is one that successfully integrates four elements' (p. 31), which they cite as:

- professional expertise ('know-how knowledge');
- the available resources;
- the patient's (informed) values;
- the research knowledge ('know-what' knowledge).

These are important factors to consider when deciding on staffing levels, skill mix, and staff preparation, for this ability to make decisions is paramount to the success of intermediate care services/schemes, as will be discussed. It is also paramount to the sense of self-esteem of the practitioner and their perception of feeling able to deal with autonomous situations and the service they are delivering, which is often quite isolated. If the developmental and support needs of staff are not addressed, staff recruitment and retention may be affected. Thus the importance of recognizing the isolation and vulnerability of staff working in intermediate care cannot be over-estimated, and the provision of staff development that strengthens advanced clinical practice, decision-making, and communication are likely to be key. Catolico et al. (1996) recommend the need to cultivate a culture among staff of systematically integrating decision-making opportunities into daily practice and that this is accompanied by productive feedback, discussion and evaluation of both the positive and negative consequences of decisions. Forums such as clinical supervision, critical incident analysis or action learning circles may be appropriate for this.

When considering this decision-making process, it is possible to identify a range of themes that often underpin this process. These are useful and important to highlight with staff so that they can relate to their own real life decisions – see Table 17.2.

Table 17.2 Themes that may often underlie decision-making

- The decision is often complex, multi-faceted and interdependent.
- There may be risks involved e.g.
    to safety;
    to people/jobs.
- There may be tensions, e.g.
    fears of reproach;
    fears of litigation;
    inter-agency values.
- Effective communication is essential.
- Knowledge is required.
- There is almost inevitably a need to take account of ethical and moral considerations.
- There will usually be a need to consider a range of practical and circumstantial influences, such as resources and their availability, and pressure.
- A level of authority is generally required.
- Consideration of the consequences of a decision needs to be accounted for.

Practitioners will also experience challenges that they have to contend with when making decisions, as in Table 17.3. These can be quite extensive, although they may replicate the themes identified above.

Table 17.3 Challenges that may influence practitioners' decision-making

- Complexity of the decision.
- The different priorities of different stakeholders and emerging conflicts, e.g.
    – value system;
    – organizational pressures, e.g. to reduce length of stay;
    – efficacy;
    – humanitarianism.
- Lack of knowledge to enable or mislead decision-making, e.g. limited referral information or miscommunication.
- Lack of supporting infrastructure to enable decision to be seen through.
- Lack of resources, e.g. people, skills, competency, confidence, equipment, time, size of case load, money, etc.
- Moral and ethical dilemmas that challenge decisions about an individual's quality of life.
- Human characteristics, e.g. personality clashes, power tactics, personal attitudes and those of others, fatigue.
- Environmental factors and logistics of acting upon decision.

Considerations for practitioners

As professionals we are faced with further factors that will influence our decision-making, as identified by Rowson (1999) and as outlined in Table 17.4.

Table 17.4 Factors influencing decision-making for professionals

The law
Social etiquette
Professional codes
Religious beliefs
Visual and aesthetic sense
Practicality and morality

Source: adapted from Rowson (1999).

For nursing and indeed all health and social care professionals there is an implicit understanding that practising to a high moral and ethical standard matters. The ethical system of a profession is based very much upon certain beliefs and values of that profession, such that differences can emerge between the thinking of different professions and disciplines that can lead to conflicts when working alongside each other. For medicine, the ethical framework drives doctors to try to treat and cure, while for nurses caring may take precedence over cure. A key social care ethic is to promote choice, and this is a concept that is really challenged within the current health and social care system, especially in relation to older people. Allowing older people choice and the time to make this choice stands in the way of priorities and the achievement of performance indicators that drive the way the health service is managed today, and can influence the way certain sums of money are awarded to Trusts.

For nurses, while the logic of ethics is important, the emotions involved in caring are implicit to their work and role, and this may create considerable challenges for them. Jolly and Brykczynska (1992) consider that caring is composed of compassion, competence, confidence, conscience and commitment. However, the conscience that cares may be in conflict with the rules that govern it, for example the UKCC Code of Conduct (1984) and now the NMC (2002). It is therefore important for nurses to acknowledge that emotionality is central to their role and may play a significant part in the factors influencing their decision-making. They may, however, face real conflicts when making decisions within the reality of day-to-day practice.

Understanding the decision-making process.

While decision-making may seem to the observer as a one-off pronouncement, on examination it may be possible to recognize an active process involving a progression of events or a course of action with a measure of systematic structure (Moore, 1996). Cooksey (1996) and Hammond (1996) have identified two types of decision-making processes: analysis and intuition.

Analysis involves a considered and conscious step-by-step process, which can be logically defended. This tends to involve information processing, use of sequential cues, use of logical rules and task-specific organization (Cooksey, 1996; Hammond, 1996).

The concept of intuition and how it occurs has been the topic of many debates (English; 1993, Farrington, 1993; Jasper, 1994). However, in the context of decision-making it is associated with the ability to recognize key elements of a situation upon which decisions need to be based. Here rapid information processing, simultaneous use of cues, recognition of patterns, evaluation of cues at a perceptual level, and use of the principle of weighted average and organization seem to be the key characteristics (Dreyfus and Dreyfus, 1986). This would seem to relate very much to the reflective and analytical skills of the practitioner and how they use and apply previous learning to new and unique situations. Farrington (1993) suggests that intuitive judgments are reached by an apparently informal and unstructured mode of reasoning without the use of analytical methods or deliberate calculation. This is borne out by Schon (1983), who suggests that in daily practice practitioners make many judgments of a quality nature for which they cannot state adequate criteria. They also, he argues, display skills for which they cannot state the rules and procedures. This decision-making process is very similar to the intuitive grasp of situations that the expert nurse displays, as described by Benner (1984). This adds to the complexity and uncertainty of many situations in which practitioners may find themselves, and contributes to the concept of 'the swampy lowlands' of much practice, as described by Schon (1983).

Hammond (1996) argues that there is a continuum running between analytical and intuitive decision-making, and that when making decisions cognitive processes may occur at any point along this continuum, depending on the circumstance and personal characteristics of the practitioner involved. This is influenced by such factors as the knowledge, education and experience of practitioners, as well as the type or culture of the health care service in which they work and the nature and context of the task. Laurie et al. (2001) consider that most decision-making involves elements of both analytical and intuitive cognitive processes, with intuitively orientated decision-making predominating when situations require a prompt decision and rapid response.

Theories and frameworks for decision-making processes

As acknowledged, there is a continuum in the way in which cognitive processes are involved in decision-making, moving from the more intuitive and less explicit processes of decision-making, to the more analytical and evident processes of decision-making. Much research has centred on understanding these processes, with a range of models or frameworks emerging. It is helpful for staff who work in challenging situations where complex decisions are often required, such as those working within intermediate care, to gain an understanding and insight into the process of decision-making. The strength of following a decision-making model is that it can provide guidance through a logical progression of thought, based on available knowledge and research, so reducing the risk of making hasty, unwise or emotionally charged judgments. In this section a range of models and frameworks will be described which may help the practitioner to identify ways of developing their own decision-making skills, relating them to some of the kinds of decisions made within the context of intermediate care.

Although many decision-making models exist, there are key components common to all. Huber (1996) identifies these as:

- identification of a problem;
- the establishment of the criteria to be used to evaluate potential solutions;
- a search for alternative solutions;
- evaluation of the alternatives.

Bernhard and Walsh (1995) suggest that the first step in decision-making requires identification of the parameters of the decision, i.e.

- the problem or need;
- the people involved;
- the setting or organization.

Schaefer (1974) refers to three phases when making decisions, where the nature of the decision process is the act of choice, following deliberation and judgment. These need to be set within the context of the key common components and steps as identified by Huber (1996) and Bernhard and Walsh (1995). These, Schaefer (1974) argues, require the fulfilment of three conditions: freedom, rationality and voluntarity.

Bernhard and Walsh (1995) also created their own model or framework of decision-making, as in Table 17.5. These stages, as with most of the decision-making frameworks or models discussed here, may not simply be followed through in the sequence as they are listed. Movement may occur back and forth with stages repeated, as information, judgments and choices emerge – so that decisions may evolve.

Table 17.5 Bernhard-Walsh Decision-making Model

- Identify the parameters of the decision situation
- Establish characteristics of the ideal solutions
- List possible solutions
- Choose the best solution
- Implement the decision
- Evaluate the results

Source: Bernhard and Walsh (1995).

Sullivan and Decker (2000) have proposed a problem-solving frame-work, which has similarities to the Bernhard–Walsh (1995) model (see Figure 17.1).

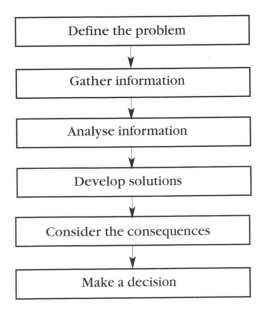

Figure 17.1 Problem-solving framework.

Source: Sullivan and Decker (2000).

Carrol and Johnson (1990) outline seven temporal stages of decision-making:

1. recognition
2. formulation

3. alternative generation
4. information search
5. judgment or choice
6. action
7. feedback

In this framework, there are two stages: those of recognition and formulation, that are not always evident as stages in other models or frameworks for decision-making. These two stages do, however, have great significance, for it is crucial for the practitioner to have the ability actually to recognize that there is a problem that needs to be addressed or decision that needs to made, and then to be able to identify the root causes or features. Bryans and McIntosh (1996) describe these two stages as pre-decisional activities, and the nature of these activities will depend upon various factors. Bryans and McIntosh (1996) suggest they help to account for the actual situation or task involved, as well as the views and perceptions of the individual practitioner in relation to their own understanding of their role. Thus it will be necessary for the practitioner to accept that they consider making the decision within the remit of their role before they engage in the decision-making process. This relates back to the conditions of freedom and voluntarity referred to by Schaefer (1974) above. The ability, experience or intuition to recognize that there is a problem is a crucial factor, and again demonstrates the complexity of decision-making and the skill required of the practitioner working in intermediate care, who often works in isolation and may be in vulnerable positions. Bryans and McIntosh (1996) go on to suggest that while these two stages are very important they are less conscious and deliberate, and therefore may not always be appreciated or articulated.

Catolico et al. (1996) refer to three principles that again influence decision-making:

- Willingness
- Frequency
- Ability

Here they talk about the willingness of the practitioner to enter into decision-making, the frequency at which they enter into decision-making situations, and their ability actually to deal with it when they do enter the process. Willingness may be influenced by the ability to recognize that there is a problem, and will therefore influence the frequency with which problems are identified and again the actual ability to deal with them. Other factors, such as personal characteristics, values, mental fatigue will also, however, play a part. Catolico et al. (1996) also highlight the place of good leadership in facilitating the willingness to enter into decision-making, and in developing the ability actually to undertake the process. It is therefore very clear that there are many factors that influence decision-making by practitioners, and this will be closely related to their understanding, insight and experience.

Ethical and moral decision-making

Wheeler (2001) suggests that there are three types of environments in which decisions are made: certain, risky, and uncertain environments. The certain environment is probably rare within health and social care services, as this requires sufficient information and/or resources to allow us to make the best decision. It is more likely that we encounter some risky environments, where information or resources may be lacking and we therefore lack complete certainty about the outcomes of various courses of action. The uncertain environment is the least comfortable within which to make decisions, as there may be very little information to inform us and again limited resources to help us, and it may not be possible to forecast the potential outcomes easily. This kind of decision is likely to depend very much upon the creative intuition and educated guesses of the practitioner, and may well be determined by their experience. Wheeler (2001) advises therefore that the practitioner should ensure that if at all possible they should have all the information they need, and can obtain, before contemplating making a decision. They should then remind themselves of the objective, reassess the priorities, consider the options and weigh up the strengths, weaknesses, opportunities and threats. Where possible, it may be that a decision can be tested out and discussed with others, but this is not always an option. They advise that having made a decision it is important to try to stick with it.

In addition to Catolico et al.'s (1996) three principles of willingness, frequency and ability that influence decision-making, there are further principles which influence decision-making, especially ethical decision-making. These can be described as the 4As and 3Ps:

Attitude

Attitude will be affected by the desire to work to a high moral standard, but will also be influenced by personal attitudes, which can be powerful in their influence.

Awareness

Unless there is an awareness of the presence of an ethical issue it will probably not be considered. There is a risk that ethical issues will not be recognized due to a particular practice becoming learned and accepted, through observing and modelling the practice of others and not being exposed to questions or challenge. This again can influence attitude and behaviour, and can be particularly problematic in institutionalized settings or contexts, where staff remain in the same situation for a long time and where they have not been exposed to a culture of questioning and challenge through staff development and education.

Analysis

Analysis relates to the processes involved in weighing up the pros and cons, etc. as involved in decision-making and discussed here.

Perspectives

Here there is a need to think about issues from the perspective of the key people, such as the patient, relatives/carers, care team and society, etc.

Principles

There are four main principles that guide our practice within ethical decision-making. These are:

- autonomy
- beneficence
- non-maleficence
- justice.

Paradigms

Here it may help to compare the problematic situation faced with another similar situation or paradigm situation that resembles it. This may help to provide some guidance on how the current problem might be addressed. Care must, however, be taken to ensure that the individual features of the current problem are considered carefully and that an inappropriate solution is not reached that does not take account of these adequately, and that is not contextualized.

Action

Action inevitably results from the above process but involves effective communication.

Moral decision-making

Brown et al. (1992) discuss five stages of moral deliberation, as demonstrated in Figure 17.2. This can be annotated with the 4As and 3Ps as described, showing how they relate to and influence the decision-making process. It is possible to see how these features could be superimposed on other frameworks outlined, so influencing and contributing to the decision-making process.

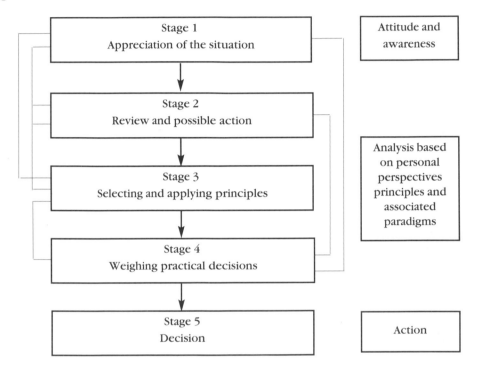

Figure 17.2 Five stages of moral deliberation and their interrelationships.

Finally, Seedhouse (2000) outlines a model/framework that is described as the 'Caring Grid' or 'Ethical Grid'. In effect this 'grid' brings together many aspects of those frameworks already outlined, collating them into one comprehensive Framework (Figure 17.3). Using the 'grid', the practitioner is asked to progress through a number of steps:

• First they are asked to consider the issue they have identified without using the grid, and to list the pros and cons of using various options for action. This should bring them to an initial position.
• They are then asked to look at the grid and either start at the outside and work in, or begin with a layer that feels most significant to them.
• They are asked to consider all levels of the grid, and to select those boxes that appear to offer the best solution. It is not necessary to consider every

box, since the importance of each varies with the context and sometimes some are of no relevance. Novice users are advised to reflect on each box and its relevance until they become familiar with the grid.

Referring to each layer:

- *The outside layer* is a level of external considerations, often raising the most important factors and, as such, may take the decisions out of the hands of the health care worker.
- *The next layer* looks at outcomes (consequences) of proposed interventions. These help to clarify priorities. This layer should be used only with the grid as a whole.
- *The next layer* focuses on duties and motive. It considers obligations

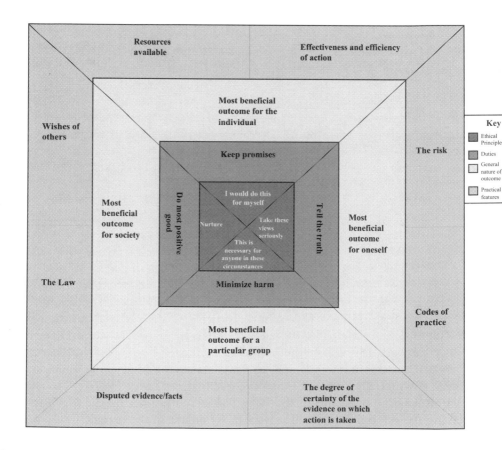

Figure 17.3 The Caring Grid: Seedhouse D. *Practical nursing philosophy: The universal ethical code.* (2000) Chichester: Wiley.

other than those immediately implied by commitment to health work.
* *The inner layer* – here at least one of these boxes should be used during deliberations, as these boxes provide a footing for making the decision.

The following section will provide some examples from practice in relation to the way decisions may be made in the use of intermediate care services/schemes. Many more important examples related to intermediate care could be provided, especially related to decisions around care and interventions. The examples cited will demonstrate how significant the many factors that influence decision-making can be, and how real-life constraints need to be taken into account both to understand how decisions are reached and to appreciate how significantly different outcomes may be reached as a result of how decisions are made.

Scenario 1

When considering the different priorities of different stakeholders, staff in intermediate care services/schemes may find themselves in dilemmas. For example, it may be that staff in A&E feel that a patient is suitable for a Rapid Response Service (RRS). The RRS staff member taking the referral may, however, feel that the patient has needs that can be provided for only in the acute hospital. But there may be other factors that are influencing the decision on both sides. The A&E staff may feel pressurized to defer admissions due to a bed crisis and feel that this patient is more suitable than others for referral to RRS. Equally, if there was not a bed crisis they may decide that the patient would benefit from admission and further investigations, etc. In either case the best needs of the patient have not taken precedence. For the RRS team, they may fully believe that the patient needs to be admitted to hospital, but again other factors may be at play. The member of staff may be inexperienced and feel that the team would be unable to meet the needs of the patient, while a more experienced practitioner may feel that the team could manage the patient. The more experienced practitioner may also have knowledge of services that could be accessed rapidly for the patient for referral, investigations, and support, or to access if needed. This may be helped by knowledge of other colleagues and established relationships with staff in these services that assist in accessing assistance, which the less experienced nurse may not have.

An alternative outcome in this scenario may have been that the nurse receiving the referral accepted the patient when in fact the service could not manage the complexity or severity of the patient's needs. Other factors could also play a part in influencing the outcome. It may have been 9.30pm – just one hour before the service finished. The referred patient could live right across the city from the RRS base, such that this could influence the decision as to whether or not to accept the patient. There may be concern that identified care or assistance might not be accessed at this time, along with concern about getting off duty in reasonable time.

Scenario 2

Within an intermediate care setting a nurse may feel that an older patient is unwell at night, and feel it would be beneficial to call a doctor. The nurse will be fully aware that the doctor may not be too pleased with such a call out, and the nurse will know that they will need to be able to justify making a request. This, however, may not always be easy because, as has been evidenced, older people do not always present with easily recognizable symptoms as discussed in Chapter 4. It may be intuitively that through experience the nurse is persuaded there is something significantly wrong, yet the rationale and reason may not be convincing or easy to comprehend by the doctor. If the doctor knows the nurse and respects and trusts them as a practitioner, they may be more easily persuaded to visit than if they do not. A similar call in the daytime may be more acceptable, especially if the GP practice makes a daily visit at some time. In this situation a less experienced nurse may have more difficulty in influencing the doctor to visit. Alternatively, the nurse may actually lack the experience to recognize that the patient is unwell, so failing to conceive that there is a problem that needs addressing, meaning that no request for a visit is made, so that perhaps a crisis or emergency may arise.

Scenario 3

Another situation could arise where the potential of a patient to benefit from rehabilitation is perceived by the team in general to be poor, but is perceived by one member of staff as being more hopeful. There may be many reasons to account for these different views. The single staff member may be influenced by an intuitive notion that the patient might well benefit based on past experience and influence. It could, however, relate to what team members expect of rehabilitation and so here differing values and philosophies come into play. The decision could also be influenced by knowledge about bed availability and known pressures from bed management or the need to address the length of stay of patients. Here the team may be influenced by the belief that the patient will take too long, or simply because it is known that there is a waiting list for the rehabilitation beds and this patient would not be perceived as high priority. Saying the patient is not suitable may sit more easily than admitting the service cannot be easily provided, but could have significant consequences for the patients and their carers.

Decision-making and delegation

Within all health and social care services, practitioners will almost inevitably be required to delegate to other more junior or unregistered staff. The development of these delegation skills can be quite challenging, and within intermediate care services/schemes this may be a particular challenge as delegation will often be to staff, some of whom may be unregistered and working alone and in isolation at some distance from their supervisor.

Conger's (1993) delegation decision-making model identifies three major components that need to be considered before making a delegation decision. These include:

- identifying the required task;
- identifying the patient problems;
- determining the most appropriate staff member to provide and delegate this care to.

Assessment of the patient's needs and all the factors and issues that have a bearing on the care needs of the patient are essential in order to begin to make a decision about delegation. Sometimes, as in the case of rapid response, much of this will initially need to be made over the phone, and will depend on accurate and honest referral information. This will first of all influence the decision as to whether to accept the patient into the service at all, and then influence the decision as to which staff member to send out to assess the situation further. Knowledge about relatives and carers and issues affecting them may also be influential, particularly when staff are going into people's own homes. Based on the assessment of the patient and the situation, the decision then needs to be made as to whom to delegate to.

Once the patients have been assessed first hand, and assuming they are then accepted, decisions will then need to be made about the ongoing care required from the service, and who will provide this. Decisions about who to delegate this to will depend on many factors such as the complexity of the care needs and the skills required for this, as well as the time required to provide this care. If the care requires extended practice then the practitioner who is asked to provide the care must be appropriately qualified and trained for this. Other factors will also need to be taken into account. Conger (1993) notes that information about the patient's circumstances, the patient's knowledge, manageability and motivation to work towards problem resolution may be influential, especially if it is in a patient's home.

It is important to develop effective skills of delegation so as to ensure that the delegator can extend their influence and capability, and manage the overall co-ordination of care and the service, through the supervision of a number of staff. This should increase productivity by sharing work out appropriately. If the delegator fails to delegate appropriately then their own time may be used inappropriately, the skills and abilities of their team colleagues may be untapped, and the overall service may be compromised. Most importantly, appropriate delegation means that colleagues have the opportunity to perform to their maximum capability and therefore should experience a sense of accomplishment and enrichment. Delegation is not only about ensuring that care is provided, but also about valuing staff and their abilities and therefore promoting and maintaining morale. Table 17.6 outlines a series of steps that may be taken when making decisions about delegation.

Table 17.6 Steps to take to ensure effective delegation

1. Plan ahead
2. Identify the skill and educational level
3. Single out suitable individuals
4. Assign responsibility
5. Set time-frames and monitor
6. Grant authority
7. Give accountability
8. Evaluate performance and feedback

Inevitably there are times when the skills and abilities of staff available do not always meet the needs of the case load. This is where the skill of the delegating practitioner comes into place, in terms of how they manage the situation. Knowing the team and their abilities will be crucial in deciding if, as a team, it can manage with careful planning, organization and prioritizing of how each team member works. This will include identifying strategies of how each team member will support each other. While not the ideal, this is the process that an accountable practitioner must explore. They should ensure that their manager is aware of the situation, and also be able to identify at what point the situation can no longer be managed without further intervention. Patients cannot easily be taken off a caseload or ward, once accepted, unless of course their needs change. Finding extra staff is generally not an easy option with the current staffing difficulties, so alternative strategies need to be found. The option often sought is to close beds, reduce the number of patients, or stop admissions. Patients will still need to be looked after somewhere so other strategies need to be explored, such as accepting less-dependent patients, reviewing the way the hours that staff work are organized, the way the work is organized, identifying priorities in care, and considering how temporary staff can be accommodated.

Sadly, with the current recruitment and retention crisis, staff have become very adept at working with these kind of strategies. They do therefore need to be able to find time to look at other ways of trying to provide an effective and efficient service. Making sure that patients are in the right place, at the right time, and with the right skills is likely to help to improve care and throughput. Identifying new services to meet a need, as has been the case with many of the new services related to intermediate care, is another strategy that is worth exploring. Other strategies worth considering may involve reducing bed numbers so as to concentrate skills and actively promote rehabilitation with the intended outcome of increasing patient throughput and therefore promote the use of beds more effectively, etc. – although this improvement will need to be demonstrable. Taking staff out to provide training or development may reduce capacity temporarily, but in the longer term may increase capacity by ensuring that staff are equipped and able to assume delegated care and to meet patient needs and to work effectively.

Involving patients in decision-making

The importance of working with and involving patients through a person-centred approach has been emphasized within this book. This means that much of the decision-making of the practitioner should be significantly influenced by the views and wishes of patients. Their work will therefore involve encouraging patients to make decisions about their care and outcomes, if they are able to and wish to. Ensuring patients are enabled to make informed decisions is no easy attribute and thus warrants exploration.

Helping patients to be involved in their care and in decision-making in an effective and helpful way is important. This will require the practitioner not only to have insight into, and understanding of, how they themselves communicate, but also to have knowledge of their patients. There is a need to be able to appreciate how the patient wishes to be involved and how best to maximize their involvement without causing them stress. The concept of knowing patients as 'Monitors' or 'Blunters' has emerged. 'Monitors' wish to be actively involved and constantly updated and consulted, while the 'Blunter' may be more compliant and indicate that they are happy to comply with whatever the professional wishes. The 'Blunter' may initially seem less challenging to care for, but this may not necessarily be the case, for trying to provide person-centred care requires the practitioner to get to know them really well, so as to ensure that patients' wishes are incorporated into goals and decisions. Equally so, the involvement of the Monitor may shift, so here again there is a need to be alert to their immediate frame of mind and needs. By establishing such a relationship, the practitioner is in a much more favourable position to work with their patient and understand how to involve them in planning their rehabilitation goals, etc., for it is essential that all the team are working to the 'same tune'.

As indicated, the practitioner also needs to appreciate the way they are communicating and involving patients. In order to make a decision, the patient often needs to have information and will depend upon the practitioner or practitioners involved in their care to provide this information to help them make an informed decision. Having comprehensively collated information within the care plans will help with these discussions, but there are a range of factors that need consideration. Kennett (1986) identifies three areas that have relevance when seeking consent to treatment.

- Who should give the information?
- What information should be given?
- Where should the information be given?

These factors also have relevance to situations where patients are being informed and assisted to make decisions.

Who should give the information?

It is evidently helpful if the patient knows the practitioner/s assisting them in their decision-making, and has established trust and a relationship. Where there are staffing problems this may not be easy, but every effort should be made to ensure this, as then there is more likely to be a good understanding of the individual patient and what their needs are. The language that is used needs to be chosen carefully so as to ensure that the patient both understands and respects their capabilities. Cartwright and O'Brien (1976) found that doctors had a less sympathetic relationship with less well educated working-class patients. This could then influence the information given and the resulting intervention. Whether this is likely to be found among other practitioners such as nurses or therapists is open to speculation, but Cartwright and O'Brien (1976) also showed that more articulate and educated older people were able to negotiate better for social care services. Thus the practitioner needs to be aware of influences such as these on the way they work with individual patients.

It is important when looking to make decisions that family members and close carers are not marginalized and excluded. Family members are important sources of information about the relatives' values and lifestyle choices and, as McCormack (2001a) suggests, can 'often confirm values expressed by patients' (p. 432). However, it is also important not to assume that they can or should make decisions about the individual patient, for it is the rights of the patient that are important. This does not mean that carers' views are not considered, particularly where decisions made will directly affect them. Similarly, where family relationships are close and involved, the care and concern invested in these relationships must not be ignored or devalued. This would be an indictment on the integrity of family networks and the bonds that often hold families closely together. McCormack (2001a) demonstrated that family members would often take a superior stance over patients when it came to decision-making and that nurses adopted a 'deferential position' to them. This, however, may result in 'the erosion of patients' rights to make individual self-determined decisions' (p. 432). What is important for the practitioner is to use the information obtained from family members to negotiate and discuss with patients when making decisions, especially those that affect the family. Thus, as McCormack (2001a) suggests, it is the individuality of each particular case that determines the most appropriate approach, where the importance of adopting an interconnected approach between practitioner and patient is overriding. This interconnectedness, McCormack argues, 'holds central the knowledge and experience that each person brings to the care situation and which is necessary for decisions that will best serve the patient's well-being' (p. 441). This involves 'the clarifying of values so as to optimize opportunities for growth and the making of authentic decisions' (p. 441). By adopting such an approach, the potential to try to maintain personhood is promoted.

What information should be given?

It is important to consider what information is given to help a patient to make a decision or choice. Quite apart from the language/jargon that may be used either intentionally or inadvertently, consideration needs to be given to how much information is given. If too much information is given, or if this is too complex, the patient may not be able to understand or follow it. Somehow there is a need to provide the patient with enough information in plain language to facilitate an informed choice, but not so much that they are confused. There is always the risk that the practitioner lacks the appropriate skills, but perhaps the most crucial concern is that the practitioner may have a view about what is best for the patient or what they 'should' want – i.e. the practitioner may have 'therapeutic good intentions'. These good intentions are then very likely to influence directly the information that is imparted, so influencing the choice made by the patient.

Thus information may be given selectively such that only limited alternatives are offered. Dyer (1994) suggests that two challenges are at work when practitioners are helping patients to make decisions. The first, she suggests, is a professional issue of communicating available choices, and this is further influenced by views about rights and risks. Thus information shared may be influenced by personal professional opinion along with our ability to relay verbally or non-verbally our approval or disapproval of the decision being reached. Information shared may be further influenced by knowledge about available resources or waiting times, etc. Our views about the risks involved and our appreciation of the rights of patients to take risks and to make choices may also influence how we share information. The practitioner needs to be able to accept the consequences of a patient's choice, even if this leads to an undesirable outcome such as an accident, deteriorating health or even death – assuming the older person can engage in the decision.

Figure 17.4 illustrates the way in which a practitioner may empower patients not only to make an informed choice, but to express that choice. It is, however, very important to acknowledge that personal views or 'therapeutic good intentions' may influence the information given – even if this is not intended. On the other hand, Figure 17.5 illustrates how the practitioner may take on a paternalistic model of care, so influencing the patient's choice.

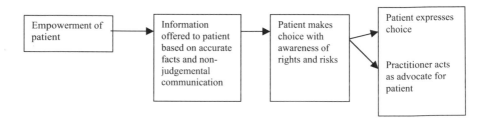

Figure 17.4 The empowerment model. (Adapted from Dyer 1994)

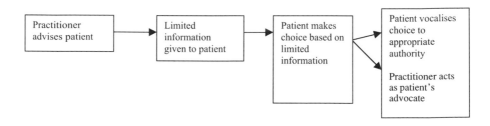

Figure 17.5 The paternalistic model. (Adapted from Dyer 1994)

Biley (1992b) suggests that there is a danger that practitioners expect or assume that an older person will not wish to participate and that they would prefer to fall in with the 'passive patient / active practitioner' relationship. Thus there is a risk that as a consequence of this expectation the older person simply complies with this since they believe the passive role is expected of them. As a result, there is a risk that this passivity becomes self-fulfilling, hence the importance of the practitioner really trying to understand the individual patient. Waterworth and Luker (1990) and McCormack (2001a) recognized this same notion in their research, such that McCormack identified that 'deference to professional opinion and decisions could be seen as the older person needing to "please" the nurse' (p. 427). Fry (1991) and Kitwood (1997) attribute this in part at least to the view that the older person lacks the capacity or ability to make decisions or choices. Experience, however, demonstrates that even when an individual has quite significant cognitive impairment, they can still often contribute actively and effectively in many decisions, if enabled and encouraged.

Evans (1992) argues that there is 'a basic contradiction in the idea of people empowering others because the very institutional structure that puts one group in a position to empower another also works to undermine the act of empowerment' (p. 142). Oliver (1989) suggests that for older people and those who are disabled, social and economic factors have as much influence in disabling and excluding them from work, social activities and the wider community as do the professional attitudes that label them as dependent and in need of empowerment. This disempowerment, Oliver (1989) argues, is further perpetuated by the enforced dependence on the social care system and access to money, and is backed up by the work of Phillipson (1998), as discussed in Chapter 5. Thus, 'although empowerment may be a useful slogan, there is a danger', as Stevenson and Parsloe (1993) point out, 'for it to act as an ill defined banner to travel under' (p. 58). So while empowerment literally means the giving of power, it might more easily be interpreted as creating opportunities that will enable and encourage the power to be taken. They argue that 'empowerment is about the processes which permeate organizations and professional thought'. 'The challenge is', they suggest, 'to create a culture in which such processes are able to thrive' (p. 58).

McCormack (2001a) was able to illustrate very effectively how nurses control information shared with patients and how they directly influenced both the direct care received, such as personal care, and the overall outcomes of care, based on their personal or 'therapeutic good intentions'. In his study examining interactions between nurses and older patients in day-to-day working practice and when nurses attended multidisciplinary meetings, he was able to illustrate that throughout the conversations recorded, patients allowed the decisions of professionals to dominate their decision-making.

It is therefore likely that, however hard the practitioner tries to be impartial and to help and advocate in a non-judgmental way for the patient, they will impart some influence as guided by their 'therapeutic good intentions' and organizational knowledge. It is, however, important to strive towards encouraging and empowering patients, but this should not be done in the naivety or 'rouse' of assuming the practitioner is not having some influence or in believing that they are acting as an advocate. A true advocate needs to be totally independent of the organization, and even then they may also find it hard to be completely non-judgemental.

Where should information be given?

Providing privacy remains a challenge for practitioners working within many settings, as environments often lack the opportunity to find personal space. Pulling a curtain round a bed does not create privacy or dignity, and yet practitioners often find such a strategy is the only one available to them. Most settings, however, do have quiet rooms that can be found and used; however, if the patient is in bed there may be factors that may make transfer to this room difficult. Difficulties may also be found in the patients' own homes, where relatives are keen to be involved and to help. Asking them to leave may not be an easy option. Evidently the practitioner should try to find ways to maximize the ability to respect the patient's privacy and dignity. If the patient cannot be moved it may be appropriate to ask others to move away in a polite and reasoned way.

Conclusion

It is very evident that decision-making and problem-solving is a complex process, and this is certainly the case within an intermediate care service/scheme. There may often be no 'right' or 'wrong' answer and it may be very difficult to make decisions or to obtain or find the right information, setting or environment or involve the right people to make decisions. Also, decision-making will be influenced by a range of factors that are specific to that particular situation, such as personal attributes and values, environmental and contextual factors, and professional mores and values. Gaining insight into the decision-making process can assist practitioners in their decision-making, together with increasing experience and adequate support and supervision.

KEY POINTS

* Practitioners working in intermediate care services/schemes will often be required to make quite complex decisions when working in isolated or autonomous situations, and therefore need to be adequately experienced and prepared to help them in their decision-making.
* Practitioners can be assisted in their decision-making and problem-solving

by recognizing and appreciating features and processes related to decision-making.

- The decision-making process will be influenced by a range of personal, situational and contextual factors that coincide at that particular moment. Use of a decision-making framework or model may assist in reaching outcomes.
- Practitioners in intermediate care will be required to delegate to colleagues who may be either junior or inexperienced and who may be working alone or in isolated settings. It is therefore important that these practitioners develop skills that enable them to delegate appropriately and are able to provide a rationale for their decisions.
- Involving patients/users in their own decision-making can be complex and challenging for practitioners. It is helped by getting to know the patient and their carers and by considering what information to give, where and when, and being there to assist them when needed. It is also often important to consider relatives' needs when making some decisions.

CHAPTER 18

Discharge planning – making it work for older people

SIÂN WADE

Introduction

The significance of managing the course or pathway of a patient's care has been discussed at intervals throughout this book. This chapter brings together these strands and focuses on the process and complexity of managing discharge or transfer of care. This latter term of 'transfer of care' has become a more accepted term in recent years, since the patient is often moving between services rather than out. This chapter will examine in some detail the concept of discharge/transfer of care, review the process and ways of managing it, and explore some of the challenges that may need to be considered and addressed in order to transfer or discharge a patient successfully.

Background

As discussed in previous chapters, there has been focused attention on admissions and the activity at the front door of hospitals, over the past few years, with a range of performance indicators and milestones being set to act as drivers for hospital managers in district general hospitals and practitioners in their work (DoH, 1998b, 2000c, 2002f). As identified, these have included such markers as reduced trolley waits, reduced waiting times for outpatient appointments and surgery, reduced lengths of stay, and a reduction of admissions, e.g. no more than a 2 per cent rise in hospital admissions for those over 75 years (DoH NHS Plan, 2000c). The subsequent preoccupation by hospitals and their staff in meeting these milestones can be attributed to the importance ascribed to their achievement and the associated funding and measures to attribute performance rating (DoH, 2000/2001).

The focus on the achievement of these contemporary milestones is in contrast to the attention given to discharge planning in the 1980s. This shift in emphasis has led to a very definite shift in the way patients move through the 'system', such that in effect patients are 'pushed through' rather than 'pulled through'. The consequences of this is that, with increased pressures and demands on beds and their availability, the rate at which the patient is transferred through the system may be escalated and this may lead to a premature and poorly planned discharge. This may mean that the needs of patients may not be appropriately met while in hospital, and these may not be adequately communicated or followed up at home. It can also lead to readmission, which may be due to poor management of aftercare arrangements, but certainly by no means always.

This emphasis on the 'front door' of activity has to some extent detracted attention from the complex and challenging activity centring on effective and successful discharge, and the pathway of care that a patient receives from the point of their admission to their transfer home or to another setting. The importance of this aspect of activity has already been referred to and discussed in earlier chapters of this book, but because of its significance within the context of intermediate care, further attention will be given to discharge planning and the concept of transfer of care in this chapter.

What are we talking about?

Booth and Davies (1991) emphasize that discharge planning is very much a process, rather than a single event. Armitage (1981) regarded discharge as 'a stage in patient care which has both a period of preparation and from which there are consequences. It cannot be examined in isolation from what has gone before or separated from what follows after the event when the patient leaves the hospital' (p. 386). Traditionally, discharge has been associated with going home from hospital. However, with the changing face of health and social care, and the increased acuity of care found in district general hospitals, the activity in acute hospitals has become one more of assessment, treatment and intervention followed by transfer on to a less acute setting or service, such as intermediate care – although there will still be many discharges/transfers directly home from the acute sector.

The challenge in achieving effective transfer/discharge can be attributed very often to the need for a number of different agencies to provide ongoing care for an individual. This is further challenged by the division of responsibilities between primary and secondary health care services and between health and social care services as discussed by Victor and Vetter (1988), and indeed those provided by voluntary agencies. A further challenge has been the mismatch between the services and resources available, and the assessed needs of individuals being discharged (Werrett et al., 2001), and indeed the presence or absence of informal carers (Jewell, 1993). In 1989 two influential documents were published which highlighted the significance of paying attention to effective discharge planning. The first was a joint statement by the British Geriatric Society and the Director of Social Services (BGS/Association of Social Services, 1989) and the second was the Department of Health Circular HC(89)5 (DoH, 1989). Both focused on the importance of starting discharge as early as possible and with the Circular (DoH, 1989) instructing health authorities to set up discharge policies for all client groups, advising that these should be monitored for their effectiveness. Discharge planning was also included in the Patients Charter in 1992 (DoH, 1992), and review by the Department of Health continues.

While attention has been given to developing care pathways over the past five to ten years, these have generally been disease focused. Here success has tended to be attributed to the predictable and fairly straightforward outcomes associated with the condition, e.g. for hip replacement, or where there is a specific diagnosis or set of symptoms (Ellis and Johnson, 1997; Middleton and Roberts, 2000). Care pathways have a very valuable part to play in relation to the journey of care many patients experience, but their potential in helping with those patients with more complex needs, particularly where multiple pathology is present, seems less easy, as discussed in Chapter 9. The recognition that there are inadequacies in meeting the discharge needs of many of these patients, especially the complex multi-factorial needs of many older people, have led to the emergence of myriad projects and services over the past few years, that could effectively be regarded as intermediate care. As discussed in earlier chapters, these services were often developed using time-limited funding. It has been only in recent years that their potential value in assisting with bed management and capacity problems has been recognized, and they have really come into their own in providing alternative future models of health and social care services. As a result, the more recent investment in intermediate care, as discussed in this book, has become a key milestone for the Department of Health within its agenda in *Delivering the NHS Plan* (DoH, 2002f) and the *National Service Framework for Older People* (DoH, 2001h). As a consequence of such service development and redevelopment, the significance of discharge planning and the monitoring of the progress of patients' care through the system has not only re-arisen but has become a significant focus of attention. Successful discharge and transfer of care is instrumental if the health service is to deal with the reduction in bed capacity that has occurred over the past decade and to manage its capacity problems effectively. If this is to be successfully achieved there is an imperative to improve and support joined-up planning and provision of services between health and social services.

Effective transfer/discharge planning can be very complex, and older people in particular 'can be very vulnerable to dislocations in the continuous patterns of care provision' (Victor et al., 1993: 1297). Traditionally health and social care systems, as discussed, have worked against each other at a time when older people, in particular, have needed them to work together, hence the attention given to the introduction of the Single Assessment Process (HSC, 2002/001: LAC (2002)1, DoH, 2002b). While the government has clearly recognized this dilemma (DoH, 2002f), and initiated reforms so that services are redesigned as barriers between health and social services start to be broken down, it is recognized that much more still needs to be done to bridge this gap. Similarly, it recognizes the gaps that still exist between hospital and community health provision. Thus, although reforms are under way there is still a long way to go.

The publication of the document *Discharge from Hospital: Pathway, Process and Practice* by the Department of Health early in 2003 (DoH, 2003) is testimony to the growing awareness of the need to shift the focus of attention from the 'front door' to the 'back door' of hospitals and services. In this document, models of good practice are provided but, as Glasby (2003) suggests, it is a long and bulky document and is difficult to read, consisting of lists and bullet points, and in effect it provides little that is new. What is really needed, Glasby argues, is detail about 'how to do it', together with support to put our good intentions into practice. It is understood that this is what the Department of Health plans to do next.

Promoting effective planning of discharge and transfer of care

It is evident that older people account for a key client group, who require skilled and co-ordinated planning for discharge and transfer of care. It is for this reason that staff working with older people in specialist and intermediate care settings/schemes probably regard transfer/discharge planning as a key activity of their service – it is in effect almost 'the name of their game' and is an implicit entity of the whole process of planned co-ordinated rehabilitation.

The need for effective liaison has been well recognized due to the multiple agencies involved in the provision of statutory health and social care services. Klop et al. in 1991 described how the division of responsibilities between different agencies created artificial boundaries that 'could result in "dislocations" in the pattern of care provision when a client either enters the system or finds themselves transferred between agencies, due to this transfer of responsibilities' (p. 409). This disparity of responsibility remains and is as powerful today as it was in the 1980s. It has in many ways become more problematic, first with the creation of Hospital Trusts and more recently with the creation of Primary Care Trusts. It is further challenged, as it always has been, by the lack of geographical co-terminosity of agencies, along with financial, legal and professional boundaries, as discussed by Glasby in Chapter 6. More recently, with the creation of the diverse range of intermediate care services/schemes, it has probably become even more complex as discussed in earlier sections, since these services/schemes often lack consistency and coherence, with individual PCTs modelling services to specific perceived local needs. This has made it even more challenging for clinical staff to keep on top of what services are provided in individual localities, what their intended purpose is and what their referral criteria are.

Reference to the concept of achieving a 'seamless discharge' was very popular in the 1980s and early 1990s, but less emphasis seems to be given to it in contemporary debates, but for the patient a sense of receiving seamless well-co-ordinated and communicated care will remain paramount. This may be because achievement of it can be extremely challenging, as discussed by Werrett et al. (2001). Werrett et al. (2001) found that the challenges of effective liaison are further compromised by the lack of, or unavailability of, a particular service, a lack of resources such as funding or skills, and poor communication. They found that staff in primary and secondary care were clearly aware of the particular training needs they had to best strive for seamless care, but these were often quite considerable. Personal experience suggests that there is sometimes a lack of appreciation by staff in each sector of the challenges faced by their colleagues. Staff in the secondary sector often fail to appreciate the very skilled capabilities of community staff and how this is sometimes compromised by the circumstances they work in, and the challenges faced in monitoring and caring for patients over the 24-hour period with limited resources and back-up. This has been known to create resentment, as has the failure by community staff to appreciate the very busy, often chaotic and pressurized circumstances that staff in hospitals and secondary care services experience.

While the importance ascribed to starting discharge planning as soon after admission as possible is still important (DoH, 1989, Circular HC(89)5), the reality of this within the current delivery of health care can be quite challenging. Patients may be very ill and may pass through a number of services at great speed. It may be difficult to collect information other than that required for their acute care needs – indeed it may be insensitive to do so at this stage. This is where ongoing assessment and collection of information is important, even if the emphasis is not immediately on the collation of this information. The introduction of single assessment and Electronic Patient Records should ensure that once information is obtained it is recorded and accessible to those involved in care in the future, and that it is not lost with the introduction of a new set of documentation in a new setting, or that the same questions are not asked on multiple occasions – see Chapter 10.

A changing picture

The picture related to transfer and discharge appears to be changing. For some patients assessment in A&E and MAU, often by designated nurses, occupational therapists, social workers or teams, may mean that the patient can be transferred directly out to an intermediate care service such as rapid response or community rehabilitation teams so as to avoid admission (Bywaters et al., 2002). Here transfer arrangements will need to be organized, but ultimate discharge is most likely to be arranged by the intermediate care service at a later stage. Where admission is planned, e.g. for surgery, then pre-admission care is increasingly incorporating discharge planning with services and equipment required after discharge, planned and ordered in advance so that they can be in place as soon as the patient is ready to go home. Where it is envisaged that discharge following admission can be achieved in a fairly straightforward way, a range of intermediate care support services are increasingly being introduced to support district general hospitals in a bid to transfer patients out as quickly as possible, so as to free up beds. Schemes such as designated occupational therapy staff or multidisciplinary teams who can outreach or work closely with community rehabilitation teams have been introduced, while supported discharge and 'hospital at home' schemes provide an alternative service. Here again, ultimate discharge arrangements are made by the team, dislocating the responsibility of arranging complex discharges from hard-pressed staff providing immediate care on acute wards. Transfer arrangements, however, will be important and will require careful attention to prevent a breakdown in ongoing care.

Where patients in acute settings are assessed and judged as needing ongoing care, e.g. significant rehabilitation or social care, it has become increasingly evident that planning for discharge is being deferred until the patient reaches their rehabilitation, intermediate or transitional/interim care service. There are a range of reasons that may account for this. With limited therapists and social workers within the acute sector, priorities need to be made and in essence attention is going to be given to those who are acutely ill or who, as suggested above, with some intervention can be speedily discharged. There is also the argument that care will need to be transferred on to another service, and so it may be wiser not to start in the acute setting. One of the problems associated with this delay is that the time lapse between referral and transfer may be quite long and can lead to regression. This time lapse may also mean that any delay at this stage will lead to further delay along the pathway of care. This dilemma seems to be a 'symptom of the times' – even though it compromises the whole drive to move patients on and eventually discharge them as speedily as possible. A delay in hospital also increases the risk of iatrogenisis (Illich, 1975) which along with regression may lead to an even greater length of stay, that could well impact upon the ultimate end destination of the patient and their quality of life. It is therefore important for acute settings to have in place a mechanism for ensuring that the needs of patients are anticipated and planned for, so that referral and transfer of care can occur as soon as is appropriate and possible. This concept of anticipation is quite skilled, and may be quite a challenge for teams, especially nurses or junior doctors who are preoccupied in giving acute and sometimes emergency care. For this reason it is probably becoming more relevant to create some kind of tracking system, such as through the creation of a designated skilled multidisciplinary team, as previously mentioned, who visit and work with the ward staff to assess patients in the acute setting. Alternatively, the creation of a virtual team may be a feasible approach as described below. It may well be that a combination of the two would be most beneficial, since there needs to be someone to co-ordinate, manage and oversee the referral and transfer. The role of the discharge liaison nurse, depending on their role, may be key in this since they interface across locations and tend to have positive communications with other health professionals and agencies (Werrett et al., 2001), although traditionally they have tended to provide more of an advisory and supportive role to staff in most settings.

In many settings it is not unusual for referral to a service to depend upon a decision by a consultant who is responsible for the care of an individual patient. For example, referral to specialist rehabilitation for older people is often dependent on the patient being referred by their consultant to a geriatrician and their team. Failure to do this denies even the opportunity for the patient to be assessed for suitability of this speciality's input. Likewise, patients may be very much dependent upon their consultant for referral to other services or specialist opinions. Very often the concept of multidisciplinary team-working does not exist in all specialities, and although ward staff can play a role in suggesting referral they may feel they have no authority, and their contribution will depend very much on how well it is received. Equally so, while some consultants, notably those in 'care of older people' specialities, are committed to working in multidisciplinary teams and reaching a collaborative decision about when a patient is fit for transfer or discharge, many clinicians in other specialities are not and here the consultant's decisions may hold sway. The consequence of this is, according to Penhale (1997), that staff either resort to subterfuge to delay the discharge, or provide a 'quick fix' by arranging as 'safe a discharge as possible' (p. 50).

Similarly, some intermediate care services will accept a patient for their service only when they have assessed the patient themselves. This can lead to delays and challenges to the decisions of others. The introduction of Single Assessment and Electronic Patient Records should enhance the identification and suitability of patients for services, helping to trigger the need for appropriate referral. The introduction of skilled, experienced multidisciplinary and/or virtual teams, as suggested, may also help to overcome these problems where peer trust is established in their ability and skill to assess and refer patients appropriately so as to enable the patient to be accepted without further assessment or delay.

Development of a tracking system or Virtual Ward

The challenges faced by hospital management in managing their bed capacity is critical, with the tough targets faced. An initiative adopted in one district general hospital involved the creation of what came to be known as a 'Virtual Ward'. Staff had expressed concern about the delays that patients seemed to experience in being transferred for rehabilitation services – specialist or intermediate care. A brief audit of those patients waiting funding for residential care helped to confirm this concern. A key finding was that older patients were repeatedly in the wrong place for their needs at a particular time in their care pathway. While it would be difficult to prove, this appeared to impede what it would seem should have been the expected outcome for the patient (Middleton and Roberts, 2000), see Case study 18.1.

Case study 18.1

Mrs S was a lady who had been managing quite well at home until she developed a urinary tract infection, which led to her admission to the district general hospital. This lady could possibly have benefited from an intermediate care service rather than admission to an acute setting, but in this case an acute admission was the only option at the time. On her fourth day in hospital she was referred to a geriatrician and accepted for the specialist rehabilitation unit; however, no beds were available in the unit due to a range of reasons, and at that time there were very few intermediate care schemes. It was some weeks before a bed was available in the rehabilitation unit, and during this time Mrs S was moved around a number of wards in the drive to manage beds. By the time she reached a rehabilitation ward, she had regressed considerably and was assessed as needing to go into residential care, yet her history suggested she should have been able to rehabilitate in a fairly short time after her admission and gone home. This raised questions about her pathway of care and indeed the services available. One could not help believing that this outcome could have been avoided if she had received the rehabilitation she needed at a more timely stage of her pathway of care. This would have released or even saved both an acute bed and a long-term care place and enabled Mrs S to go home and continue to live relatively independantly.

This case study was not unique in the audit. While it was evident that there were a number of key factors specific to the organization that contributed to this scenario, which could not be solved by one intervention – it was clear that there were lessons to be learnt and action to be taken.

Among other initiatives, this was to lead to the establishment of the 'Virtual Ward'. In effect, a system was established whereby a team of staff who worked on the wards was identified to participate in the tracking and progress of certain identified patients, from their point of access either in A&E/MAU or their next destination/s – be this back home, to an intermediate care service or to another ward. It involved working with the IT department, as a key component of the system was the creation of a website that would allow patients who were classified with certain conditions or reasons for presenting at the hospital to be tagged on the system (not electronic tagging of the patient). A range of coding classifications were identified, as outlined in Table 18.1.

Table 18.1 Patient groups identified for Virtual Ward

- People who had fallen so that they could be tracked to ensure that they accessed a falls clinic when appropriate

- Patients who were perceived as having complex needs and who might benefit from a comprehensive geriatric assessment (with the Single Assessment Process these patients may be more easily identified anyway)

- Patients perceived as needing rehabilitation so that action could be taken to try to assess them and transfer them to the right setting as soon as it is appropriate

- Patients who had had, or were suspected of having had, a stroke

---

The system created would allow patients to be tracked to whatever setting they went to, by tagging their name on the information technology system. To support this initiative it was necessary to create an e-mail site for team members so that they could communicate with each other, providing information and recommending actions related to specific patients that they felt was important. Initial agreement was reached as to who should be involved in the 'virtual team' although this was probably only a starting point and was not deemed to be exclusive (Table 18.2). At the time of planning there was a nurse employed to work within A&E and MAU, a role that, as previously discussed, has proved to be successful in a number of hospital settings – although the actual roles may vary (Khanna and Geller, 1992; Bridges et al., 2000). While the role and remit of this nurse in A&E and MAU was wide-ranging it was envisaged as having a key part in the success of the Virtual Ward.

Table 18.2 The virtual team

- A&E nurse for older and vulnerable adults
- Discharge liaison sisters
- Therapists
- Geriatricians
- Social workers
- Bed management
- Ward managers
- Link ward discharge nurses

The overall effect of the system was for any team member to identify a patient that they felt would benefit, or would benefit in time, from a service. As suggested, these might include services such as rehabilitation or a falls clinic, etc. The virtual team members would then be aware of the patient and where they were in the system, and could keep patients monitored – trying to ensure that they received the correct therapy on their current ward and were referred in a timely way to the appropriate service, e.g. specialist rehabilitation, intermediate care schemes, falls clinic, etc. Such a tool would be only a guide and aid, and each patient would need to be assessed individually according to their specific needs. Also it would assess only the circumstances, as of that time. In conjunction with this work a screening tool was drawn up that would help team members to assess and refer patients deemed suitable for the various specialist setting or intermediate care rehabilitation schemes available. For this to work an agreement had to be reached for certain team members to be allowed to assess patient suitability and to refer the patient to another service without others coming in to reassess. While the team would include geriatricians, who up to that date had to have seen and accepted the patient for their service, their remit to refer was no longer exclusive. Such a system could contribute to comprehensive assessment and could eventually form part of the Single Assessment Process.

To make this kind of system work requires a number of factors to be addressed. There is a need to work closely with bed management to ensure that patients are transferred to the right wards, for although bed management will try to ensure the appropriate transfer of patients, crisis can lead to unexpected moves which do not best meet patients' needs. In particular, this means ensuring that only patients who would benefit from transfer to a specialist care and rehabilitation setting for older people are transferred to this setting, and those who will benefit from intermediate care are transferred to the appropriate intermediate care service. There is also a need to make sure that the specialist care and rehabilitation setting provides an effective service (which depends on resources, skills, environment and indeed the right patients being there), and for there to be clarity about the resources available in intermediate care services/schemes. There is a need to have and to be aware of the range of intermediate care services/schemes that are available for patients to be referred to, and for clarity about the resources of the intermediate care service/scheme, as well as having access to equipment in a timely and accessible way. There also needs to be adequate intermediate care support.

One of the biggest challenges facing acute hospitals at present are those patients who need time before they can rehabilitate, e.g. patients in plaster of Paris, as well as terminally ill patients and those patients who have been assessed as unable to benefit from further rehabilitation, and who are awaiting funding or placement. The needs of these patients are very poorly addressed, as has already been identified in Chapter 4. These patients may not meet the criteria for rehabilitation or intermediate care beds or schemes, and if they are transferred to any of these they may be perceived as preventing the bed or place being used for its designated purpose. While it is important that patients are given every chance to maximize their potential for rehabilitation, there will inevitably be some frail older people for whom rehabilitation is no longer realistic. It may well be that they have already benefited from rehabilitation opportunities in the past and been enabled to remain at home for some considerable time. However, at some point, for some individuals, this situation at home can no longer be sustained and the long-term care requirements of these patients need to be addressed.

As discussed, these patients currently seem to fall into a 'black hole', and they may remain on an acute ward, which is not suitable for them, or their placement may become very 'hit and miss'. They need, and have a right to, skilled care. Where there is no identified setting or funding for their care, it is this client group that is likely to lead to the beds not being used for the purpose they are intended for, and for them not necessarily to be in the best setting for them.

The process of transfer/discharge planning

As suggested, the skill of ensuring the appropriate transfer or discharge of older people with complex care needs increasingly falls very much to specialist care settings and intermediate care services, so staff in these settings need to ensure that they develop appropriate skills. It is important that staff develop a comprehensive understanding of the process involved in planning and preparing for transfer or discharge of care. This process can be effectively displayed diagrammatically as a flow chart, and Jewell (1993) provide a useful example of this (Fig 18.1).

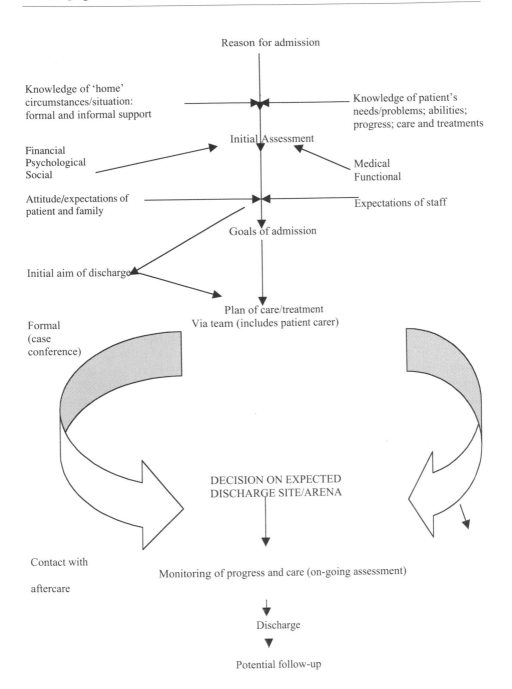

Figure 18.1 The discharge process.
Source: adapted from Jewell (1993).

The importance of effective assessment, teamwork and communication cannot be over-estimated. Skeet (1970) suggested that there was a distinct lack of communication between multidisciplinary teams and patients regarding discharge. This was in 1970 and yet numerous research and studies undertaken since then have re-enforced communication as a problem (Patton, 1980; DoH, 1989, circular (HC(89)5); Victor and Vetter, 1988; Jewell, 1993, Victor et al., 1993; Tripp and Caan, 1999; Werrett et al., 2001).

A range of early studies highlighted the failure to assess the home circumstances of patients, especially older patients, so that a social 'diagnosis' and accurate evaluation of need were difficult to make (Skeet, 1970; Amos, 1973; Hockey, 1968; Bowling and Betts, 1984). This is of significance since older patients are likely to need a greater level of aftercare following admission than they did before (Bowling and Betts, 1984; Victor and Vetting, 1988). It could be argued that this has improved over the years with a greater emphasis on the place of a home visit. However, the effectiveness of home visits has been questioned (Bore, 1994) for, as Clarke and Dyer (1998) contend, they provid only a 'snapshot in time' (p. 38) where safety is often a priority, and at a time when the patient is often in a state of anxiety. Clarke and Dyer (1998) go on to discuss how the episodic nature of a home visit means that the occupational therapist has little opportunity to monitor or evaluate their input. Patients often find themselves with equipment they can't use, don't need or won't use, while recognizing the need for additional or alternative interventions, but not knowing to whom they can turn for help to access these. The recent development of community rehabilitation teams and other intermediate care services go some way to resolve these concerns, but as yet there is no parity or consistency in the provision of these services.

Another challenge related to home visits occurs when there is pressure on beds in hospital so that a home visit may not be managed as well as it could be. Here a hospital discharge may be driven more by the exigencies of emptying beds (Means and Smith, 1994; Wistow, 1995), than best meeting patients' needs.

These studies reinforce the importance of the need to identify collaborative goals with patients within the process of rehabilitation so as to work effectively towards agreed discharge plans. Many of these were early studies, but a study by Clarke and Dyer (1998) and that by Tripp and Caan in 1999 suggested that involvement of patients in collaborative goal-planning still remained problematic in the late 1990s. Tripp and Caan's (1999) study showed that patients had not been involved in identifying their goals of rehabilitation, such that the goals of professionals could well differ from those of the patients, and thus militate against the opportunity to negotiate appropriate outcomes with the patient. They also identified the implicit need to involve patients and to include relatives/carers in discussions about discharge plans. This supports the value of effective multidisciplinary, inter-disciplinary or trans-disciplinary working in reaching negotiated and collaborative goals that are meaningful for patients and effectively communicated, as discussed in Chapter 16. Personal experience still suggests this is an aspiration that is poorly met in many rehabilitation areas.

Victor et al. (1993) clearly found that patients and their carers remained peripheral to the transfer/discharge process, as did Tripp and Caan (1999). Waterworth and Luker (1990) found that patients were often reluctant to become involved in decisions about their care but, as discussed in Chapter 17, every effort should be made to involve them as much as they feel able and to try to help them to recognize that this is valued. This should be part of the inherent culture of the service.The importance of documenting any conversations with patients and their carers is imperative if their views and concerns are to be reflected in planning for the future. Failure to share or transfer documentation on to new settings again compromises the opportunity to ensure that all information that is collected is shared in relation to discharge planning, and supports the imperative of introducing single assessment. Currently, however, communication between staff members is not only compromised by the lack of shared documentation, but also by the lack of information technology skills of staff, as identified by nurses in Werrett et al.'s study (2001) and by the lack of a compatible information technology infrastructure across agencies and Trusts.

As noted, in 1989 the Department of Health released its circular HC(89) 5 entitled 'Discharge of patients from hospital'. In this document three key areas were emphasized as needing to be addressed for effective discharge or transfer of care, as outlined in Table 18.3.

Table 18.3 Three key areas for effective discharge or transfer of care planning

1. A multidisciplinary approach to discharge
2. The importance of starting discharge planning as soon as possible
3. The active involvement and centrality of patient/carers in the discharge process

Source: DoH (1989).

The importance of each of these key areas has already been reflected in discussions to date.

Waters and Booth (1991) also identified a number of key areas that they felt needed to be addressed when planning discharge, and these are noted in Table 18.4.

Table 18.4 Recommendations for effective discharge planning

1. Starting discharge preparation as soon as possible
2. The centrality of patients and carers in the discharge planning process
3. A named member of the multidisciplinary team should hold responsibility for discharge planning
4. Where appropriate, written information should be provided about lifestyle, diet and medical symptoms
5. All discharge preparation should be based on effective multidisciplinary working, including both hospital and community staff
6. The provision of written discharge procedures

Source: Waters and Booth (1991).

This highlights the importance of having a named member of the team who is responsible for co-ordinating and ensuring a successful discharge. Because discharge planning involves a range of team members and staff from across agencies it is difficult to pinpoint any one person who is responsible, as demonstrated in the study of Victor et al. (1993). Despite this, it is often the nurse, who is present over the 24-hour period, who is perceived as co-ordinating the plans and being responsible. Ultimately it is either the consultant or GP who accepts the final responsibility, or within nurse-led settings may delegate this, once medical problems have been resolved. They will not, however, co-ordinate the planning and, according to Victor et al. (1993), they would not see themselves as responsible for this. Victor et al.'s (1993) study also revealed that it was unclear as to who was responsible and made a plea for this ambiguity to be clarified. The introduction of the concept of the 'named nurse' in the 1990s (or primary nurse/key worker role) may well have been an indicator that they should take responsibility. In general, however, nurses do not have the infrastructure or resources in terms of managerial authority to make decisions or the resources to implement them, let alone the knowledge of services, agencies and resources available (Werrett et al., 2001). Increasingly, much of the responsibility has fallen to care managers following the introduction of the Community Care Act (DoH, 1990a). Responsibility, however, does often fall to the patient's key nurse to co-ordinate and collate the information, although all team members play a part and make contributions towards the plans, often with the support of discharge liaison nurses where available. It may well be that the nurse is the most appropriate person, but to be effective this must involve teamwork where effective decision-making is made involving the knowledge and perspective of each team member.

Booth and Davies (1991) conclude that the nurse should co-ordinate the care, but emphasize the importance of communication and documentation. Because of the complexity of the planning and the roles played by so many people, the importance of documentation is paramount. This again calls for both effective team-working and also collaborative care planning and records, so that a quick reference to the documentation can provide a clear picture of the progress to date with clarity about who is doing or has done what. Booth and Davies (1991) recommend a multidisciplinary checklist of the information that should be transferred with patients when they transfer or go home, as outlined in Table 18.5. This ties in with the importance of patient education prior to discharge, e.g. on the side effects of drugs, dietary needs, activity and pain management, along with real discussion about aftercare. This was found to be poor in both early studies (Skeet, 1970) and more recent studies (Booth and Davies, 1991; Klop et al., 1991. Even if this has been provided, it may not have been given in written form for the patient

Table 18.5 Health and education needs assessment checklist

Activities of living
Mobility around the house and presence of stairs
Getting up in the morning
Dressing/undressing
Washing and bathing
Footcare
Eating, drinking: preparation of meals
Shopping
Maintenance of continence
Sexuality
Stress management/relaxation
Communication, e.g. care of hearing aid
Comfort needs and keeping warm

Social needs
Presence of carers/relatives or arrangements
Support of carers, e.g. lifting techniques and how to prevent pressure sores
Relief for carers (respite care)
Companionship
Advice on financial needs and any benefits
Advice on how to obtain information
Self-help groups
Security needs
Worship needs

Nursing/medical needs
Understanding of diagnosis
Understanding of medication
Nursing procedures, e.g. dressings
Arrangements for emergencies
Medical and nursing follow-up

or recorded as given. The provision of booklets in which written information can be provided for patients is another addition that supports the spoken word, and can be very valuable for patients and their carers as a backup and reassurance of both the care/services arranged and of any advice given. This may be pre-written or collated according to individual patients' needs.

There is also a need to have a checklist for staff so that a record is available of who has arranged what. This might include who has the key to the home, if there will be someone there to meet them, when and what transport has been arranged, and if medications have been ordered and arrived, etc.

Once the patient has moved to a new setting or returned home, inadequate information is often available to staff involved in providing ongoing care. Transfer summaries and future plans of care or action are often poor or non-existent, and there may be long delays before GPs receive discharge letters. With the introduction of the Single Assessment Process and Electronic Patient Records, all these aspects should be covered in a more structured way and, all being well, this will help to improve the experience of patients transferred between services and agencies – providing that the information is recorded.

In addition to the skills of planning effective discharge and transfer of care, there is also an important and often neglected role for staff in helping to prepare those patients transferring to a care home, as discussed in Chapter 15. Here the patient is facing a major life-changing transition, often fraught with emotional challenges, and there is an implicit need for staff members to demonstrate skill and empathy in facilitating this transfer.

Other considerations

There are a range of other issues or concerns that centre round the process of discharge planning and transfer of care. One of these concerns the procedure adopted when patients are admitted to hospital as an emergency and who have already established community services provided at home. While liaison of discharge planning may be problematic, the procedure used to ensure that these community services are informed of an admission is even more problematic. Patients may often be admitted via a 999 call and then transferred through a range of settings before eventually reaching a ward. There does not always appear to be a system by which these services are contacted and informed of their patients' admission and so achievement of this may be rather 'hit and miss'. This was a criticism put forward by primary care providers in Victor et al.'s study (1993). If the patient is very ill the focus on their social circumstances may not be a priority, but it seems that some kind of protocol is needed. Again, a checklist asking what services are involved and triggering the need to ensure that they are aware of the admission could help. It is also useful and important to keep in mind that if a range of services is already involved in supporting a patient at home, this can be reinstated on discharge, so long as this is within two weeks of admission. If, however, discharge is delayed, the funding and whole provision will need to be reassessed and funding resought – inevitably leading to some delay. Of course, it is not unusual for reassessment to be necessary as a result of changed care needs, but this will not always be the case.

The pressures faced by social services in funding care are ongoing and seem to be escalating, as the government tries to find ways not only of avoiding admission to hospital and speeding up discharge, but also in preventing admission to long-term care. Social services funding has been a long-term concern within the equation of health and social care. The introduction of intermediate care has been one means to try to address this, but it is by no means sufficient. There has been a failure to address the issue of interim or transitional care in many areas, so that patients who are waiting for funding, or indeed a place in a care home, may have to wait in an acute/district general hospital bed. This goes back to the discussion in Chapters 1 and 3, where the older person is criticized for 'blocking a bed'.

The introduction of health flexibilities, where money is pooled from different health and social services budgets into a mutually accessible budget to provide services, may go some way to resolve some of these challenges (Glasby and Littlechild, 2000b; DoH, 2002f). Here the source of the funding contributions lose their specific identity, and the funds can be used to assist in meeting the needs of certain patients. This system has its potential, but it does have to be set up carefully and requires legal involvement to reach agreements and monitoring strategies. The creation of Care Trusts, where health and social services are brought together in one local organization for specific client groups has been heralded as another way of resolving some of the issues concerning clients needs (Glasby and Littlechild, 2000b), and they do seem to have potential. Fundamentally, however, there still needs to be the resources there to fund these schemes. Currently the funding going into health care seems to be disproportionately greater than that going into social services, as has been identified by a study commissioned by Help the Aged (2002). This, together with the government guidance to target resources on those in most acute need, has resulted in cuts in preventive help. Another scheme to be adopted by the government originates from Sweden and Denmark and is referred to as the Scandinavian Model. This involves cross-charging and requires that social services cover the cost of beds blocked in hospitals through delayed discharges. This was a recommendation made by the Wanless Review and may be legislated for (DoH, 2002f – *Delivering the NHS Plan*).

It was suggested that the cash announced for social services in the Budget in March 2002 would include the funding to cover this cost. It was intended that councils should use these resources to expand care at home and to ensure that older people are able to leave hospital once their treatment is completed and they are deemed medically fit and safety needs have been considered. The government believes that if local councils reduce the number of 'blocked beds' in hospital, they will have the freedom to use these resources to invest in alternative social care services, and that the initiative will provide an incentive to ensure that patients do not experience long delays in their discharge. How this will work in reality will be interesting to see but, as Glasby (2002) suggests, the concept is flawed, since the charges will threaten to distort social services priorities. While attention is focused on discharging, there could be a growth in admissions as preventive measures to stop admission are compromised. This is potentially likely to increase the problems associated with the flow of patients once a patient has been admitted, so compounding current problems. It would seem very much more desirable to invest in preventing admissions more proactively, with investment here, as discussed in Chapter 3. The government has claimed it is going to match this social services initiative with incentive charges on NHS hospitals, making them responsible for the costs of emergency readmissions, so as to try to prevent patients being discharged prematurely. Again, it will be interesting to see how the distinction is made between a 'failed discharge' and a genuine deterioration in health of a frail older person whose medical stability is compromised.

Another problem facing Hospital Trusts occurs where a patient has been assessed as medically stable and able to go home or be transferred e.g. to a care home, but who declines to go, or whose relative declines to agree to transfer. This is a challenge that has been experienced by a number of Trusts over the years, and indeed a number of the cases have made headline news. The challenge has been addressed in a number of ways, but is increasingly being addressed more assertively. In Oxfordshire a joint policy was drawn up between social services and the then health authority, and supported by all the Trusts and a range of voluntary and patient representation groups (OHA/OSS, 2002). The resulting document provides standards that have to be followed in facilitating the transfer of the patient and which, if unsuccessful, eventually leads to a referral to legal services with legal action commencing.

The situation with regard to the care home industry may become more challenging as the closure of care homes escalates. This is in the face of insufficient funding and fees that have not progressed with the rate of inflation, difficulty in recruiting and retaining staff, and the need to meet the new care home standards. Many homes are finding these standards almost impossible to meet (DoH, 2001a), although some have been be relaxed for those homes already in existence. Avoidance of this may well depend upon the ability of social services to increase their fees, as suggested within *Delivering the NHS Plan* (DoH, 2002f).

A final issue that is of relevance here relates to those patients who for some reason find their discharge home compromised due to housing issues. This may be due to the need for adaptations or for rehousing and may be due to a range of reasons. There is inevitably a small but significant group of such people who are assessed as medically fit to be discharged, but who become caught in the health care system. There seem to be very few options available for these people while they need to wait, and often this does seem to be in a hospital bed. This issue goes back partly to the lack of transitional/interim care beds for some patients. It does, however, seem that the process by which housing problems are resolved often seem to be intractable, and that it is an area that needs to be worked on – it is certainly acknowledged as a issue within *Delivering the NHS Plan* (DoH, 2002f).

Conclusion

The attention and focus on the importance of discharge and transfer of care planning have waxed and waned over the years. In reality it cannot be ignored if patients are to receive appropriate ongoing care and follow-up when needed. Nor can it be ignored within the contemporary challenges of effective bed management and use of bed capacity. New ways of working and new services are currently being developed continuously through joined up planning and provision to try to support the delivery of services that meet the health and social care needs of patients. The process of planning for complex ongoing care is challenging, but if managed in a structured and organized way that keeps the patient/client at the centre of the plans, and ensures effective communication among the diverse team members involved, it is well within the capacity of staff involved in care, and most certainly of staff in intermediate care services.

KEY POINTS

- Well-planned and co-ordinated discharge/transfer of care is essential if many older people with complex or complicated needs are to experience smooth and seamless care.
- Discharge planning is very much a process, rather than a single event. It can be regarded as a stage in patient care that involves a period of preparation and from which there are consequences. It cannot be examined in isolation from what has gone before, and relates directly to what follows afterwards.

- Discharge planning/transfer of care should start at admission, if not before; however, the reality of this within current health care delivery can be challenging.
- Managing effective discharge planning/transfer of care is unequivocally implicit in effective bed management of trolley waits, waiting lists and appointments times.
- Arranging effective discharge/transfer of care can be challenging due to divisions in responsibility and the range of different agencies often involved in providing care and support – this can result in dislocations in the pattern of care received. It has become increasingly challenging with the increase in the range of services a patient may be able to access.

CHAPTER 19
Conclusion

This book has set out to explore the potential of intermediate care for older people within health and social care delivery in the twenty-first century. It has endeavoured to explore the concept of intermediate care and the context within which it has emerged. Intermediate care seems to be developing as an additional range of services to support the traditional and established health and social care service model or framework we have become familiar with. With the rapid advances made in health care and the remarkable increase in health-related technology – along with the changing population profile – it has become evident that this changing picture can no longer be sustained within this established model or framework of health and social care. The activity now undertaken within the acute sector is one much more of assessment, diagnostics, treatment and intervention. On-going recovery no longer 'fits into this mould' and with the changing population of older people requiring time to recover and rehabilitate following illness, this element of care is perhaps better provided 'closer to home' whenever possible. This need not, however, mean that the care, services and support received are second rate. As has been argued within this book, if this 'closer to home' care is developed and managed appropriately older people could well receive an excellent service – a Rolls-Royce service in fact.

In Chapter 4 the effects of ageing and how it can affect older people reveals why it is that older people in particular have been affected by this changing picture of health and social care. Older people are more likely to experience complex and multiple pathology, and primary ageing means that functional reserve is often compromised, so that a longer time is required for recovery and/or rehabilitation. As a result of acute illness, chronic problems may emerge which means that some older people will need ongoing help and support – at least for a period of time. Chapter 5 has tried to provide some background to the emergence of societal views towards older people, and in particular how their care needs have often been viewed, and as a result marginalized within the health care services. The changing picture of activity in acute health care delivery, as described above, seems to have compounded the situation for older people, often singling them out as presenting as a 'problem'.

This concept of older people being a 'problem' has been totally unnecessary, and could have been avoided had the health and social care economy pre-empted and acknowledged the 'inevitable' and responded proactively to the predictable changing population profile and its needs. The fact that the population has long been predicted with life-expectancy increasing consistently over recent years has indicated clearly the longer-term impact. The effects of ageing, as discussed, and the fact that older people need time to recover has also been a well-known fact. Yet despite this, the concept of intermediate care has been slow in coming. Indeed, as discussed in Chapter 1, the history of this kind of service has been very chequered, with repeated evidence of resistance to recognize the value and potential for this kind of model of care. It seems sad, therefore, that it has in effect taken a crisis in terms of bed management and capacity problems in the acute sector for the potential of intermediate care to be realized.

There has been a preoccupation with centralization and technology. While concentrating this level of activity centrally has probably been the correct move, it could be argued that 'heads have remained buried in the sand' when the predicted demographic trends and the associated changing needs were clearly evolving at the same time. Had a more visionary view been taken of the direction that health and social care delivery might best move in order to respond to these demographic changes and needs, the concept of 'care in the middle' or intermediate care could have become established in a more organized and measured way. In particular, needs-responsive models of care for older people could have been better planned and developed. Instead, it seems that intermediate care has had to develop as a 'bolt on' or 'add on' service trying to integrate into an already well-established and enshrined traditional norm of health and social care delivery. The challenge of this has not only been from a structural and organizational perspective but also from a cultural perspective, and in particular from the perspective of professionals who seem to have remained wedded to traditional ways of working. It is also having to develop at considerable speed rather than, as suggested, in a planned and measured way, and it could be argued that in some ways it has come too late, and we are 'trying to shut the stable door when the horse has already bolted'.

All this is occurring at a time when community services have recently been taken over by PCTs and when PCTs have been preoccupied and immersed in organizational change. As such, these are still immature organizations which have not only lacked experience in commissioning new services but, it could be argued, have not always perceived this kind care, i.e. intermediate care as part of their remit (after all, it is 'in the middle'). Some PCTs have taken it on with enthusiasm and commitment, while for others little enthusiasm has been evident.

In the process of demonstrating the opportunities related to intermediate care there have emerged a range of tensions, barriers and challenges, that if not addressed or resolved could in fact 'sabotage' the potential of intermediate care in providing a needs-responsive model of care for older people. The result of this could be that it becomes a lost opportunity, and indeed a replication of the much maligned 'Cinderella services'. If developments are to be successful and effective, as discussed in Chapter 6, it will require a concerted effort on behalf of all participating agencies to look above and beyond their own individual agendas and work collaboratively so as to reach workable compromises – so as to achieve positive outcomes for older people. While this by no means prevents the potential of intermediate care emerging, it adds to the challenges faced, hindering the ease and speed with which these developments can progress.

A range of strategies and approaches that may help have been introduced in this book and, if adopted, may help to overcome some of the challenges. Intermediate care offers the opportunity to provide a person-centred and individualized service for older people – recognizing the importance of personhood and enabling practitioners to 'get inside the person' so as to respond in a way that tries to listen to and respond to their needs and wishes. It provides a means of providing support and care in a more equitable way across localities, while also acknowledging that 'a one size fits all' approach is not appropriate.

Involvement of older people is essential if services are to respond appropriately, and Thewlis in Chapter 7 has described one way in which they can be actively involved and the voice of the real user can be heard. The development of care pathways and use of the Single Assessment Process, as discussed in Chapters 8 and 9, also provide tools that should help, while comprehensive evaluation is important in demonstrating successes, and also limitations that can then be addressed. Effective multi/interdisciplinary working is essential if the holistic needs of older people are to be provided for, and this needs to be addressed proactively if it is to be achieved appropriately. Above all, staff development will be crucial, and at a time when recruitment and retention of staff is critical, 'thinking outside the box' and looking for lateral solutions will need to be high on the agenda. Looking to new roles to facilitate this agenda provides many opportunities, while strong leadership will be at the crux of developments.

This book has tried to demonstrate how, if managed and developed well, intermediate care could provide a very effective service, particularly for older people. The potential to develop and redesign gerontological services for older people is considerable. If the potential opportunities can be grasped wholeheartedly then a holistic, responsive and whole-systems service could emerge, which would provide a Rolls-Royce service for older people. The challenge, however, is huge, as identified throughout this book. Considerable work, and indeed tenacity and determination, will be required. This is at a time of adversity, when there are enormous pressures on health and social care workers, and for many it seems as if there is very little if no additional funding evident.

When undertaking this work it is important to keep in mind that development needs to be locally responsive and driven, while recognizing the need to fit into the whole system and also to try to ensure equity. There needs to be a genuine commitment to older people, keeping a 'can do' attitude that is not risk averse, and which is flexible and pragmatic so that the needs of older people have some chance of making progress. At the heart of all this work it is helpful to keep in mind the tenets of respect, redesign and renewal, recognizing the needs of older people. It is also perhaps useful to keep in mind a recent quote derived, apparently, from the Department of Health: 'If I tell you about the present, and it sounds like the future then you are living in the past.' This sums up the importance of grasping the opportunities out there in a positive and constructive way, so as to rise to and respond to what older people want and need within what has inevitably become a changing health and social care economy.

Writing a book about service development is very much more simple than the reality of actually doing it. No attempt is made here to deny this. This book has provided an opportunity to begin to explore the issues around intermediate care and the associated agenda and to set the scene for further debate and developments so as to better meet the health and social care needs of older people.

Glossary

Age discrimination A judgement or decision made solely on the basis of a person's age.

Ageism This is regarded as the systematic stereotyping and discrimination against people simply on the basis of their age. Ageism is found in negative, derogatory or inappropriate behaviour by individuals and institutions.

Bed management A term used to describe the way bed capacity is used and managed. It may be within a single setting such as a hospital or across a whole health and social care system taking a 'whole systems approach'.

Bio-availability The rate and extent to which a drug is absorbed from a given pharmaceutical preparation and becomes available at its site of action.

Capacity management A contemporary term referring to the way that bed stock is used and managed within the health and social care economy, e.g the number of beds in a hospital or number of hospitals, or the number of beds and places available to a health and social care locality.

Care pathway The pathway of care that a patient may expect to experience, together with predetermined services/diagnostics, etc. They are usually organized around case types, specific disease categories, levels of dependence and by access routes (e.g. elective or emergency). For this reason they present as a challenge in the care of an older person with complex or multiple care needs.

Cinderella service A term used to describe services that have been marginalized within health and social care, in relation to a range of factors, e.g. resources, environments, recognition, representation. Services that have historically been regarded as Cinderella services include mental health, care of older people, learning disabilities, community care.

Community assessment rehabilitation team / community rehabilitation team (CART/CRT) A peripatetic multidisciplinary team of staff whose main remit is to promote rehabiliation. They may visit in the home, in nursing or care homes, or both. They may specialize e.g in neuro rehabilitation or provide more general rehabilitation.

Convalescence A period of time over which an individual recovers from sickness. This is usually spontaneous without active intervention.

Coping A strategy adopted by an individual to contend or deal with stressors or events.

Discharge planning / transfer of care This is very much a process, rather than a single event. Discharge is regarded as a stage in patient care. It involves a period of preparation which will then have consequences. It cannot be examined in isolation, but is integrally tied to what has gone before and to what follows after the event. Traditionally, discharge has been associated with going home from hospital. However, with the changing face of health and social care, patients may be transferred through a range of services.

Discrimination Drawing or making distinctions between or from others on the basis of a specific feature, e.g. age.

Electronic patient records (EPR) A system by which records of patients are held electronically and are accessible to a range of professions and disciplines who are given the right to access (by PIN), and who may also be able to add information. Patients will also be able to access elements of these.

Functionalism Structural functionalists are interested in the structure of societies and in the ways in which changes in one part of a society may set up a chain reaction leading to changes elsewhere.

Functional reserve This occurs in many biological systems where there is some spare capacity, such that a steady deterioration in the function of the system may proceed before there is actual evidence of this reduced functional capacity.

Half-life of drugs The time required for the concentration of a drug in the plasma to decrease to one-half of its initial value.

Homeostasis The maintenance of stability of the environment, despite variations in either internal or external environment.

Hospice at home Similar to 'hospital at home', only in this case the level and intensity of care is of a similar level to that provided in a hospice.

Hospital at home A level of care that enables a patient to be transferred from hospital but still receive the kind and intensity of care that is normally provided in hospital.

Integrated care pathway A pathway that determines locally agreed, multidisciplinary practice based on guidelines, and evidence where available, for a specific patient/client group. It forms all or part of the clinical record, documents the care given, and facilitates the evaluation of outcomes for continuous quality improvement.

Interdisciplinary team-working Here collaboration between team members is the key to success. Rather than each discipline identifying treatment goals, as occurs in multidisciplinary working, the team identifies goals – with the patient – and strives to avoid duplication and conflict in goals.

Intermediate care Has been described using a range of definitions, but in principle it is a range of services that prevent admission to acute hospital beds or speeds up discharge from such beds. In recent years the HSC/LAC definition has been widely adopted in the development or redesign of services.

Interim or transitional care A term used to describe the care required by individuals who are waiting to transfer to another service but who are unable to do so for various reasons. It tends to be associated with patients who have reached their peak or will benefit from another service and are ready to transfer, but awaiting other care resources, e.g. home care, funding for a care home or a place in a care home.

LIFT A form of public–private partnership announced in the government's NHS Plan (DoH, 2000c) and designed to provide the capital and expertise necessary to improve primary care buildings.

Lipophilic drugs Drugs which are attracted to fats and are fat soluble.

Multidisciplinary team-working Multidisciplinary teams combine the efforts of various disciplines where each discipline submits findings and recommendations related to a patient's care. They set out their own discipline-specific goals and work within their own discipline boundaries to achieve these goals. Discipline-specific progress is communicated with other team members directly or indirectly.

Nurse-led This refers to care that is led and provided primarily by nurses, and usually relates to the care of patients who are regarded as medically stable and can be cared for or managed by nurses, where there is no immediate on-site medical cover available. Settings or services entitled as nurse-led tend to be multidisciplinary and could in fact be led by any member of the team – although this is unlikely to be a doctor by the nature of the name.

Primary ageing Normal ageing; the gradual ageing that will occur in all members of a species. It is intrinsic, inevitable, deleterious and universal, although the rate of these changes will vary from individual to individual.

Person-centred Being person-centred and providing person-centred care involves shifting the power base from the health care professional to the older person and by so doing listening to the voice and aspirations of the older person and their carers and putting these at the centre of care and the goals of care.

Personhood Personhood and the value of person ascribe to people of all ages the authenticity of being alive and having lived and of valuing this.

Pharmacodynamics The way in which the drug affects the body, i.e. the effects at the intracellular site.

Pharmacokinetics The way in which the body affects the drugs with time or the extent to which drug response is dependent on the time course of drug concentration in the body.

Pharmacotherapy Use of a number of different drugs in the treatment of illness.

Polypharmacy Taking multiple drug regimes, often taken to be four or more medications and closely associated with older people due to the increased likelihood of multiple pathology.

Quality of care This is a term that can be defined in many ways but in essence describes care that meets the wishes and expectations of the older person receiving care so that their experience of care is good from their perspective.

Quality of life This is a term that has many definitions, but in general it is finding out what is important for the older person in enabling them to feel a sense of self-esteem and satisfaction with their life and what they are doing.

Rapid access clinic (RAC) A clinic to which older people can be referred by their GP for rapid access to be seen and assessed by a consultant geriatrician and multidisciplinary team – usually within a specified period of time (24–72 hours), often accessing other services and diagnostics rapidly.

Rapid Response Team (RRT) A team of staff who can respond to care needs in the community within a designated time scale – often having access to other services. The service is usually provided for only a time-limited period – anything from 5 days to 6 weeks.

Rehabilitation A wide range of definitions are available. In principle it is about focusing on re-enablement, facilitating and trying to recapture motivation so as to help people to adapt to changes in their life and circumstances. It must be of therapeutic value to the older person with the ultimate aim of maximizing social well-being. It is a process aiming to restore personal autonomy in those aspects of daily living considered most relevant by patients and service users and their families. It is a function of services rather than a service in its own right.

Seamless care A complex concept that has been used extensively to signify that the person using or moving through a range of services experiences a smooth transition, whereby staff seem to be sufficiently familiar with their care needs that staff do not need to revisit and reassess ground that has already been covered.

Secondary ageing Disease-related ageing that does not occur in all individuals.

Single Assessment Process The Single Assessment Process is seen as a means of ensuring that a more standardized assessment process is in place and that the same assessment process is used across all agencies. It is a process of assessment that is intended to allow assessment to be an incremental process that avoids duplication or replication and that is shared by all those involved in the assessment process within one document, and accessible eventually with Electronic Patient Records. It has been identified for older people, but there seems no reason why it should not be used for all people who would benefit from this kind of assessment.

Sociology Described as the science of the development and nature and laws of human society. It is, however, viewed from very different standpoints by different sociologists and is a wide and complicated subject.

Supported discharge A process by which a patient is discharged perhaps sooner than they would otherwise have been, because extra support services can be provided – usually for a time limited period.

Therapeutic index of a drug The dose at which the available drug is effective in its action and is neither sub-therapeutic in its effects nor toxic.

Transdisciplinary Here one member of the team is selected as the primary therapist/key worker. This person varies, depending upon the patient's needs. The other team members contribute information and advice through this identified person. In this way the team plans implementation to reduce joint collaboration when one team member can effectively accomplish the task, regardless of the discipline. Transdisciplinary working involves a certain amount of boundary blurring between disciplines and implies cross-training and flexibility in accomplishing the task.

Transition A passage from one life phase, condition or status to another; a process that forms a bridge from one reality that has been disrupted to a newly constructed or surfacing reality. A key feature is that there is no going back and there is a need to accept the change and find a way of incorporating it into one's life course.

Whole-systems approach This tends to refer to the management of health and social care across the whole range of services and Trusts so as to try to provide an integrated service where services interface seamlessly.

References

Age Concern (1999a) Ready to Go Home: Rehabilitation Re-discovered. London: HMSO.

Age Concern (1999b) Turning Your Back on Us: Older People and the NHS. London: Age Concern.

Age Concern (2000) Involving Older People: Good Practice Guide. London: Age Concern.

Akid M (2001) The last resort. Nursing Times 97(46): 12-13.

Alfono GJ, Hall LE (1969) The Loeb centre for nursing and rehabilitation: a professional approach to nursing practice. Nursing Clinically in North America 4: 487-93.

Alforo-LaFevere R (1994) Teaching nurses critical thinking. Academic Medical Surgical Nursing News 4-8.

Allatt P (1992) The dis-ease of social change: time and labour markets in the lives of young adults and their families. In R. Frankenberg, Time Health and Medicine. London: Sage.

Altshul A (1972) Patient-nurse interactions. University of Edinburgh Department of Nursing Studies, Monograph No. 3. Edinburgh.

Amos G (1973) Care is Rare. Liverpool: Age Concern.

Antonovsky A (1984) The sense of coherence as a determinant of health. In JP Matarazzo (ed.), Behavioural Health. New York: Wiley.

Apps C (1997) Beyond the NVQ - course breaks new ground for care workers. Working with Older People (July): 27-9.

Arber S, Ginn J (1991) Gender and Later Life: A Sociological Analysis of Resources and Constraints. London: Sage.

Areskog NH (1988) The need for multiprofessional health education within under-graduate studies (editorial). Medical Education 22: 251-2.

Armitage S (1981) Negotiating the discharge of medical patients. Journal of Advanced Nursing 6: 385-9.

Armstrong-Esther CA, Brown KD, McAfee JG (1994) Elderly patients: still clean and sitting quietly. Journal of Advanced Nursing 19: 264-71.

Arrol B (2001) Older people's experience of discrimination by the NHS. Ageing and Health 7: 7-8.

Audit Commission (1992) Lying in Wait: The Use of Medical Beds in Acute Hospitals. London: HMSO.

Audit Commission (1995) United They Stand: Co-ordinating the Care for Elderly Patients with Hip Fractures. London: HMSO.

Audit Commission (1997) The Coming of Age: Improving Care Services for Older People. London: Audit Commission.

Audit Commission (2000) The Way to Go Home: Rehabilitation and Remedial services for older people. London: Audit Commission.

Avorn J, Langer E (1982) Induced disability in nursing home patients: a controlled trial. Journal of the American Geriatrics Society 30(6): 397–400.

Bagust A, Place M, Posnett J (1999) Dynamics of bed use in accommodating emergency admissions: stochastic simulation model. British Medical Journal 319: 155–8.

Baltes, M. Barton EM (1979) Behaviour analysis of ageing: a review of the operant model and research. International Journal of Behavioural Development. 2(30); 297–320.

Banks-Smith J, Dowswell T, Gillam S, Shipman C (2001) Primary care groups and trusts. Nursing Times 97(45): 30–2.

Barber T (2001) Privacy and dignity: why you can't ignore it. Nursing Times, 97 (47) 23–15.

Barnes M (1997) Care, Communities and Citizens. London: Longman

Barnes M, Bennett-Emslie G (1997) 'If they would listen ...' An evaluation of the Fife User Panels Project. Edinburgh: Age Concern Scotland.

Barnes M, Walker A (1996) Consumerism versus empowerment: a principled approach to the involvement of older service users, Policy and Politics 24(4).

Baumann A, Deber R (1989) Decision Making and Problem Solving in Nursing – An Overview and Analysis of Relevant Literature. Literature Review Monograph. Toronto, University of Toronto.

Becker G (1994) Age bias in stroke rehabilitation – effects on adult status. Journal of Ageing Studies 8(3): 271–90.

Beckingham AC, DuGas BW (1993) Promoting healthy aging: a nursing and community perspective. St Louis, Mo: Mosby.

Begley S (2002) Timelines in Intermediate Care-Giving: A Constructivist Grounded Theory Approach (Unpublished PhD dissertation) Chalfont St Giles, Buckinghamshire: Chilterns University College.

Bend J, Solomon SA (1999). The attitudes of patients to integrated medical care. Age and Ageing 28: 271–3.

Bengston VL, Rosenthal C, Burton LM (1990) Families and ageing: diversity and heterogeneity. In Binstock R, George L (eds), Handbook of Ageing and the Social Sciences, 3rd edn. New York: Academic Press.

Benner, P (1984) From Novice to Expert: Excellence and Power in Clinical Nursing Practice. Menlo Park, Calif: Addison-Wesley.

Bennett G, Ebrahim S (1995) Health Care in Old Age, 2nd edn. London: Arnold.

Bernhard LA, Walsh M (1995) Leadership – The key to professionalization of nursing. The Nurse Leader and the Decision Making Process. St Louis, Mo: Mosby, ch 8.

Better Government for Older People (2000) All Our Futures: The Report of the Better Government for Older People Steering Committee. Better Government for Older People. www.bettergovernmentforolderpeople.gov.uk/

Biley F (1992a) In defence of the passive patient. Nursing Times 88(21): 58.

Biley F (1992b) Some determinants that affect patient participation in decision making about nursing care. Journal of Advanced Nursing 17: 414–21.

Birchall R, Waters K (1996) What do elderly people do in hospital. Journal of Clinical Nursing 5: 171–6.

Bird C, Cottrell N (1990) A prescription for self help. Nursing Times 81(43): 52–7.

Black A, Durrow P (1998) What is intermediate care? Conference paper, Harrogate Conferences, Durrow Management Services. andyblack_durrow£££compuserve

Black C, Black D, Alberti G (2000) Intermediate Care: Statement from the Royal College of Physicians. Presented at the British Geriatrics Society Conference, 30 November 2000. Royal College of Physicians.

Black D, Pearson M (2002) Average length of stay, delayed discharge, and hospital congestion. British Medical Journal 325: 610-11.

Blunden R (1998) Terms of Engagement: Engaging Older People in the Development of Community Services. London, King's Fund.

Bond J (1999) Living arrangements of older people. In Bond J, Coleman P, Peace S (1999) Ageing in Society: An Introduction to Social Gerontology. London: Sage Publications.

Bond J, Coleman P, Peace S (eds) (1999) Ageing in Society: An Introduction to Social Gerontology. London: Sage Publications.

Booth J, Davies C (1991) Happy to be home? Professional Nurse, March: 330-2.

Bore J (1994) Occupational therapy home visits: a satisfactory service? British Journal of Occupational Therapy 57(3): 85-9.

Bowling A, Betts G (1984) Communications on discharge. Nursing Times 80(32): 31-2.

Brändstädter J, Greve W (1994) In Lundh U, Nolan M (1996) Ageing and quality of life 2: Understanding successful ageing. British Journal of Nursing 5(21): 1291-5.

Bridges J, Meyer J, Barnes L (2000) Specialising in older people. Nursing Times 96(30): 42.

British Geriatric Society and Association of Directors of Social Services (1989) Discharge to the Community of Elderly Patients in hospital. London, BGS/ADSS.

British Geriatric Society (1998) Intermediate Care: Medical Guidance for Purchasers and Providers. Compendium document 4.

British Geriatrics Society (2002) Consultant Recruitment Survey - May 2002. BGS Newsletter, September. London: BGS.

Brocklehurst JC (ed.) (1978) Textbook of Geriatric Medicine and Gerontology, 2nd edn. Edinburgh: Churchill Livingstone.

Brown J, Kitson A, McKnight T (1992) Challenges in Caring: Explorations in Nursing Ethics. London: Chapman & Hall.

Bryans A, McIntosh J (1996) Decision making in community nursing: an analysis of the stages of decision making as they relate to community nursing assessment practice. Journal of Advanced Nursing 24(1): 24-30.

Buchan J, Ball J (1991) Caring Costs: Nursing Costs and Benefits. Brighton: The Institute of Manpower Studies.

Bulmer C (1998) Clinical decisions: defining meaning through focus groups. Nursing Standard 12(20): 34-6.

Butler RN (1975) Why Survive Being Old in America? New York: Harper & Row.

Bytheway B (1995) Ageism. Buckingham: Open University.

Bywaters P, McLeod E, Cooke M (2002) A diversionary tactic? Social work in an emergency assessment unit. Nursing Older People 14(8): 19-21.

Campbell ME (1971) Study of attitudes of nursing personnel toward the geriatric patient. Nursing Research 20: 147-51.

Carrol JS, Johnson EJ (1990) Decision Research: A Field Guide. Newbury Park, California, Sage.

Carter T, Beresford P (2000) Age and Change Models of involvement for older people. YPS for Joseph Rowntree Foundation.

Cartwright AD, O'Brien M (1976) Social class variables in health care and in the nature of general practice consultations. In Stacey M (ed.), The Sociology of the National Health Service, Sociological Review Monograph 22, pp. 77-96.

Casey A (1995) Partnership nursing: influences on involvement of informal carers. Journal of Advanced Nursing 22: 1508-62.

Castledine G (1994) The role of the nurse in the 21st century. British Journal of Nursing 3: 621–2.

Catolico O, Navas M, Sommer C, Collins M (1996) Quality of decision-making by registered nurses. Journal of Nursing Staff Development 12(3): 149–54.

Cawley JC (1983) Haematology. London: Heinemann.

Challis D, Darton R (1990) Evaluation research and experiment in social gerontology. In S Peace, Researching Social Gerontology. London: Sage.

Challis D, Knapp M, Davies B (1988) Cost effectiveness evaluation in social care. In J Lishman (ed.), Research Highlights in Social Work 8: Evaluation, 2nd edn. London: Jessica Kingsley.

Charmaz K (1983) Loss of self: a fundamental form of suffering in the chronically ill. Sociology of Health and Illness 5: 168–95.

Chenitze WC (1983) Entry into a nursing home as status passage: a theory to guide nursing practice. Geriatric Nursing 4(2): 92–7.

Clarke H, Dyer S (1998) Equipped for home from hospital. Health Care in Later Life 3(1): 36–45.

Clinical Standards Advisory Group (1998) Community Health Care for Elderly People. London: Clinical Standards Advisory Group.

Cocchi A, Franceschini G, Antonelli-Incalzi F, Farani G (1988) Clinico-pathological correlations in the diagnosis of acute myocardial infarction in the elderly. Age and Ageing 17: 87–93.

Col N, Fanale JE, Kronholm P (1990) The role of medication in non-compliance and adverse drug reactions in hospitalisations of the elderly. Archives of Internal Medicine 150: 841–5.

Coleman P, Bond J (1999) Ageing in the twentieth century. In J Bond, P Coleman, S Peace (1999) Ageing in Society: An Introduction to Social Gerontology. London: Sage Publications. Ch. 1.

Colucciello ML (1997) Clinical pathways in sub-acute settings, Journal of Nursing Management 28(6): 52–4.

Conger CO, Marshall ES (1998) Recreating life: toward a theory of relationship development in acute home care. Qualitative Health Research 8(4): 526–46.

Conger MM (1993) Delegation decision-making. Journal of Staff Development 9(3): 131–5.

Connell RW (1987) Gender and Power. Cambridge: Polity Press.

Cook G (1996) Risk taking in rehabilitative care: professional and legal considerations. Health Care in Later Life 1(1): 5–13.

Cook WL (1993) Interdependence and the interpersonal sense of control: an analysis of family relationships. Journal of Personality and Social Psychology 64(4): 587–601.

Cooksey RW (1996) Judgement analysis: theory, methods and applications. London: Academic Press.

Coombes R (2001) Same old story about elderly care. Nursing Times 97(14): 12.

Corbin JM, Strauss AL (1988) Unending Work and Care: Managing Chronic Illness at Home. San Francisco: Jossey Bass.

Cormie J, Warren L (2001) Working with Older People: Guidelines for Running Discussion Groups and Influencing Practice. London, Policy Press.

Cowgill D (1974) Ageing and modernization: a revision of the theory. In Gubrium JF (ed.), Late Life: Communities and Environmental Policy. Springfield, Ill: C.C. Thomas. pp 123–46.

Cowgill D, Holmes LD (eds) (1972) Ageing and Modernization. New York: Appleton-Century-Crofts.

Cowie R, Douglas-Cowie E, Stewart P (1987) The experience of becoming deaf. In Kyle JG (ed.), Adjustment to Acquired Hearing Loss. Bristol: Centre for Deaf Studies, pp. 65-80.

Cox C (1983) Sociology: An Introduction for Nurses, Midwives and Health Visitors. London: Butterworths.

CSP (2001) CSP Position Statement: Rehabilitation and Intermediate Care. London: Chartered Society of Physiotherapy.

Cummings E, Henry W (1961) Growing Old: The Process of Disengagement. New York: Basic Books.

Cunningham S (1996) The biological basis of cancer. British Journal of Nursing 5(14): 869-74.

Cunningham WR, Brookbank JW (1988) Gerontology: The Psychology, Biology and Sociology of Aging. New York: Harper & Row.

Davis RW (1968) Psychological aspects of geriatric nursing. American Journal of Nursing 68: 802-4.

Dellasega C, Nolan M (1997) Admission to care: facilitating role transition amongst family carers. Journal of Advanced Nursing 6: 443-51.

Dennis M, Langhorne P (1994) So stroke units save lives: where do we go from here? British Journal of Medicine 309: 1273-77.

Denzin NK (1989) The Research Act: A Theoretical Introduction to Sociological Methods (3rd edn), Prentice Hall: Englewood Cliffs.

Department of Health (1989) Discharge of Patients from Hospital (guidance booklet accompanying Circular HC(89)5, LAC (89) 7. London: HMSO.

Department of Health (1990a) Community Care in the Next Decade and Beyond: Policy Guidance. London: HMSO.

Department of Health (1990b) The NHS and Community Care Act. London: HMSO.

Department of Health (1992) The Patient's Charter. London: HMSO.

Department of Health (1997) The New NHS: Modern, Dependable. London: HMSO.

Department of Health (1998a) A First Class Service: Quality in the New NHS. London: DoH.

Department of Health (1998b) Modernising Health and Social Services: National Priorities Guidance 1999-2000-2001-2002. London: HMSO.

Department of Health (1998c) Modernising Social Services: Promoting Independence, Improving Protection, Reviewing Standards. London: HMSO.

Department of Health (1999a) Making a Difference: Strengthening the Nursing, Midwifery and Health Visiting Contribution to Health and Health Care. London: HMSO.

Department of Health (1999b) The National Beds Inquiry. London: DoH.

Department of Health (1999c) Royal Commission: With Respect to Old Age: Long Term Care - Rights and Responsibilities. London: HMSO.

Department of Health (2000b) The National Beds Inquiry. London: DoH.

Department of Health (2000c) The NHS Plan: A Plan for Investment, A Plan for Reform. London, DoH. Website: www.nsh.uk/nhsplan.

Department of Health (2000d) Shaping the Future NHS: Long-term Planning for Hospitals and Related Services. Consultation Document on the Findings of the Beds Inquiry. London: HMSO, DoH.

Department of Health (2000/2001) NHS Performance Ratings: Acute Trusts. London: DoH.

Department of Health (2001a) Care Homes for Older People: National minimum standards. Care Standards Act 2000. London: HMSO.

Department of Health (2001b) The Care Standards Act 2000 (commencement no. (England) and transitional and savings provisions) order 2001. London: DoH.

Department of Health (2001c) Caring for Older People: A Nursing Priority: Integrating Knowledge, Practice and Values. London: DoH.

Department of Health (2001d) Frequencies of inspection and regulatory fees: a consultation paper. London: DoH.

Department of Health (2001e) HSC 2001/01: LAC (19 January 2001) 1. Intermediate Care Circular. London: DoH. Website: www.doh.gov.uk/coinh.htm

Department of Health (2001f) Improving the Flow of Emergency Admissions, The Modernization Agency, London.

Department of Health (2001g) The National Care Standards Commission (Registration) Regulations: Consultation Document. London: DoH.

Department of Health (2001h) The National Service Framework for Older People; Modern Standards and Service Models. London: DoH.

Department of Health (2001i) Older People's National Service Framework: Standard 3: Intermediate Care. London: DoH.

Department of Health (2001j) The Single Assessment Process. London: DoH. www.doh.gov.uk/scg/sap/locimp.htm

Department of Health (2002a) Extended Independent Prescribing within the NHS in England: A Guide for Implementation. London: DoH.

Department of Health (2002b) HSC 2002/001: LAC (2002) 1. Guidance on the Single Assessment Process for older people (and associated Annexes) Jan. 2002. London: DoH. www.doh.gov.uk/scg/sap/locimp.htm

Department of Health (2002c) Implementing the NHS Plan. London: DoH.

Department of Health (2002d) Intermediate Care: Moving Forward. London: DoH.

Department of Health (2002e) Intermediate Care Services: Glossary of terms: Definition of Intermediate care services. www.doh.gov.uk/intermediatecare/icmovingforward.htm

Department of Health (2002f) The NHS Plan: Delivering the NHS Plan. London: DoH.

Department of Health (2002g) The Single Assessment Process: Assessment Tools and Scales. London: DoH.

Department of Health (2003) Discharge from Hospital: Pathway, Process and Practice. London: DoH.

Department of Health NHS Executive (1999) The NHS Performance Assessment Framework. London: DoH.

Donabedian A (1980) Explorations in Quality Assessment and Monitoring. Vol. 1. The Definition of Quality and Approaches to its Assessment. Anna Arbor, Michigan: Health Administration Press.

Downie G, Mackenzie J, Williams A (1999) Pharmacology and Drug Management for Nurses, 2nd edn. Edinburgh: Churchill Livingstone.

Draper P (1997) Nursing Perspectives on Quality of Life. London: Routledge.

Dreyfus HL, Dreyfus SE (1986) Mind over Machine. New York: Free Press.

Dunbar A (1996) Altered presentation of illness in old age. Nursing Standard 10(44): 49-52.

Dyer S (1994) Power to the People. Elderly Care, Sept/Oct: 6(5): 30-1.

Earl-Slater A (1995) Coventry's fast response service cuts hospital stays. British Journal of Healthcare Management 1(12): 596-9.

Eddy DM (1986) Before and after attitudes toward ageing in a BSN program. Journal of Gerontological Nursing 12(5): 30-4.

Ellis, B.W. and Johnson, S. (1997) A clinical view of pathways of care in disease management. International Journal of Health Care Quality Assurance, 10 (2): 61-66.

Elzinga A (1990) The knowledge aspect of professionalization: the case of science-based nursing education in Sweden. In R Torstendhal, M Burrage (eds), The Formation of Professions. London: Sage, pp. 150-73.

Emrys-Roberts M (1991) The Cottage Hospitals, 1859-1990: Arrival, Survival and Revival. Motcombe, Dorset: Tern.

Endacott R et al. (1999) Towards a faculty of emergency nursing. Emergency Nurse 7(5): 10-16.

Enderby P (1998) Therapy Outcome Measures, Florence Ky, USA: Singular Publishing Group Inc.

English I (1993) Intuition as a function of the expert nurse: a critique of Benner's novice to expert model. Journal of Advanced Nursing 18: 387-93.

English National Board for Nursing, Midwifery and Health Visiting (2001a) Education and Training Implications of the National Service Framework for Older People (Department of Health 2001). London: ENB.

English National Board for Nursing, Midwifery and Health Visiting (2001b) Exploring the Role and Contribution of the Nurse in the Multi-Professional Rehabilitation Team. London: ENB.

Erikson EH (1965) Childhood and Society. Penguin, London: Harmondsworth. First published 1950.

Erikson EH (1980) Identity and the Life Cycle: A Reissue. New York: W.W. Norton.

Estes C (1979) The Ageing Enterprise. San Francisco: Jossey Bass.

Evans EN (1992) Liberation theology, empowerment theory and social work practice with the oppressed. International Social Work 35: 135-47.

Ewing AB (2002) Altered drug response in the elderly. In D Armour, C Cairns (eds), Medicines in the Elderly. London: Pharmaceutical Press. Ch. 2.

Exton-Smith AN (1985) The elderly patient – special characteristics of disease in old age. In AN Exton-Smith, ME Weschler (eds), Practical Geriatric Medicine. Edinburgh: Churchill Livingstone.

Eysenck HJ (1990) Type A behaviour and coronary disease: the third stage. Journal of Social Behaviour and Personality 5(1): 25-44.

Falkingham J, Victor C (1991) The myth of the Woopie: incomes, the elderly and targeting the elderly. Ageing and Society 11: 471-93.

Farrell M, Schmitt MH, Heinemann GD (2001) Informal roles and the stages of interdisciplinary team development. Journal of Interprofessional Care 15(3): 31-45.

Farrington A (1993) Intuition and expert clinical practice. British Journal of Nursing 2(4): 228-32.

Faull C (2000) A Pilot Project of a New Service in Birmingham. Research Report for the Cancer and Palliative Care Commissioners in Birmingham, St Mary's Hospice.

Finlayson B, Dixon J, Meadows S, Blair G (2002) Mind the gap: the extent of the NHS nursing shortage. British Medical Journal 325: 538-41.

Forkner DJ (1996) Clinical pathways: benefits and liabilities. Journal of Nursing Management 27(11): 35-8.

Fosbinder D (1994) Patient perceptions of nursing care. Journal of Advanced Nursing 20: 1085-93.

Fotherby MD, Panayiotou B, Potter JF (1993) Age-related differences in simultaneous interarm measurements. Postgraduate Medical Journal 69(809): 194-6.

Fox S, Wold J (1996) Baccalaureate student gerontological nursing experiences: raising consciousness levels and affecting attitudes. Journal of Nursing Education 35(8): 348-55.

Frankenberg R (1992) Your time or mine: temporal contradictions of biomedical practice. In R Frankenberg (ed.), Health, Time and Medicine. London: Sage.

Frey GA (1990) A framework for promoting organizational change. Families in Society, the Journal of Contemporary Human Studies 71(3): 142-7.

Fry S (1991) Health care and decision-making. In Jecker (ed.), Ageing and Ethics. Clifton, New Jersey: Humana Press.

Gibson D (1994) Time for clients: temporal aspects of community psychiatric nursing. Journal of Advanced Nursing 20: 110-16.

Glasby J (2002) A highly charged debate. Nursing Older People 14(4): 6.

Glasby J (2003) A backward step? Nursing the Older Person 15(2): 6.

Glasby J, Littlechild R (2000a) Fighting fires? - emergency hospital admission and the concept of prevention, Journal of Management in Medicine 14(2): 109-18.

Glasby J, Littlechild R (2000b) The Health and Social Care Divide: The Experiences of Older People. Birmingham, PEPAR Publications.

Glasby J, Littlechild R (2001) Inappropriate hospital admissions: patient participation in research. British Journal of Nursing 10(11), 738-74.

Godchaux CW, Travioli J, Hughes A (1997) A continuum of care model. Nursing Management 28(11): 73-6.

Goffman E (1961) Asylums: Essays on the Social Situation of Mental Patients and Other Inmates. London: Doubleday & Co.

Goldberg EM, Connelly N (1982) The Effectiveness of Social Care for the Elderly: An Overview of Recent and Current Evaluative Research. London: Heinemann Educational.

Gould D (2002) Health-related infection and hand hygiene: I. Nursing Times 98(38): 48-51.

Griffith P, Wilson-Barnett J (2000) The effectiveness of 'nursing beds': a review of the literature. Journal of Advanced Nursing 27: 1184-92.

Griffith P, Wilson-Barnett J, Richardson G, Spilsbury K, Miller F, Harris R (2000) The effectiveness of intermediate care in a nursing-led in-patient unit. International Journal of Nursing Studies 37: 153-61.

Griffith-Kenny JW, Christensen. P.J. (1986) The Nursing Process: Application of Theories, Frameworks and Models. St Louis: Mosby.

Griffiths P, Harris R, Richardson G et al. (2001) Substitution of a nursing-led inpatient unit for acute services: randomised controlled trial of outcomes and cost of nursing-led intermediate care. Age and Ageing (30): 483-8.

Grimley Evans J (2001) Huge strides in care. In Healthy Oxfordshire: Older People in Oxfordshire: Annual Report of the Directors of Public Health. Oxfordshire: Health Oxfordshire.

Grimley Evans J, Tallis RC (2001) A new beginning of care for elderly people. British Medical Journal 322: 807-8.

Gulland, A. (2002) Making advances. Nursing Times 98(33): 10.

Hammond KR (1996) Human Judgement and Social Policy. Irreducible Uncertainty, Inevitable Error, Unavoidable Injustice. New York: Oxford University Press.

Hanford L, Easterbrook L, Stevenson J (1999) Rehabilitation for Older People: The Emerging Policy Agenda. London: King's Fund.

Health Advisory Service (1998, 2000) 'Not Because They are Old': An Independent Inquiry into Care of Older People on Acute Wards in General Hospitals. London: Health Advisory Board.

Health Services Circular (2000/016) Local Authority Circular (2000/14), Winter 2000/01. Capacity Planning for Health and Social Care: Emergency and Social Care.

Health Services Management Centre (2001) Getting into Their Stride: Interim Report of a National Evaluation of Primary Care Groups, May 2001, University of Birmingham, School of Public Policy.

Heath H (2002) Editorial: Sensitivity is key to effective partnership. Nursing Older People 14(7): 3.

Heath H, Webster C (1999) Pharmacology and medications. In Heath H, Schofield I (eds), Healthy Ageing: Nursing Older People. London: Mosby.

Heath I (2000) Editorial: Dereliction of duty in an ageist society. British Journal of Medicine 320: 1422.

Helgeson VS (1992) Moderators of the relation between perceived control and adjustment to chronic illness. Journal of Personality and Social Psychology 63(4): 656-6.

Heller BR, Walsh FJ (1976) Changing nursing students' attitudes towards the aged: an experimental study. Journal of Nursing Education 15: 9-17.

Help the Aged (2000) Dignity on the ward: Promoting Excellence in Care, Promoting Practice in Acute Hospital Care for Older People. University of Sheffield, School of Nursing and Midwifery.

Help the Aged (2002) Nothing Personal: Rationing Social Care for Older People. London: Help the Aged.

Henry S, LeBreck D, Holzemer W (1989) The effects of verbalization of cognitive processes on clinical decision-making. Research Nursing Health 12: 187-93.

Hensher M, Fulop N, Coast J, Jefferys E (1999) Better out than in? Alternatives to acute hospital care. British Medical Journal 319: 1127-30.

Henwood M, Hardy B, Hudson B, Wistow G. (1997) Inter-agency collaboration: hospital discharge and continuing care sub-study. Leeds: Nuffield Institute for Health Community Care Division.

Herbert R (1986) The biology of ageing: maintenance of homeostasis. Geriatric Nursing, May/June; 14-16.

Herbert R (1992) The normal ageing process reviewed. International Nursing Review 39(3): 93-6.

Hetu R, Jones L, Getty L (1993) The impact of acquired hearing impairment on intimate relationships: implications for rehabilitation. Audiology 32: 363-8.

Hill SN, Milnes JP, Rowe J et al. (1987) Nursing the immobile: a preliminary study. International Journal of Nursing Studies 24(2): 123-8.

Hinshaw A, Atwood JR (1982) A patient satisfaction instrument: precision by replication. Nursing Research 31(3): 170-5.

Hockey l (1968) Care in the Balance. London: Queens Institute of District Nursing.

Hoeman S (ed.) (1996) Rehabilitation Nursing: Process and Application. St Louis, Mo: Mosby.

Holmes TH, Rahe RH (1967) The Social Readjustment Rating Scale. Journal of Psychosomatic Research 11: 213-18.

HOPe (2000) Our Future Health: Older people's priorities for health and social care. London: Help the Aged.

Horne D (1998) Getting Better? Inspection of Hospital Discharge (Care Management) Arrangements for Older People. London: DoH.

House of Commons Debates (1997) Hansard, 9 December, Col 802.

Houston AM, Cowley S (2002) An empowerment approach to needs assessment in health visiting. Journal of Clinical Nursing 11: 640-50.

Howe D (1987) An Introduction to Social Work Theory. Aldershot: Wildwood House.

Huber D (1996) Leadership and Nursing Care Management. Philadelphia: W.B. Saunders.

Hudson B (2000) Inter-agency collaboration: a sceptical view. In A Brechin, H Brown, MA Eby (eds), Critical Practice in Health and Social Care. Milton Keynes: Open University Press.

Hudson B, Hardy B, Henwood M, Wistow G (1997) Inter-Agency Collaboration: Final Report. Leeds, Nuffield Institute for Health Community Care Division.

Hudson SA, Boyter AC (1997) Pharmaceutical care of the elderly. Pharmaceutical Journal 259: 685-8.

Hughes B (1995) Older People and Community Care. Buckingham: Open University Press.

Hurst R (2002) Managing hypertension: measurement prevention. Nursing Times 98(38): 38-40.

Illich I (1975) Medical Nemesis. London: Calder & Boyers.

Jasper M (1994) Expert: a discussion of the implications of the concept as used in nursing. Journal of Advanced Nursing 20: 769-76.

Jeon YH, Madjar I (1998) Caring for a family member with chronic mental illness. Qualitative Health Research 8(5): 694-706.

Jewell S (1993) Discovery of the discharge process: a study of patients discharge from a care unit for elderly people. Journal of Advanced Nursing 18: 1288-96.

Johns C (1991) The Burford Nursing Development Unit Holistic Model of Nursing Practice. Journal of Advanced Nursing 16: 1090-98.

Johnson M (1988) Biographical influences on mental health and old age. In Mental Health Problems in Old Age. Milton Keynes: Open University. Ch. 17.

Jolly A (1991) Taking blood pressure. Nursing Times 87(15): 40-3.

Jolly M, Brykczynska G (1992) Caring - a dying art? In Nursing Care: The Challenge to Change. London: Edward Arnold. Ch 1.

Jones AJ (1988) Clinical reasoning in nursing. Journal of Advanced nursing 13: 185-92.

Kellett UM, Mannion J (1999) Meaning in Caring: Reconceptualizing the nurse–family carer. Relationship in Community Practice. Journal of Advanced Nursing 29(3): 697-703.

Kelly J (1995) Pharmadynamics and drug therapy. Professional Nurse 10(12): 792-6.

Kennett A (1986) Informed consent: a patient's right. Professional Nurse 2(3): 75-7.

Khanna PM, Geller J (1992) Clinical implications in the elderly. Top Emergency Medicine 14(3): 1-9.

King TI (1995) Gerontological courses for undergrads. The Canadian Nurse (May): 27-31.

Kings Fund (2001) Intermediate Care Co-ordinators: Exploring the Role. London: Kings Fund Institute.

Kirby J (2000) It's back to basics for the new nursing units. SAGA, Dec.

Kitwood T (1997) Dementia reconsidered: the person comes first. Buckingham: Open University Press.

Kivnick HQ, Murray SV (1997) Vital involvement: an overlooked source of identity in frail elders. Journal of Ageing and Identity 2(3): 205-25.

Klop R, Van Wijmen FCB, Philipsen H (1991) Patients rights and the admission and discharge process. Journal of Advanced Nursing 16: 408-12.

Knopp N (2000) Professional influence on care package design for elderly people with health and social needs. (unpublished paper, University of Hertfordshire).

Knowles L, Sarver V (1985) Attitudes affect quality care. Journal of Gerontological Nursing 11(8): 35-6.

Lancaster J (2001) Evaluation Report: So you want to be a nurse/therapy consultant. A paper arising from the National Leadership Projects. Modernization Agency, DoH.

Laurie S, Salantera S, Chalmers K, Ekman L, Kim H, Käppeli S, MacLeod M (2001) An exploratory study of clinical decision-making in five countries. Journal of Nursing Scholarship 33(1): 83-90.

Lazarus, Folkman (1984) In RL Atkinson, RC Atkinson, EE Smith, ER Hilgard (1985) Introduction to Psychology. San Diego, Harcourt Brace Jovanovich.

Lazenbath A (2002) The Evaluation Handbook for Health Professionals. London: Routledge.

Lees L (2001) Rapid response teams: towards a uniform definition. Website article, Department of Health, NHS Magazine: www.nhs.uk/nhsmagasine.

Lees L, Crouch P (1999) Intermediate Care Working Group; Point Prevalence Study appendices from City Hospital, Birmingham. In Department of Health (2000) The National Beds Inquiry. London: DoH.

Legge A (1996) Age no barrier to treatment. Backup News 27: Autumn 11.

Leininger M (1985) Qualitative Research Methods in Nursing. Philadelphia, W.B. Saunders.

Levi L, Frankenhauser M, Gardell B (1983) Work stress related to social structures and processes. Cited in I Norman (1997) Supporting paid carers. In I Norman, S Redfern (eds), Mental Health Care for Elderly People. London: Churchill Livingstone.

Levkoff S, Cleary P, Wetle T, Besdine R (1988) Illness behaviour in the aged: implications for clinicians. Journal of the American Geriatrics Society 36: 622-9.

Lewis J (2001) Older people and the health–social care boundary in the U.K.: half a century of hidden policy conflict. Social Policy and Administration 35(4): 343-59.

Leyland S (1994) Osteoporosis. Elderly Care 6(1): 41-5.

Lipman T, Deatrick J (1997) Preparing advanced practice nurses for clinical decision making in speciality practice. Nurse Educator 22(2): 47-50.

Littlechild R, Glasby J (2000) Older people as 'participating patients'. In H Kemshall, R Littlechild (eds) User Involvement and Participation in Social Care. London: Jessica Kingsley.

Lyder C, Molony S (1999) Topics in gastrointestinal care. In Molony S, Waszynski C, Lyder C (eds), Gerontological Nursing: An Advanced Practice Approach. Stamford, Conn: Appleton and Lange. Ch. 7.

Lynott RJ (1983) Alzheimer's disease and institutionalization: the ongoing construction of a decision. Journal of Family Issues 4: 559-74.

McCormack B (1992) The developing role of community hospitals: an essential part of a quality service. Quality Health Care 2: 253-8.

McCormack B (2001a) Autonomy and the relationship between nurses and older people. Ageing and Society 21(4): 417-46.

McCormack B (2001b) Clinical effectiveness and clinical teams: effective practice with older people. Nursing Older People 13(5): 14-17.

McGavock HA (1996) A review of literature on drug adherence. London: Royal Pharmaceutical Society of Great Britain.

McGrath J, Davis A (1992) Rehabilitation: where are we going and how do we get there? Clinical Rehabilitation 6: 225-35.

McHale J (2002) Extended prescribing: the legal implications. Nursing Times 98(32): 36-8.

MacMahon D (2001) Intermediate care - a challenge to the speciality of geriatric medicine or its renaissance. Age and Ageing 30(S3): 19-23.

McMurray A (1990) Community Health Nursing. London: Churchill Livingstone.

Macphee G, Brodie M (1992) Drugs and the elderly. Medicine International: The Medicines Group Journal: 4258-63.

Mahoney C (2001) That time of year again. Nursing Times 97(42): 10.

Main A, Lees L (2000) Older People's Joint Working Party; Outcome Measures Tool. (Unpublished) Birmingham Health Authority.

Manley K (1997) A conceptual framework for advanced practice: an action research project: operationalising an advanced practitioner/consultant nurse role. Journal of Clinical Nursing 6 (3): 1179-90.

Marinker M (1997) Personal paper: writing prescriptions is easy. British Medical Journal 314: 747-8.

Marks L (1997) Home and Hospital Care: 'Redrawing the Boundaries'. London: The King's Fund Institute.

Marquis, Huston (1996) Leadership Roles and Management functions in Nursing Theory and Application. 2nd edn. Pennsylvania: Lippencott Co.

Martin F. (2001) Intermediate care for older people - the new Cinderella non-speciality. Ageing and Health: Institute of Ageing and Health.

Means R, Smith R (1985) Development of Welfare Services for Elderly People. London: Croom Helm.

Means R, Smith R (1994) Community Care: Policy and Practice. Basingstoke: Macmillan.

Medina J (1996) The Clock of Ages. Cambridge: Cambridge University Press.

Middleton S, Roberts A (2000) Integrated Care Pathways: A Practical Approach to Implementation. Oxford: Butterworth-Heinemann.

Miller S, Combes C (1989) Information, Coping and Control in Patients Undergoing Surgery; and Stressful Medical Procedures. In A Steptoe, A Apples (eds), Stress, Personal Control and Health. Chichester: Wiley.

Milner J, O'Brien (2002) Assessment in Social Work (2nd edn). Houndmills: Macmillan.

Moore PA (1996) Decision making in professional practice. British Journal of Nursing 5(10): 635-40.

Morgan D, Reed J, Palmer A (1997) Moving from hospital into a care home - the nurse's role in supporting older people. Journal of Clinical Nursing 6: 463-71.

Morris J, Bowman C, Carr D (2000) Discriminating for the ageing population - the positive approach. Journal of Royal College of Physicians of London 34(4): 353-54.

National Care Pathways Association, cited in Middleton S, Roberts A (2000) Introduction: What are integrated care pathways? In Integrated Care Pathways: A Practical Approach to Implementation. Oxford: Butterworth/Heinemann. Ch. 1.

Nazarko L (1997) Improving hospital discharge arrangements for older people. Nursing Standard 11(40): 44-7.

Newman M (1979) Theory and Development in Nursing. Philadelphia: Davis.

Newman P (1998) A literature review: aspects of intermediate care. Commissioned by

South Thames in collaboration with Anglia and Oxford Regional Office: jane.carri-erdoh.gsi.gov.uk

NHS Estates (2000) Facilities for Rehabilitation. London: HMSO.

NHS Executive (1999) Nurse, Midwife and Health Visitor Consultant: Establishing posts and making appointments. Health Service Circular 1999/217. London: DoH.

NHS Executive (2000a) The NHS Plan: A Plan for Investment. A Plan for Reform. 2000/0455. London: DoH.

NHS Executive (2000b) NHS Plan News. London: DoH.

NHS Modernization Agency (2002) Keynote Address, Modernizing Older People's Services Conference, Brighton Metropole, 5 November.

Nilsson M, Ekman S, Sarvimäki A (1998) Ageing with joy or resigning to old age: older people's experiences of quality of life in old age. Health Care in Later Life 3(2): 94-100.

Nocan A, Baldwin S (1998) Trends in Rehabilitation Policy: A Review of the Literature. London: Kings Fund and Audit Commission.

Nolan M, Davies S, Grant G (eds) (2001) Working with Older People and Their Families: Key Issues in Policy and Practice. Buckingham: Open University Press.

Norman I (1997) Supporting paid carers. In I Norman, S Redfern (eds), Mental Health Care for Elderly People. London: Churchill Livingstone.

Nursing and Midwifery Council (2002) Code of Professional Conduct; London, NMC.

Nursing Older People (2002) News in focus – fast-track scheme scoops award. Nursing Older People 14(7): 5.

O'Connor J (1996) From Women in the Welfare State to Gendering Welfare State Regimes. Ed. R.J. Brym. London: Sage.

O'Connor SE (1996) Stroke units: centres of nursing innovation. British Journal of Nursing 5(2): 105.

Oliver M (1989) Social work with disabled people. Social Work Today, 6 April: 21.

OPCS (2001) Population Trends. Office of Population Censuses and Surveys. London: HMSO.

Orem DE (1980) Nursing Concept of Practice. New York: McGraw-Hill.

Oxford Pocket Dictionary (1999) The Oxford Pocket Dictionary, 10th edn. Oxford: Clarendon Press.

Oxford Radcliffe Hospitals Trust (2002) Evaluating a Health Service, Oxford, Clinical Governance Support Unit.

Oxfordshire Health Authority and Oxfordshire Social Services (May 2002) Oxfordshire Acute and Community Hospitals Transfer of Care (Discharge) Inter Agency Standards. Oxfordshire Health Authority and Oxfordshire Social Services.

Paniagua H (1995) The scope of advanced practice: action potential for practice nurses. British Journal of Nursing 4(5): 269-74.

Parry-Jones B, Soulsby J (2001) Needs-led assessment: the challenges and the reality. Health and Social Care in the Community 9(6): 414-28.

Passuth P, Bengston V (1996) Sociological theories of ageing: current perspectives and future directions. In J Quadagno D Street (eds), Ageing for the Twenty-First Century. New York: St Martin's Press.

Patmore, C, Qureshi, H, Nicholas, E (1999) Tuning in to Feedback Community Care, 24-30 June: pp. 28-9.

Patton M (1980) Qualitative Evaluation Methods. London: Sage.

Pearce L (2002) Nursing Leaders. RCN magazine, Autumn.

Pearson A, Punton S, Duran I (1992) Nursing Beds: An Evaluation of the Effects of Therapeutic Nursing. Harrow: Scutari Press.

Pembrey S (1983) Nursing care: professional progress. Journal of Advanced Nursing 9(6): 539–47.

Penhale B (1997) Towards effective discharge planning. Health Care in Later Life 2(1): 46–55.

Penner LA, Ludenia K, Mead G (1983) Staff attitudes: image or reality. Journal of Gerontological Nursing 10: 110–17.

Peters DJ (1995) Human experience in disablement: the impetus of the ICIDH. Disability and Rehabilitation 17(3214): 23–44.

Philipose V, Tate J, Jacobs S (1991) Review of nursing literature: evolution of gerontological education in nursing. Nursing Health Care 12(10): 524–30.

Phillipson C (1982) Capitalism and the Construction of Old Age. London: Macmillan.

Phillipson C (1998) Reconstructing Old Age: New Agendas in Social Theory and Practice. London: Sage.

Phillipson C, Walker A (1986) Ageing and Social Policy: A Critical Assessment. Aldershot: Gower.

Philp I (2001) Independence way: intermediate care. Health Service Journal 35(4): 22–3.

Playle J, Keeley P (1998) Non-compliance and professional power. Journal of Advanced Nursing 27: 304–11.

Polit DF, Hungler BP (1999) Nursing Principles and Methods. Philadelphia: Lippincott Co.

Porteous D (1976) Home the Territorial Core. Geographical Review 66: 383–90.

Pound P, Gompertz P, Ebrahim S (1994) Patients' satisfaction with stroke services. Clinical Rehabilitation 8: 7–17.

Queens Nursing Institute (2002) District Nursing: The Invisible Workforce. London: Queens Nursing Institute.

Rafael ARF (1996) Power and caring: dialectic in nursing. Advances in Nursing Science 19(1): 3–17.

Redfern S. and Norman, I. (1999) Quality of Nursing Care perceived by patients and their nurses: an application of the clinical incident technique: parts 1 and 2. Journal of Clinical Nursing, 8: 407–21.

Reid, B and Metcalfe, A. (2001) Room as the top. Health Service Journal, 12th July.

Richards, S.Z. Coast, J. Gunnell, D.J. et al (1998) Randomised controlled trials comparing effectiveness and acceptability of an early discharge, hospital at home scheme for cute hospital care. British Medical Journal, 316; 1796–801.

Ridley SA (1998) Intermediate care: possibilities, requirements and solutions. Journal of Anaesthesia 53: 654–64.

Riseborough, M (1996) Listening to and Involving Older Tenants: Anchor Tenant Views on Anchor and Tenant Involvement. Kidlington, Anchor Trust

Robertson CE (1990) Falls in the elderly: an accident and emergency perspective. In Age Concern Scotland, Falls – Whose Concern. Scotland: Age Concern Scotland.

Robinson J, Barstone G (1996) Rehabilitation: a Development Challenge. London: Kings Fund.

Rodgers BL (1989) Concepts, analysis and the development of nursing knowledge: the evolutionary cycle. Journal of Advanced Nursing 14(4): 330–35.

Rodwell, C.M. (1996) An Analysis of the Concept of Empowerment. Journal of Advanced Nursing,.22; 305–313.

Rosbotham-Williams (2002) Integrating health care services for older people. Nursing Times 98(32): 40–41.

Rowles, G. (1983) Place and Personal Identity in Old Age: Observations from Appalachia. Journal of Environmental Psychology,.3; 299–313.

Rowntree Report (1980) Old People: Report of a Survey Committee on the Problems of Ageing and the Care of Old People. New York: Arno Press.

Rowson (1999) An Introduction To Personal And Professional Ethics; Morality Explained. New York: Jessica Kingsley.

Royal College of Nursing (1992) A Scandal Waiting to Happen. London: RCN.

Royal College of Nursing (1993) The Value and Skills of Working with Older People. London: RCN.

Royal College of Nursing (1996) Nursing Homes: Nursing Values. London: RCN.

Royal College of Nursing (1997) What a Difference a Nurse Makes. An RCN report on the benefits of expert nursing to clinical outcomes in the continuing care of older people. London: RCN.

Royal College of Nursing (1999) The Value and Skill of Working with Older People. London: RCN.

Royal College of Nursing (2000) Rehabilitating older people: the role of the nurse. London, RCN.

Royal College of Nursing and British Geriatrics Society (2001) Older People's Specialist Nurse: A Joint Statement from the Royal College of Nursing and the British Geriatrics Society. London: RCN and BGS.

Royal College of Physicians (1997) Medication for older people: summary and recommendations of a report of a working party of the Royal College of Physicians. Journal of the Royal College of Physicians of London 31(3): 254–56.

Royal College of Physicians (2000a) The Health and Social Care of Older People in Care Homes: A Comprehensive Interdisciplinary Approach. Report of Joint Working Party. London: RCP.

Royal College of Physicians (2000b) Management of the Older Medical Patient: Teamwork in the Journey of Care. London: RCP.

Royal College of Physicians – Royal Pharmaceutical Society of Great Britain (1998) From Compliance to Concordance: Towards Shared Goals in Medicine Taking. London: RCP

Royal College of Physicians, Royal College of Nursing and British Geriatric Society (2000) The Health and Care of Older People in Care Homes: A Comprehensive Interdisciplinary Approach. Report of a Joint Working Party of the Royal College of Physicians of London, the Royal College of Nursing and the British Geriatric Society. London: RCP.

Royal Commission Report (1998) With Respect to Old Age. London: The Stationary Office.

Royal Pharmaceutical Society (1997) From Compliance to Concordance. London: Royal Pharmaceutical Society of Great Britain.

Rudd AG, Wolfe CAD, Tilling K, Beech R (1997) Randomised controlled trial to evaluate early discharge scheme for patients with stroke. British Medical Journal 315: 1039–44.

Rutman D, Freedman J (1988) Anticipating relocation: coping strategies and the meaning of home for older people. Canadian Journal for Ageing 7(1): 17–31.

Ryan W (1971) Blaming the Victim. New York: Vintage.

Salmon P (1993) Interactions of nurses with elderly patients: relationships to nurses' attitudes and to formal activity periods. Journal of Advanced Nursing 18: 14–19.

Salomon G (1986) Hearing problems and the elderly. Danish Medical Bulletin 33 (Supplement 3): 1–23.

Sarafino EP (1998) Health Psychology: Biopsychosocial Interactions, New York: John Wiley & Sons.

Saxton DF, Hyland PA (1979) Planning and implementing nursing intervention: Stress and Adaptation applied to Patient Care. 2nd revised edn. St Louis: Mosby.

Schaefer J (1974) The interrelatedness of the decision making process and the nursing process. American Journal of Nursing 74(10): 1852–5.

Schon D (1983) The Reflective Practitioner. London: Temple Smith.

Seedhouse D (2000) Practical Nursing Philosophy: The Universal Ethical Code. Chichester: Wiley.

Seligman MEP (1975) Helplessness: On Depression, Development and Death. San Francisco: Freeman.

Sellick K (1985) Interdisciplinary health teams: a question of attitude. The Australian Journal of Advanced Nursing 3: Sept–Nov: 38.

Seymore J (1998) The unsound barrier. Nursing Times 94(20): 56–8.

Shanus E (1979) The family as a social support system in old age. The Gerontologist 19(1): 169–74.

Sheffler S (1995) Do clinical experiences affect nursing students attitudes towards the elderly? Journal of Nursing Education 34(7): 312–16.

Shepherd M (1998) The risks of polypharmacy. Nursing Times 94(32): 60–2.

Shepperd S, Illiffe S (1998a) The effectiveness of hospital at home compared with in-patient hospital care: a systematic review. Journal of Public Health Medicine 20(3): 344–50.

Shepperd S, Illiffe S (1998b) The effectiveness of hospital at home compared to in-patient hospital care. Protocol for Cochrane Library. In L Bero, R Grilli, J Grimshaw, A Oxman (eds) Cochrane Library. Oxford: Update Software.

Shepperd S, Illiffe S (1998c) Randomised controlled trial comparing hospital at home care with inpatient hospital care, Part 1: Three month follow up of health outcomes. British Medical Journal 316: 1786–91.

Shepperd S, Harwood D, Jenkinson C et al. (1998) Randomised controlled trial comparing hospital at home with care with in-patient care. 1:3 month follow up of health outcomes. British Medical Journal 31(9): 1786–91.

Shetty H, Woodhouse K (1994) Geriatrics. In R Walker, C Edwards (eds), Clinical Pharmacy and Therapeutics. Edinburgh: Churchill Livingstone. Ch. 8.

Short MS (1997) Charting by exception on a clinical pathway, Journal of Nursing Management 28(8): 45–6.

Shulman J (1985) Making the best use of drugs: drug compliance. Geriatric Nursing Sept/Oct: 16–17.

Sinclair A, Dickinson E (1998) Effective Practice in Rehabilitation: The Evidence of Systematic Reviews. London: Kings Fund.

Skeet M (1970) Home from Hospital. Dan Mason, Nursing Research Committee, Florence Nightingale, Memorial Committee. London: Macmillan.

Slevin O (1991) Ageist attitudes among young adults: implications for a caring profession. Journal of Advanced Nursing 16: 1197–1205.

Snape J (1986) Nurses' attitudes to care of the elderly. Journal of Advanced Nursing 11: 569–72.

Social Services Inspectorate (1997) The Cornerstones of Care: Inspection of Care Planning for Older People. London: DoH.

Somerfield K (1999) Laboratory values and implications. In H Heath, I Schofield (eds), Healthy Ageing: Nursing Older People. London: Mosby.

Spencer J, Davidson H, White V (1997) Helping clients develop hopes for the future. American Journal of Occupational Therapy 51(3): 191–8.

Squires A (1988) (ed.) Rehabilitation of the Older Patient. London: Chapman & Hall.

Squires A, Hastings M (2002) Rehabilitation and the Older Patient: A Handbook for the Interdisciplinary Team, 3rd edn. London: Nelson Thornes Ltd.

Stacey M. (1993) The Sociology of Health and Healing, 2nd edn. London, Routledge.

Stanley L (1993) An auto/biography in sociology. Sociology 27(1): 41–52.

Steiner A (1997) Intermediate Care: A Conceptual Framework and Review of the Literature. London: King's Fund.

Steiner A (2000) Post-acute intermediate care: evaluation of a nurse-led unit. Presentation at the British Society of Gerontology Conference, Oxford 2000: Old Age in a New Age, 10 September.

Steiner A (2001) Intermediate care – a good thing? Age and Ageing 30(S3): 33–9.

Steiner A, Vaughan B (1997) Intermediate care: a discussion paper arising from the King's Fund Seminar, October 1996. Intermediate Care Series 1. London: King's Fund.

Steiner A, Walsh B, Wiles B, Ward J (2000) Post-acute intermediate care: evaluation of a nurse-led unit. In A Dickinson H Bartlett, S Wade (eds), Old Age in a New Age. Proceedings of the British Society of Gerontology 29th Annual Conference. School of Health Care, Oxford Brookes University, pp. 319–23.

Steiner A, Walsh B, Pickering R, Wiles R, Ward J, Brooking J (2001) Therapeutic nursing or unblocking beds? A randomised controlled trial of post-acute intermediate care beds. British Medical Journal 322: 453–9.

Stevens J, Crouch M (1995) Who cares about care in nursing education? Journal of Nursing Studies 32(3): 233–347.

Stevenson O, Parsloe P (1993) Community Care and Empowerment. York: Joseph Rowntree Foundation.

Stevernick N, Lindeiberg S, Ornel J (1998) Towards understanding successful ageing: patterned changes in resources and goals. Ageing and Society 18(4): 441–68.

Strehler BL (1977) Time, Cells and Ageing. New York: Academic Press.

Suchman EA (1967) Evaluative Research. New York: Russel Sage Foundation.

Sullivan EJ, Decker PJ (2000) Effective Management in Nursing. Englewood Cliffs, NJ: Prentice Hall.

Swift C (1988) Disease and Disability in the elderly – prospects for interventions. In A Squires (ed.) Rehabilitation of the Older Patient. London: Chapman & Hall. Ch. 1.

Tarlow B (1996) Caring: a negotiated process that varies. In S Gordon, P Benner, N Noddings (eds), Caregiving: Readings in knowledge, Practice, Ethics and Politics. Philadelphia, PA: University of Pennsylvania Press.

Thewlis P (2001) Lilac from the Garden Day Services for Older People in Rural Oxfordshire: A Study of Needs and Innovations. Age Concern, Oxfordshire.

Thewlis P (2002) Older people making a difference seminar report: income and health. Age Concern, Oxfordshire.

Thomas D (1995) Flexible Learning Strategies in Higher Education. London: Cassell.

Thompson C, McCaughan D, Sheldon T, Raynor P (2002) The value of research in clinical decision-making. Nursing Times 98(42): 30–4.

Thompson SC, Sobolew-Shubin A, Galbraith ME, Schwankovsky L, Cruzen D. (1993) Maintaining perceptions of control: finding perceived control in low control circumstances. Journal of Personality and Social Psychology 64(2): 293–304.

Thorne B (1984) Person-centred therapy. In W Dryden (ed.) Individual Therapy in Britain. London: Harper & Row.

Thornton P (2000) Older people speaking out developing opportunities for influence. YPS for Joseph Rowntree Foundation.

Tolson D (1991) Making sense of ... hearing aids. Nursing Times 87(18): 36–8.

Tolson D, Stevens D (1997) Age-related hearing loss in the dependent elderly population: a model for nursing care. International Journal of Nursing Practice 3: 224–30.

Tolson D, Nolan M (2000) Gerontological nursing 4: age-related hearing explored. British Journal of Nursing 9(4): 205–8.

Townsend P (1962, 1964) The Last Refuge: A Survey of Residential Institutions and Homes for the Aged in England and Wales. London: Routledge and Kegan Paul.

Treharne G (1990) Attitudes towards the care of older people: are they getting better? Journal of Advanced Nursing 15(7): 777–81.

Tripp I, Caan W (1999) Is post-rehabilitation discharge of older people successful? British Journal of Therapy and Rehabilitation 6(10): 500–4.

Twigg, J. (1999) The Spatial Ordering of Care: Public and Private in Bathing Support at Home. Sociology of Health and Illness, Jul. 21 (4) 381–400.

United Kingdom Central Council for Nursing, Midwifery and Health Visiting (1984) Code of Professional conduct for the nurse, midwife and health visitor. (2nd ed). London: UKCC.

United Kingdom Central Council for Nursing, Midwifery and Health Visiting (1997) The Continuing Care of Older People. London: UKCC.

United Kingdom Central Council for Nursing, Midwifery and Health Visiting (2001) The Register 37: 6. London: UKCC.

University of York Centre for Health Economics (1992) Skill Mix and the Effectiveness of Nursing Care. University of York Centre for Health Economics.

Vaughan B (1998) United Kingdom: caring differently; intermediate care – an alternative approach to service provision in response to client need and workforce changes in the NHS. International Journal of Nursing Practice 4(1): 62–7.

Vaughan B, Lathlean J (eds) (1999) Intermediate Care – Models in Practice. London: King's Fund Publishing.

Vaughan B, Steiner A, Hanford L (1999) Intermediate Care: The Shape of the Team. Intermediate Care Series 5. London: King's Fund.

Victor CR (1994) Old Age in Modern Society. London: Chapman & Hall.

Victor CR, Vetter NJ (1988) Preparing the elderly for discharge home: a neglected aspect of care. Age and Ageing 17: 155–63.

Victor CR, Young E, Hudson M, Wallace P (1993) Whose responsibility is it anyway? Hospital admission and discharge of older people in an inner-London District Health Authority. Journal of Advanced Nursing 18: 1297–1304.

Wade D (1996) Designing district disability services – the Oxford experience. Clinical Rehabilitation 4: 147–58.

Wade OL (1996) The Romance of Remedies. Durham: Durham Academic Press.

Wade S (1992) Measuring communication. Journal of Community Nursing 6(2): 4–8.

Wade S (1995a) Beycrest Centre for elderly care in Toronto (editorial). British Journal of Therapy and Rehabilitation 2(7): 343–5.

Wade S (1995b) Partnership in care: a critical review. Nursing Standard 9(48).

Wade S (1999) Promoting quality of care for older people: developing positive attitudes to working with older people. Journal of Nursing Management 7: 339–47.

Wade S (2000) Nursing older people: the key to success. Nursing Times 96(2): 42-44.

Wade S (2001) Combating ageism: an imperative for contemporary health care. Reviews in Clinical Gerontology 11: 285-94.

Walker LO, Avant KC (1995) Strategies for Theory Construction in Nursing, 3rd edn. Norwalk, Conn: Appleton & Lange.

Wallace S (1992) Gerontological content in nursing education: a need or a luxury. Perspectives 16(4): 14-17.

Wanless D (2002) The Wanless Report: Securing our Future. Taking a Long-Term View. London: HM Treasury.

Waters K (1994) Getting dressed in the early morning: styles of staff/patient interaction on rehabilitation wards for elderly people. Journal of Advanced Nursing 19: 239-48.

Waters K, Booth J (1991) Home and dry. Nursing Times 16(87): 3.

Waterworth S, Luker K (1990) Reluctant collaborators: do patients want to be involved in decisions concerning care. Journal of Advanced Nursing 15: 971-6.

Watson G, Glaser E (1964) Critical Thinking Appraisal Manual. New York: Harcourt & Brace.

Watson J (1988) Nursing: Human Science and Caring. New York: National League of Nursing.

Watson R (1995) Hypothermia. Elderly Care 5(6): 41-3.

Watson R (2001) Nursing older people: assessment of older people using medication. Nursing Older People 13(7): 29-30.

Werrett J, Helm R, Carnell R (2001) The primary and secondary care interface: the educational needs of nursing staff for the provision of seamless care. Journal of Advanced Nursing 34(5): 629-38.

Wheeler J (2001) Thinking your way to successful problem-solving. Nursing Times 97(37): 36-7.

Wheeler R (1986) Housing policy and elderly people. In C Phillipson, A Walker (eds), Ageing and Social Policy: A Critical Assessment. Aldershot: Gower.

Wild D (2002) The single assessment process. Primary Health Care 12(11): 20-1.

Wiles R, Postle K, Steiner A (2001) Nurse-led intermediate care: an opportunity to develop enhanced roles for nurses? Journal of Advanced Nursing 34(6): 813-21.

Williams B, Grant G (1998) Defining 'people-centredness': making the implicit explicit. Health and Social Care in the Community 7(6): 475-82.

Williams J, Last S (1998) Intermediate care: smoothing the road to recovery. Nursing Times 94(9): 52-4.

Wistow G (1995) Aspirations and realities: community care at the crossroads. Health and Social Care in the Community 3: 227-40.

Woodrow P (2002) Ageing: Issues for Physical, Psychological and Social Health. London: Whurr.

Worth A (2001) Assessment of the needs of older people by district nurses and social workers: a changing culture? Journal of Interprofessional Care 15(3): 257-66.

Young H (1990) Management of relocation to a nursing home. Holistic Nursing Practice 4(3): 74-83.

Young J (1996) Rehabilitation and older people. British Medical Journal 313: 677-81.

Young J, Brown A, Foster A, Clare J (1999) An overview of rehabilitation for older people. Reviews in Clinical Gerontology 9: 183-96.

Index